My Health Technology *for* Seniors

Lonzell Watson

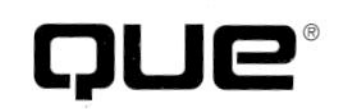

800 East 96th Street,
Indianapolis, Indiana 46240 USA

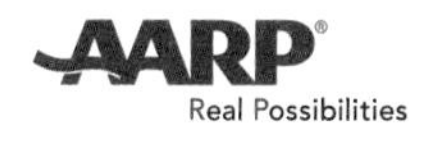

My Health Technology for Seniors

ISBN-13: 978-0-7897-5821-7
ISBN-10: 0-7897-5821-0

Library of Congress Control Number: 2015960645

Printed in the United States of America
First Printing: March 2016

Trademarks

Warning and Disclaimer

Special Sales

For information about buying this title in bulk quantities, or for special sales opportunities (which may include electronic versions; custom cover designs; and content particular to your business, training goals, marketing focus, or branding interests), please contact our corporate sales department at corpsales@pearsoned.com or (800) 382-3419.

For government sales inquiries, please contact governmentsales@pearsoned.com.

For questions about sales outside the U.S., please contact international@pearsoned.com.

Editor-in-Chief
Greg Wiegand

Acquisitions Editor
Michelle Newcomb

Marketing Manager
Dan Powell

Director, AARP Books
Jodi Lipson

Development Editor
Brandon Cackowski-Schnell

Managing Editor
Kristy Hart

Senior Project Editor
Lori Lyons

Copy Editor
Paula Lowell

Senior Indexer
Cheryl Lenser

Proofreader
Gill Editorial Services

Technical Editor
Jeri Usbay

Editorial Assistant
Cindy Teeters

Cover Designer
Mark Shirar

Compositor
Nonie Ratcliff

Contents at a Glance

Table of Contents

About the Author

Lonzell Watson, recently honored by the University of Kentucky's 2014-15 College of Communication and Information Outstanding Alumnus Award, has been fascinated with technology ever since he disassembled his first Commodore 64 computer in grade school and then attempted to put it back together. He went on to work a 100-mile paper route for an entire year, just to buy his first Apple computer, and he has been writing about technology ever since. Lonzell helped pay his way through college making house calls to individuals who were 50 years of age and older, helping them learn how to use common software programs, how to use their hardware, how to buy new computers, and even helping them set up home networks. Lonzell went on to work as an IT consultant for clients including the J. Peterman Company, Time Warner Communications, and Verizon Wireless.

Lonzell is the award-winning author of *Teach Yourself Visually iPad*, for which he won the 2010 International Award of Excellence from the Society for Technical Communication. This work also earned Lonzell the Distinguished Technical Communication award and Best of Show 2010 from the STC. Lonzell was also presented the Award of Excellence for *Teach Yourself Visually iPhoto '09* in 2009. He is the author of other popular titles, including *My Samsung Galaxy Tab*, *My Amazon Fire Phone*, *Teach Yourself Visually iPad 2*, *My HTC EVO 3D*, the *Canon VIXIA HD Digital Field Guide*, *Final Cut Pro 6 for Digital Video Editor's Only*, and *Teach Yourself Visually Digital Video*.

Currently, Lonzell is the owner of Creative Intelligence LLC, an instructional design and technical writing company, whose courseware is being used to train the CIA, FBI, NASA, and all branches of the U.S. Armed Forces. With a master's degree in Instructional Design and Development, Lonzell has taught Digital Asset Creation to graduate students at Bellevue University, has been a frequent contributor to StudioMonthly.com, and an author for one of the leading online learning companies, Lynda.com. Lonzell's writing has been syndicated, with hundreds of published tutorials and tips that help demystify consumer electronics and software.

Find out more at the author's website: www.creativeintel.com.

About AARP and AARP TEK

AARP is a nonprofit, nonpartisan organization, with a membership of nearly 38 million, that helps people turn their goals and dreams into *real possibilities*™, strengthens communities, and fights for the issues that matter most to families such as healthcare, employment and income security, retirement planning, affordable utilities, and protection from financial abuse. Learn more at aarp.org.

The AARP TEK (Technology Education & Knowledge) program aims to accelerate AARP's mission of turning dreams into *real possibilities*™ by providing step-by-step lessons in a variety of formats to accommodate different learning styles, levels of experience, and interests. Expertly guided hands-on workshops delivered in communities nationwide help instill confidence and enrich lives of the 50+ by equipping them with skills for staying connected to the people and passions in their lives. Lessons are taught on touchscreen tablets and smartphones—common tools for connection, education, entertainment, and productivity. For self-paced lessons, videos, articles, and other resources, visit aarptek.org.

Dedication

To anyone living with Alzheimer's and to those fighting cancer—two fights I have seen up close and personal. Thank you for showing me what it means to live life to its fullest, regardless of the circumstances. I love you, S.

Acknowledgments

I would like to give special thanks to Michelle Newcomb, without whom this project would not have been possible, and thank you to Brandon Cackowski-Schnell, Todd Brakke, Lori Lyons, Paula Lowell, Nonie Ratcliff, Karen Davis, Jeri Usbay, and Marcy Schneidewind. Thank you to Jodi Lipson at AARP for working with me to create such a unique, wonderful, and much-needed resource for the times we live in. Thank you to all the people who worked with me in bringing this book into fruition. Thank you to Moses Zonana of the CleverCap, Ian Twinn at Withings, Michelle Jeong and Gary Rotman of Reminder Rosie, and Jeffrey Eisenberg from HydraCoach. Thank you to all the inventors and developers whose works are featured in this book, and for helping to make living a healthier lifestyle easier, every day. I would like to give a heart-felt thank you to my wife Robyn. Without your support, none of this would be possible.

We Want to Hear from You!

As the reader of this book, *you* are our most important critic and commentator. We value your opinion and want to know what we're doing right, what we could do better, what areas you'd like to see us publish in, and any other words of wisdom you're willing to pass our way.

We welcome your comments. You can email or write to let us know what you did or didn't like about this book—as well as what we can do to make our books better.

Please note that we cannot help you with technical problems related to the topic of this book.

When you write, please be sure to include this book's title and author as well as your name and email address. We will carefully review your comments and share them with the author and editors who worked on the book.

Email: feedback@quepublishing.com

Mail: Que Publishing
ATTN: Reader Feedback
800 East 96th Street
Indianapolis, IN 46240 USA

Reader Services

Register your copy of *My Health Technology for Seniors* at quepublishing.com for convenient access to downloads, updates, and corrections as they become available. To start the registration process, go to quepublishing.com/register and log in or create an account*. Enter the product ISBN, 9780789758217, and click Submit. Once the process is complete, you will find any available bonus content under Registered Products.

**Be sure to check the box that you would like to hear from us to receive exclusive discounts on future editions of this product.*

Introduction

Whether you're looking to get in better shape, prevent an illness, or manage a chronic condition, I hope you'll find that this book offers resources that help you be the best version of yourself. Advancements in health care technology are impacting how we approach our own personal health and fitness, and the way we receive medical care. We now enjoy a more active role in our health care management by using websites, apps, and smart tools to monitor our exercise, improve our diet, interact with our doctors, and even track how well we are responding to a treatment. The best thing about these technological leaps is that they are helping us to prevent illnesses and not just manage them.

You won't find a bunch of technical jargon in this book. The practical use of a resource is considered first and foremost. Any brief dives into the technical weeds will be for a better understanding of how a product can best be used in your personal life. It also might be to ensure a product is compatible with the phone, tablet, or computer you already have. Regardless, its application will have a clear purpose: "What can this technology do for me?"

This book is organized using three principles: prevention, management, and safety. In Chapter 1, "Choosing the Right Technology to Support Your Health Goals," we begin looking at prevention. Chapter 1 discusses the world of smartphones, fitness trackers, and apps, and how you can use them to aid in a healthy lifestyle. It provides tips on how to find the best smartphone and fitness tracker for you, if you decide you want one to begin with.

Chapter 2, "Maintaining a Healthy, Balanced Diet," showcases resources that help you make healthier food choices, track your body weight and measurements from your phone, and find options for getting groceries delivered to your door.

If you're looking to get in better shape, lose some weight, or maintain your current weight, Chapter 3, "Keeping Active and Fit," shows you how to put personal health and fitness technology to use in your life. You'll see how to use some of the most popular apps and fitness trackers to set goals for your daily workouts, or track simple activities such as walking or doing chores. This chapter also gets into options for professionally designed workout regimens—no gym required. You'll even learn how to work on your posture.

Chapter 4, "Sleeping Better and Managing Stress," helps you take a more holistic approach to health by showcasing some resources for getting a better night's sleep and managing stress. You'll see options that can help you fall asleep faster and wake up less groggy. You might want to have a pair of headphones or earbuds on hand for this chapter, as you'll see how easy it is to incorporate meditation and some happy time into your day.

Chapter 5, "Staying on Top of Your Medicine," begins looking at the management principle. This chapter provides plenty of options that can help you stay on top of a medication regimen—both simple and complex. You'll discover options from talking clock reminders and smart pill bottles, to simple reminders appearing on your phone.

Chapter 6, "Using Social Engagement as Health Support Systems," shows you how to stay socially engaged with family, friends, and even caregivers. Whether you have a busy lifestyle, distance challenges, or disability, you'll discover some resources that help you gain the benefits of staying in touch with those who matter the most. If you have a challenging or rare health condition, you are shown options to help you connect with others living with the same condition. You'll also learn about some great transportation services.

Chapter 7, "Finding Solutions to Manage Specific Conditions," offers solutions and resources that help manage chronic health conditions, including diabetes, high blood pressure, obesity, asthma, COPD, and more.

Chapter 8, "Being Prepared for an Emergency," discusses safety principles, including the use of personal and family medical alert systems ranging from simple GPS pendants to ICE (In Case of Emergency) apps on your smartphone, to comprehensive, subscription-based systems.

Chapter 9, "Connecting with Your Health Care Professionals and Saving Money," shows you the convenience of consulting with your doctor from home and receiving diagnoses, recommended treatments, and prescriptions. You also see how to save money on costly health procedures and pay less for medication. This chapter also dives into resources for letting loved ones and health care professionals know your wishes, should something happen to you.

Although this book covers some of the most popular health care technology products and services, it is not a comprehensive list of what's out there, and new products are always being developed. As you read, think of this book as a field guide to get you going, an opportunity to learn of some helpful products you might not have known about, and gain some perspective as to what personal health care technology can do for you. Some of the resources discussed are best used with guidance from a health care professional; your doctor can provide further insight into your own personal health situation, so you can get the most from everything discussed here.

I sincerely hope this book finds you in good health, and as you turn through its pages, you find something that helps improve your quality of life.

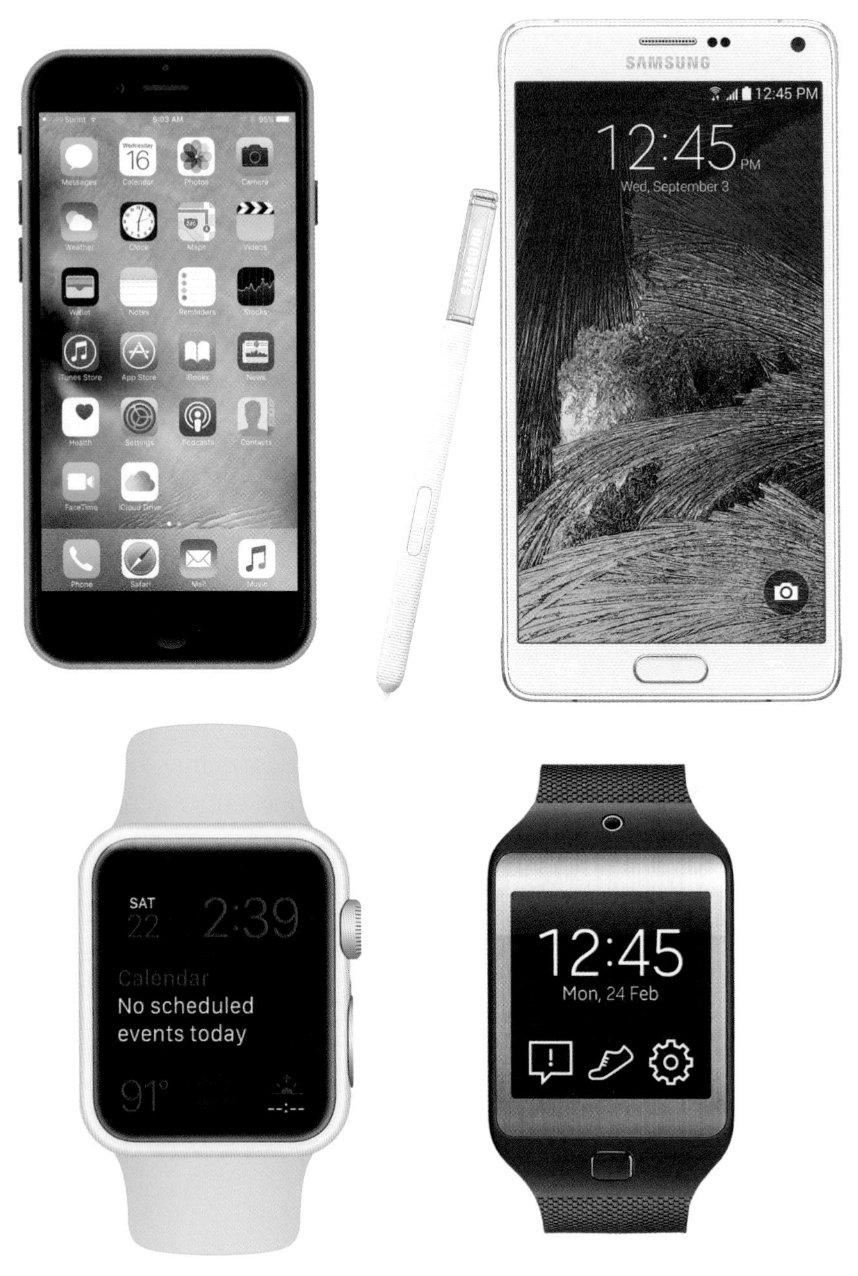

Get to know the technology available to you to help live a more healthy, active, and independent lifestyle.

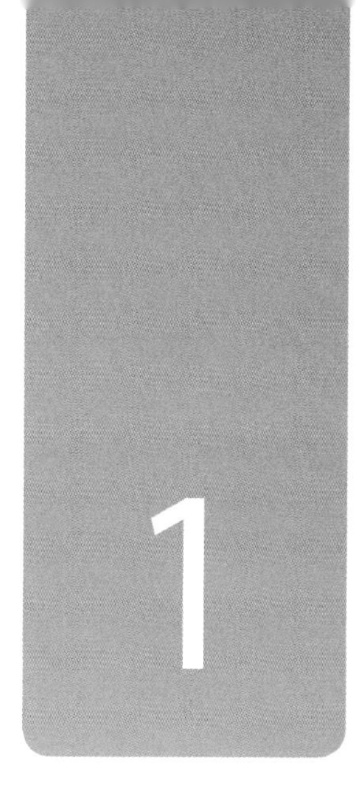

In this chapter, you explore some of the most popular smartphones and wearables (smartwatches, fitness trackers, pendants, and bracelets) and how they can assist you in living a healthy and independent lifestyle. You also learn how to find the best health apps, discover web-based health solutions for health care and management, and explore health technology for the household.

- → Using a Smartphone to Aid in a Healthy Lifestyle
- → Finding Health Apps for Your Device
- → Exploring Web-Based Solutions
- → Taking a Look at What Wearables Can Do for You
- → Exploring Technology for Your Household

Choosing the Right Technology to Support Your Health Goals

A multitude of health care gadgets in the market today claim they can help you lead a healthier lifestyle. Maybe you have such a device on your person right now—perhaps a smartphone or a fitness tracker. The market for healthcare technology is booming, and wading through the many choices to find what's right for you can prove to be a chore for anyone. The great thing about this entire quest is that it starts with you. What are your health goals? What do you require to be the healthiest version of you and to remain independent, whatever your current health condition? Knowing what's available can help you align specific health technologies with what you need.

Many devices and software applications are available that can help you live with vitality by tracking physical fitness, aiding in diet and nutrition, and monitoring vital signs. A bounty of options is available to help you manage medications, stay socially engaged with family and friends, and acquire care online. Resources exist for emotional health, such as apps to aid in meditation and to learn healthy sleep patterns. Later in this chapter we also cover options for emergency detection and response, and ways to potentially prevent accidents in the home.

Using a Smartphone to Aid in a Healthy Lifestyle

Owning a smartphone is having a mobile computer that fits into your pocket or purse. Smartphones have moved so far beyond their original application as a means to place a call that most reviews spend very little time at all discussing a phone's call capabilities. A smartphone gives you access to many of the health technologies that are available to you. Many of the devices covered in this book are made to interact with your cellphone and supply you information that was once only accessible through a care provider or personal trainer. The many *apps* (specialized programs for mobile devices) available for smartphones can help you perform tasks such as count calories, monitor the steps you've taken, set fitness goals, manage blood pressure, help with medication adherence, and much, much more. Every day, manufacturers are creating accessories that interface with smartphones, including smartwatches and fitness trackers for better health tracking, spirometers for asthma and COPD patients, and even a device called the CellScope to identify inner ear infections.

Many health resources are made for specific smartphones. Just like a Mac or Windows desktop computer, smartphones run operating systems. The most popular operating systems are Android (Google), iOS (Apple), and Windows, with Android and Apple being the clear frontrunners among users and product developers. Many apps have been developed to run on multiple platforms, as discussed later in the "Finding Health Apps for Your Device" section of this chapter. If you have recently purchased a smartphone, the types of apps and accessories you can use will—at least to some degree—be determined by your phone. If you are in the market for a smartphone, then thinking of it in terms of buying into a specific ecosystem (device-compatible accessories, apps, and services) is a good idea. With that being said, let's take a closer look at some of the phones.

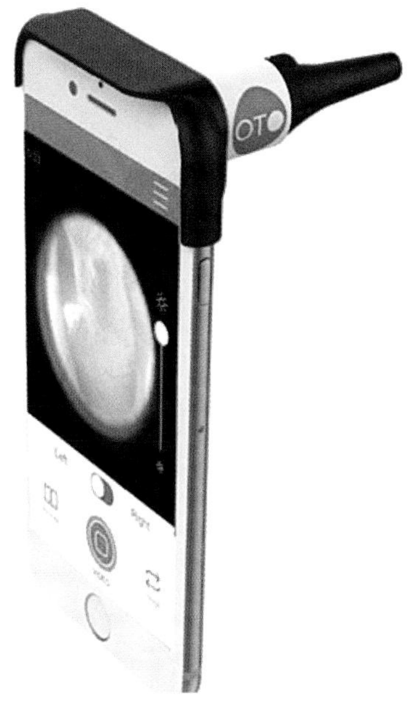

A CellScope attached to an iPhone

Mac and PC Compatibility

When choosing a smartphone, don't worry about how well it connects with your current computer—Android phones and iPhones are both compatible with Macs and PCs.

Explore Android Devices

Android phones are the most used phones around the world. Many manufacturers, including Google, HTC, Huawei, LG, Motorola, and Samsung, produce Android phones. In contrast, only Apple produces the iPhone. Android phones also come in a variety of price ranges, so you can get a good phone without paying a premium price.

Samsung

Samsung is the leading manufacturer in sales of Android devices.

An important thing to keep in mind is that the many manufacturers of Android devices like to include their own "bells and whistles" on top of the Android interface. On Samsung devices, this proprietary software is called TouchWiz. HTC's is called Sense. The various cell phone carriers that support these devices like to add their own stuff, too, like the AT&T Family Map. What this means for you is that, out of the box, what you see on two Android phones running the same underlying software version, but made by different manufacturers or on different carriers, might be organized differently or have other visual differences. Nexus phones, by Google, are the only exception to this and run Android as it was originally designed.

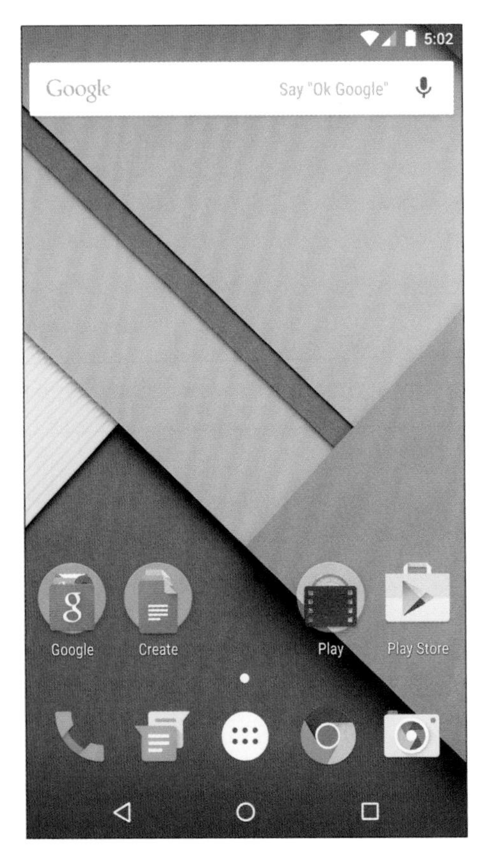

Nexus 6 screen running Android 5.1.1

These software differences allow manufacturers and carriers to differentiate themselves and offer tools and services that consumers might find helpful or easier to use, but this increase in choices can make choosing a smartphone more complicated. The best way to figure out which phone is right for you is to get your hands on several and test them out. Big box stores and your local cellular carriers have demos of various models set up to let you "test drive" some of the most popular devices. See what other people are saying about a phone you might be interested in and read product reviews online. Cnet.com and engadget.com, for example, do a great job on smartphone reviews.

Save Money on Your Cell Phone Plan

Visit the AARP website as well as tech sites to read articles on how to choose the best cell phone plan for you at the best price. Keep in mind that each cell phone provider has a list of particular phones they support. After you have done your research and you find a phone that you really like, make sure it's covered by the cellular provider you prefer. Consumer Cellular (www.consumercellular.com/AARP) offers special benefits for AARP members.

To get the most from your Android phone as a resource for a healthy lifestyle, make sure you are running a recent version of the Android operating system. It doesn't have to be the newest version, but recent. Most of the health apps and accessories are developed for more recent phones. Android names its software versions after tasty treats such as Jelly Bean and Ice Cream Sandwich; as of the writing of this book, the latest line of Android smartwatches are compatible with Android 4.3 (Jelly Bean) or higher.

Check Your Version of Android

If you have an Android phone and are unaware of the current operating system version, perform the following steps.

1. Tap Settings (an icon shaped like a gear).
2. Swipe down, and then tap About Phone.
3. Look for the version number under Android Version.

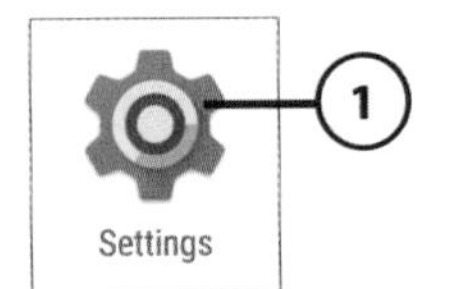

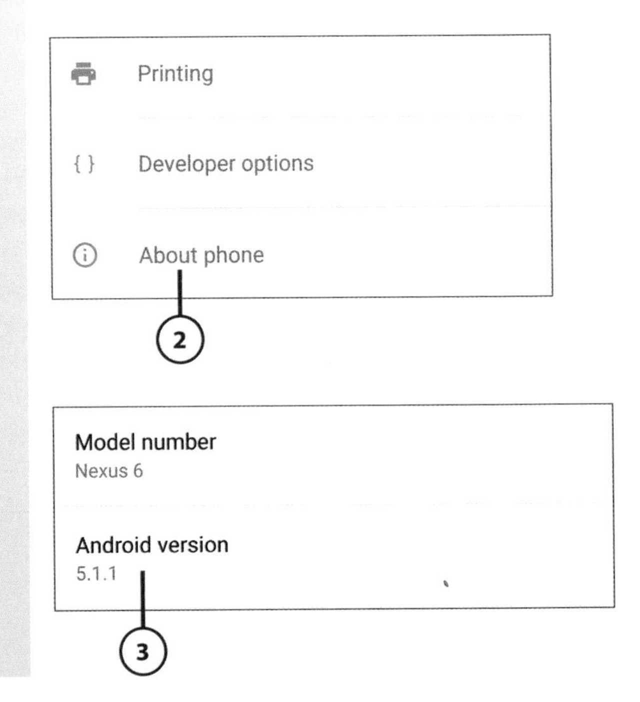

Choose an Android Phone

So, which Android phone should you get? Preferably, you want a later model. It doesn't have to be the latest, but one that will be eligible for updates for some time to come. More storage space enables you to download more apps along with your other media such as photos and videos. Here are a few phones that will give you access to great health apps and accessories for quite some time.

Definitely do not limit yourself to what is suggested here. Plenty of wonderful phones are out there, like the LG G4 that I do not put in the list. Search online and join the AARP community to ask questions and read product reviews to make the most informed decision. This is just a list to get you started.

- **Samsung Galaxy Note 4 and Note 5:** These are two of the highest-end Android phones that you can get, and they are pricier than some other options. If you have an aversion to big phones, these phones might not be the right fit for you. Their large screens and stylus features, however, make them wonderful devices for high-end users who like to do a lot of work on their phones.

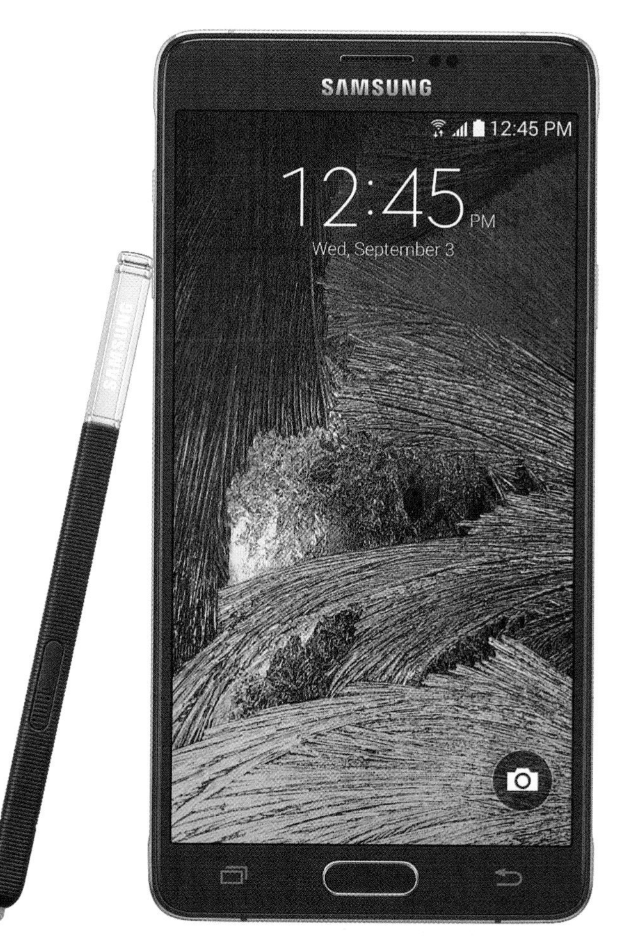

Samsung Galaxy Note 4

- **Samsung Galaxy S5 and S6:** The S5 and the S6 are two more powerful smartphones that can interface with the current collection of Android-compatible apps and accessories. These two do not come with a stylus.

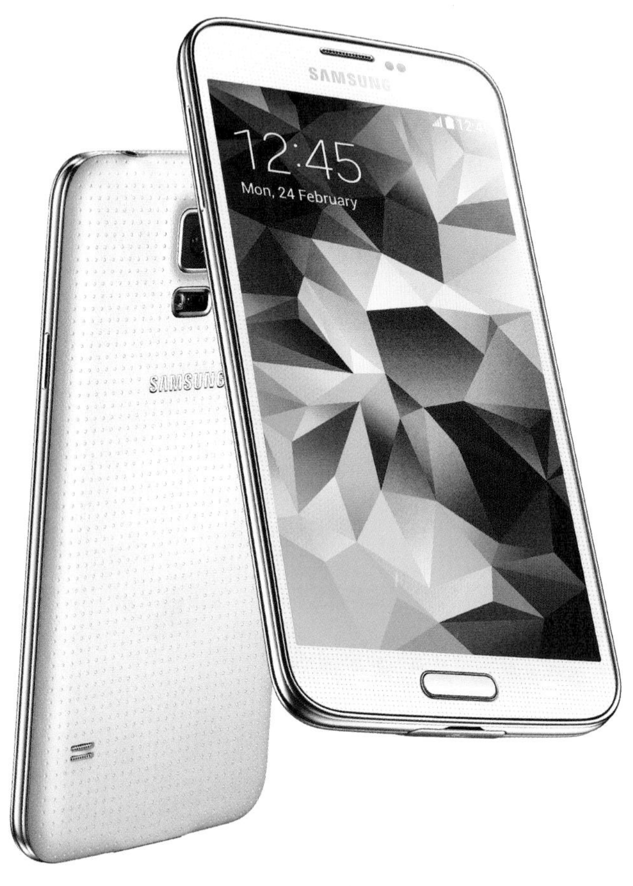

Samsung Galaxy S5

Easy Mode

If you feel there is just too much information onscreen, the Samsung Galaxy S5 and S6 have an Easy Mode you can use to simplify the screen and enlarge the icons. Easy Mode rearranges things and removes some options altogether. Don't worry—you can still access these options when needed.

- **Nexus 5 and Nexus 6:** These Nexus phones are Google devices. If you want to be first in line to get new updates, these phones are for you. The Nexus 5 has been the more popular of the two due to its smaller screen size and price point. The Nexus 6 boasts a six-inch display, which makes it one of the biggest smartphones on the market.

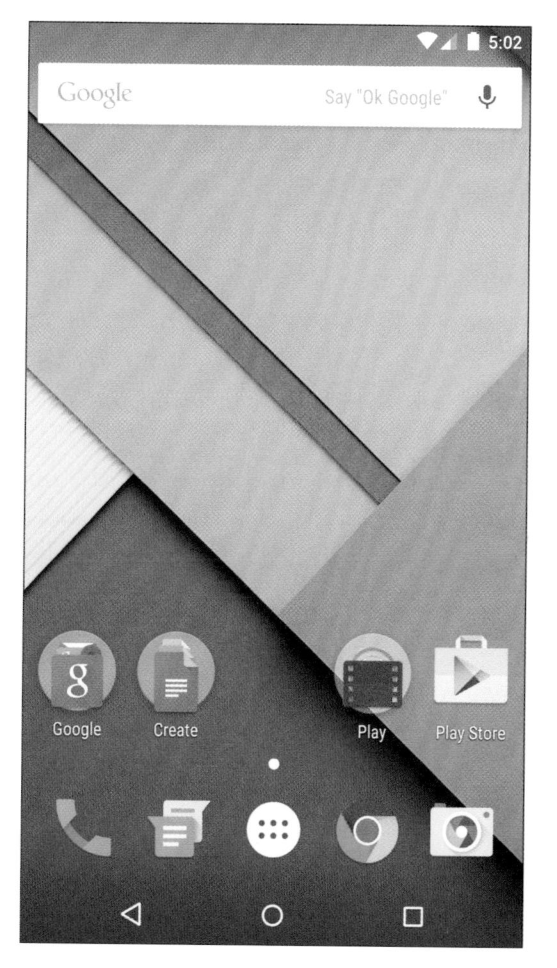

Google Nexus 6

Consider an Apple iPhone

Apple creates its own operating system (iOS) and manufactures its own hardware. Just as with the Android phones, the older devices stop receiving updates; such as is the case with the iPhone 4. When a device stops receiving updates for its operating system, its ability to run the latest, greatest health apps and use new accessories withers on the vine. The Apple Watch, a handy and expensive health device, is only compatible with the iPhone 5 model or later. When an iOS release is rolled out by Apple, it is immediately available to all supported phones. To get the most from your iPhone as a resource for a healthy lifestyle, get one of the iPhone 5 models (5, 5C, or 5S) or newer.

It's easy to know which iPhone model you have if you purchased it yourself, but how can you determine the model if someone gives one to you, or you buy a used one? It isn't very easy for you to find out. There is no signage that reads "You are holding an iPhone 5." First, the model number can be found on the lower back of the phone. Good, right? Except that this number alone doesn't tell you very much, and the etching is so small, it's hard for anyone to read without a magnifying glass. After you locate the model number, go to https://support.apple.com/en-us/HT201296 and find your model number in the list. This webpage can inform you of the iPhone model you have.

The iPhone is one of most sought-after phones on the market, and it comes with a premium price. Good deals can be had if you purchase an older, but supported, device such as the iPhone 5. They are currently up to 6S and 6S Plus.

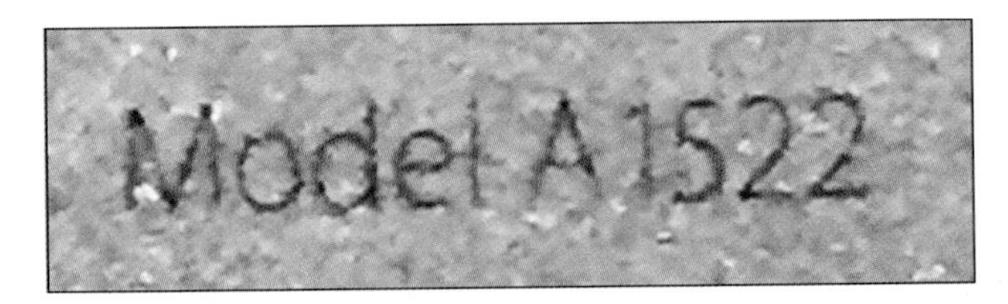

Model number for iPhone 6 Plus

So, which iPhone should you get? For starters, definitely don't go any older than iPhone 5, or you won't be able to take advantage of many health apps and accessories:

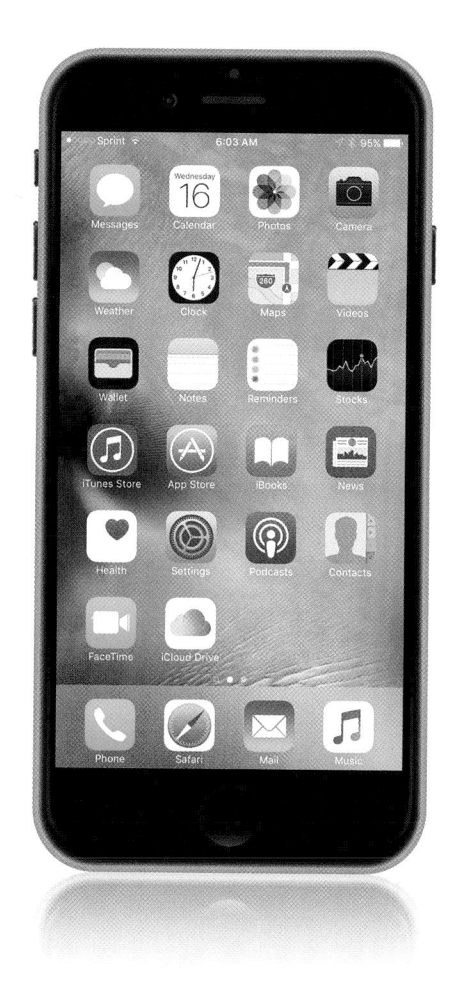

iPhone 6S Plus

iPhone 5S: This is the latest iteration produced in the iPhone 5 models that can be found at a good price but still has the latest iPhone 5 specifications. Keep in mind that this phone's display is only 4 inches. If you require a larger viewing space, consider moving up in class.

iPhone 6S and iPhone 6S Plus: The iPhone 6S and 6S Plus are two of the most sought-after phones in the world and it comes at a premium price. The iPhone 6 comes in two models: iPhone 6 with a 4.7-inch display and the iPhone 6 Plus that comes with a 5.5-inch display.

Check Your Version of iOS

If you have an iPhone and you don't know the current operating system version, perform the following steps.

1. Tap Settings (an icon shaped like a gear).
2. Tap General.

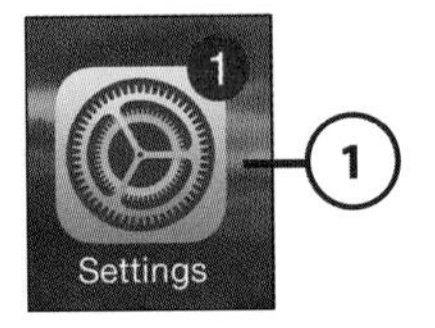

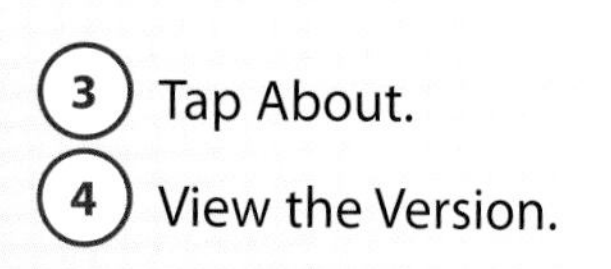

3. Tap About.
4. View the Version.

Settings General

About (3)

Software Update 1

General About

Name

Network AT&T

Songs Loading...

Videos Loading...

Photos Loading...

Applications 96

Capacity 55.4 GB

Available 1.9 GB

Version 8.4.1 (12H321) (4)

Carrier AT&T 20.0

Model MGAU2LL/A

Keep in Touch with the Jitterbug Touch3

The company GreatCall designs phones that are uniquely attuned with its customers' needs. If you are looking for a more simplified smartphone, consider the Jitterbug Touch3. It has no extraneous interface clutter or functions that you might not use. GreatCall has listened to its customer base, tested its product in the field, and taken constructive feedback to create a phone that is focused on the essentials.

The Jitterbug Touch3 is built by Samsung, designed by GreatCall, and runs Android 4.3. It has a 4-inch screen and large buttons for easy readability. You can send texts and emails, capture and share photos, download apps, and browse the Internet, like with any smartphone. This phone is preloaded with GreatCall's exclusive health and safety apps: The 5Star app enables you to immediately connect with highly trained agents in case of an emergency. The Urgent Care app provides you unlimited 24/7 access to registered nurses and board-certified doctors. You can use the GreatCall Link app to keep in contact with family and friends about your well-being. This simple, fun phone has everything you need. You won't have to dig through menu after menu or flip through screens. At the same time, if you want to do more with your phone, you still have access to more than 700,000 Google Play Store apps.

App Compatibility with Other Devices

The 5Star, Urgent Care, and Link apps are available for download on any Android phone or iPhone.

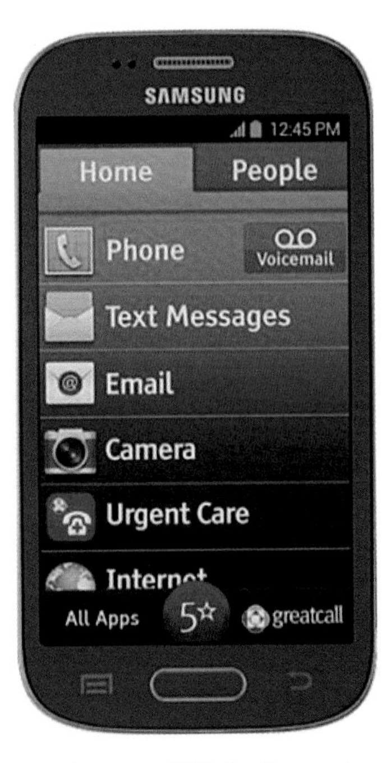

Jitterbug Touch3 by GreatCall

Consider the Snapfōn ezTWO3G

For those looking for a practical phone that has a more simplistic approach but still has in-demand features, the Snapfōn might be the phone you have been looking for. The ezTWO3G is an unlocked phone, which means you can use it on a variety of networks worldwide. As of this writing, this phone is not compatible with Verizon or Sprint. It has big buttons with a keyboard that speaks numbers as you dial them to ensure accuracy. It has an intuitive interface, and its functions are easy to set up. Purchase this device on the Snapfōn website or on Amazon.com, and then activate it at snapfon.com.

The key feature on this phone is an emergency S.O.S button located on the back of the device. You can set up the ezTWO3G to include up to four names and numbers as emergency contacts to call when you press the S.O.S button. After pressing the button, you can talk to your designated contact through the speakerphone. A text message is also sent to your emergency contact. Press and hold the S.O.S button for five seconds to sound an alarm. Snapfōn also offers a 24/7 monitoring system option. An sosPlus agent can dispatch emergency services, alert family members, conference in emergency services, and stay on the line until the situation has been resolved.

With an sosPlus account, you can also pre-emptively input important information that agents can access in case of an emergency. The collected information can include a list of all medications you take, known allergies, medical condition, emergency contacts, your doctor, and past surgical history. You can also give instruction on what to do if you are nonresponsive in case of an emergency.

The Snapfōn ezTWO3G is a great way to be independent and still keep in touch while safeguarding yourself and helping loved ones in case of an emergency. With this in mind, know that this phone will not enable you to take advantage of many of the apps and devices discussed later in this book.

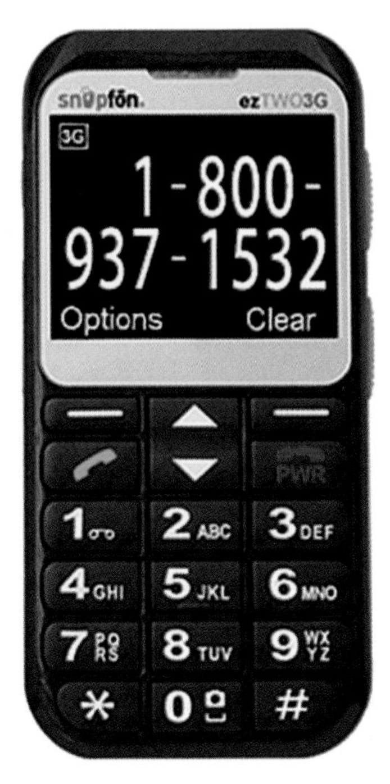

© 2004-2016, Snapfōn® and Visikey® by SeniorTech, LLC

Snapfōn ezTWO3G

>>>Go Further

TAKING A LOOK AT SOME SNAPFŌN GENERAL FEATURES

You can't download apps on the Snapfōn ezTWO3G, but it does share some of the most used features of the common cellphone such as Bluetooth (wireless connectivity), 250 phonebook contacts, text messaging, eight speed-dial locations, keypad lock, a built-in camera, and English and Spanish languages. This phone also has a flashlight that you can easily activate from its side so you can watch your step in low-lit places.

Finding Health Apps for Your Device

For our purposes, the strength of the smartphones and wearable devices discussed in this book lies in the health-related software that is developed for them. The devices come with some inventive fitness apps right out of the box, but you can expand many of their capabilities even further by downloading new apps. Some of the phones and wearables discussed in this book do not have the capability to install additional apps. Those devices will be identified as we discuss them, but for those that can, the selection is plentiful and growing every day, and warrants some guidance on where to start.

Many ways exist to find health-related apps for your device. Where you find them depends largely on which ecosphere you land in: Android or Apple. Within the Android ecosphere, in some circumstances, where you find apps will also depend on which type of device you have. For example, Samsung has its own app store. Some fitness trackers, including the Pebble, have their own accompanying apps that you can use as a portal to find more apps. First, let's start with the most basic of searches.

Perform a Google Search

Open your preferred Internet browser—which may include Internet Explorer, Safari, Chrome, Firefox, or Microsoft Edge—and type **google.com** in the address bar at the top of the page. Press the Enter button on your PC or the Return button on your Mac. Type a term into the search field, such as **Best health apps for Android (or iPhone)**. You can be more specific and search **Best fitness app for Android (or iPhone)**. Press Enter or Return on the keyboard, and the results are displayed. This is a great way to find a review of the software by someone other than the manufacturer and determine whether it's the right app for you. Be aware that some of these sites are sponsored by the developers and might not convey completely objective views.

If you currently don't have a smartphone and are deciding between Android and iPhone, just do a general search; for example, "Best fitness app." Most reviews include which platform is compatible with the app. The good news is that the most popular apps are available for both Android and Apple devices. If you happen to find a few apps that seem perfect for you but only run on a specific platform, that might be the deciding factor for you.

Choose from a Bounty of Apps

The lion's share of health apps are made for the most popular devices, including Android and Apple, and activity trackers such as Pebble, just to name a few.

Find a Forum

Search online or join the AARP community to connect with others on similar interests. Ask questions to see whether anyone recommends a specific app. Personal experience with an app coupled with the ability to ask questions is a great way to make an informed decision. Many communities are online, but beware that experienced product users might not moderate all of these forums, and the advice you receive can be questionable.

Ask Your Doctor

Your doctor's office is a great place to ask for suggestions related to a good activity app, blood pressure app, and so on. It is also a great place to find out whether you're healthy enough to do a certain activity or whether an app is actually effective or not.

Browse the Play Store

For those who already land in the Android ecosphere or who are planning to get an Android phone, the Google Play Store makes it easy for you to browse content that you can download to your phone. If this is your first time shopping the Google Play Store, you will find the interface quite intuitive. You can access the Google Play Store on your Android phone by tapping on the Play Store icon on your device. A great way to become acquainted with Google Play Store is just to start browsing.

1. Tap the Play Store icon on the screen.
2. Tap Apps.
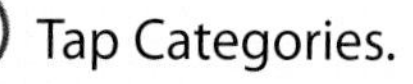
3. Tap Categories.
4. Swipe down the screen using your finger, and then tap Health & Fitness. A whole list of featured health and fitness apps appears.

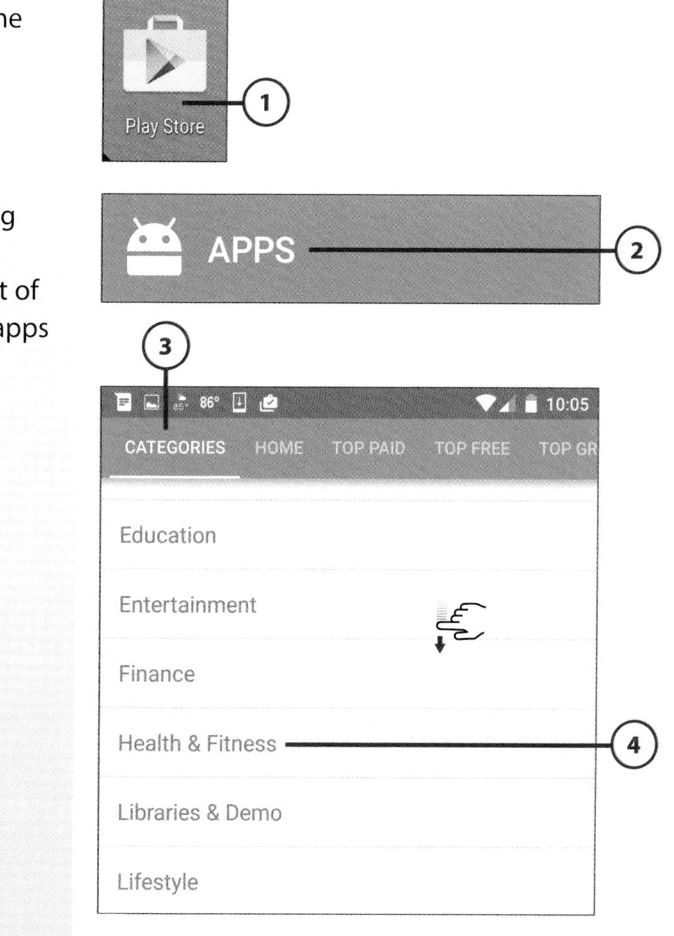

5. Swipe up and down the screen to view the results. You'll be happy to see that many of the apps are free. You can tap an app to go to the description page and read more information about an app, see screenshots, and even purchase or install the app for free.
6. Tap the search field (the magnifying glass) at the top of the page, and then type to search for a specific app. Suggestions begin to appear underneath the search field.
7. Tap a search suggestion to select it. The product detail page opens.

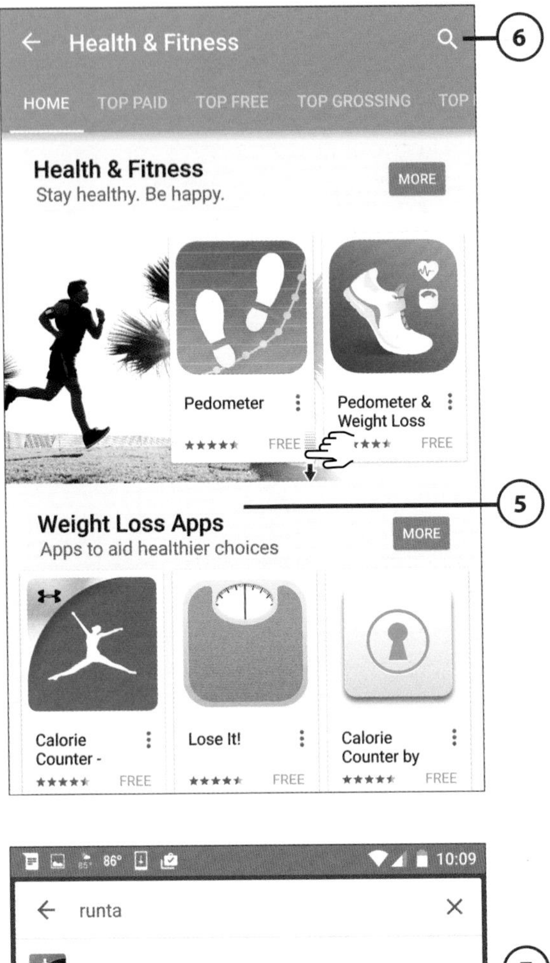

8. Tap Read More to learn more about the product. If you are already signed in with your Google account, you can either purchase the app or install it for free via the description page. If the option to download or purchase is not available, sign in to your Google account and then revisit the app page.

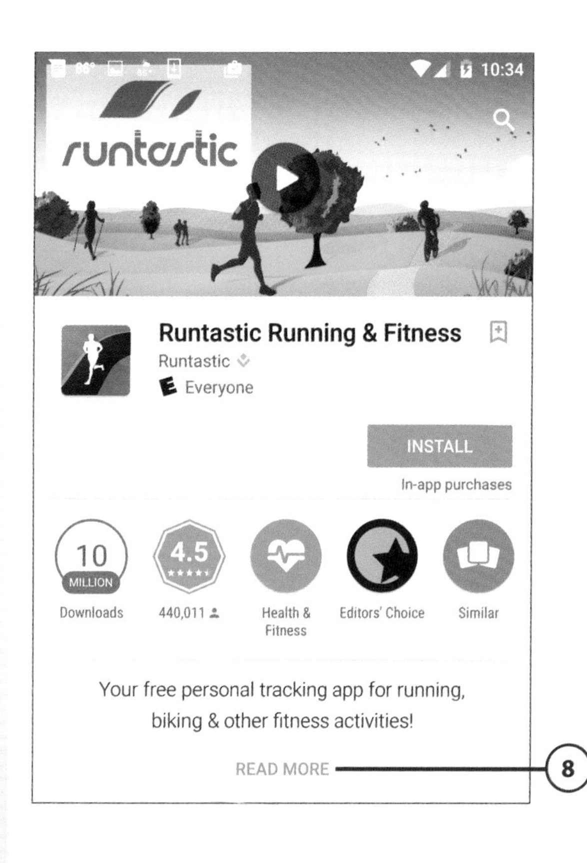

More About Product Descriptions

The description page for an app is full of useful information so you can make an educated decision on whether you want to purchase the app. Sample screenshots of the app are featured on this page along with customer reviews and information about the developer.

Tips for Searching the Play Store

Type **Android Wear Fitness** to search for apps that can be installed on your Android Wear smartwatch. You learn about the Android Wear line of smartwatches later in the "Taking a Look at What Wearables Can Do for You" section.

Use the Gear Manager App

The Samsung Gear Manager app is strictly for Samsung phones and wearables. The app enables you to sync your Galaxy Gear watch to your phone, but also acts as a portal to watch apps. You must install the app from the Samsung Apps store. The Galaxy Apps store is full of apps for you to browse that are optimized for your Gear device.

1. Tap Apps.
2. Tap Gear Manager.
3. Tap Samsung Gear Apps.
4. Select a category or tap the search icon to search for a specific app.
5. Tap an app to go to the description page and read more about the product. You can purchase or select Free to download the app for free via the description page. Before you can download anything from the Samsung Galaxy App Store, you first must sign in to your Galaxy App account.

Gear Fit Manager

The Samsung Gear Fit has a Gear Fit Manager app that enables you to install apps and configure your device.

It's Not All Good

Transferring Galaxy Apps to a New Phone

You can download apps from the Galaxy Apps store to your phone and to your Gear smart-watch. Apps found in Samsung's Galaxy Apps store are designed for use on Samsung Galaxy devices. If you download apps from the Galaxy Apps store and then later switch to a non-Samsung Android phone, those apps will not transfer to the new phone.

Use the Android Wear App

The Android Wear app's purpose is much like that of the Gear Manager app. It enables you to sync your Android Wear to your phone, and it is a portal for downloading apps to your Android Wear smartwatch. You must first download the Android Wear app from the Google Play Store. The Android Wear app is also available from the App Store, allowing you to connect to an iPhone. Later in this chapter you'll learn more about the Android Wear operating system and how it can be a deciding factor in choosing a smartwatch and smartphone. You don't have to exclusively use the Android Wear App to browse the available apps. You can easily perform a search for "Android Wear Apps" in the Google Play Store to narrow down the search for your smartwatch. With that being said, the Android Wear App offers a quick way to filter the search for your particular smartwatch.

After you have synced your phone to your watch, follow these directions to download the app and search for fitness apps.

1. Tap the Android Wear app.
2. Tap More beside Essential watch apps.

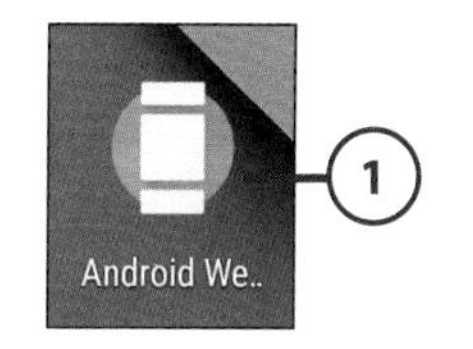

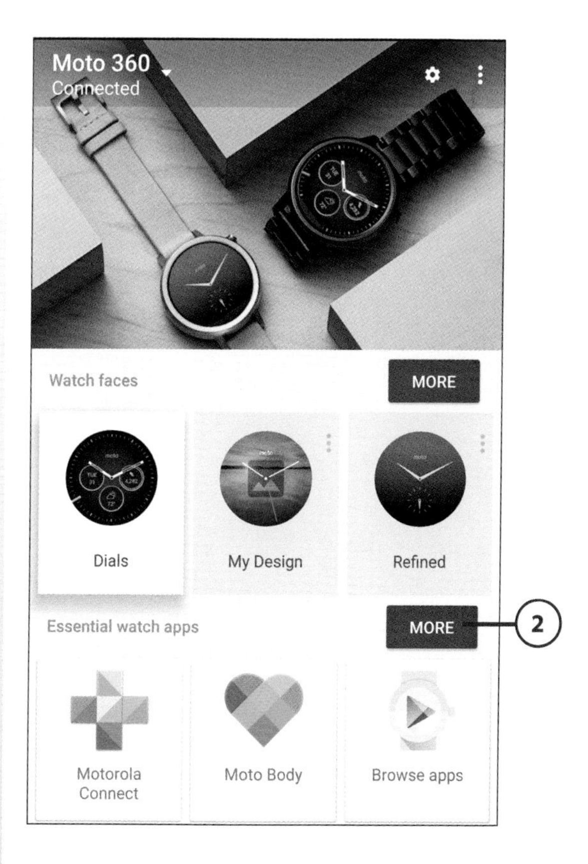

3. Tap Accept to agree to the Google Play Terms of Service.
4. Swipe down the page with your finger to find the Health Goals category of apps, and tap on an app you want to review, or tap an app from another category.

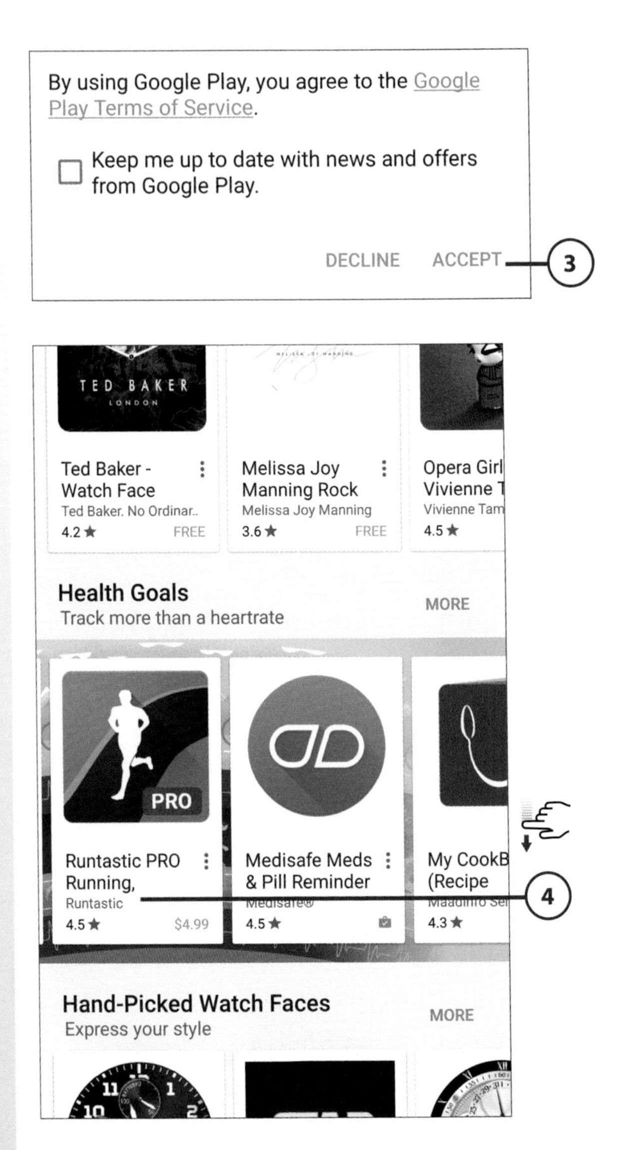

5. Tap Read More to learn more about the app from the description page. You can also purchase or install the app for free on the description page. Before you can download anything, you must first sign in to your Google account.

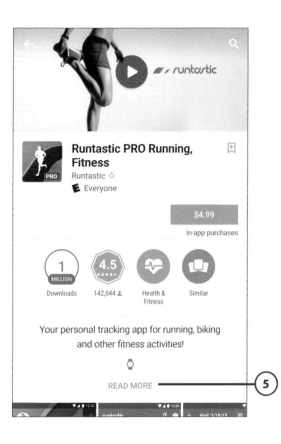

Browse the App Store

This option is for those who have already landed in the Apple ecosphere or are planning to get an Apple phone. The App Store also makes it easy for you to browse content that you can download to your phone or wearable. You can access the App Store on your Apple phone by tapping on the App Store icon on the Home screen. Follow these steps to browse the many options that the App store offers.

1. Tap the App Store icon.
2. Tap Explore.
3. Swipe down the screen using your finger, and then tap Health & Fitness. A list of popular health and fitness apps appears, along with subcategories.
4. Tap a subcategory. An entire page filled with related apps appears.

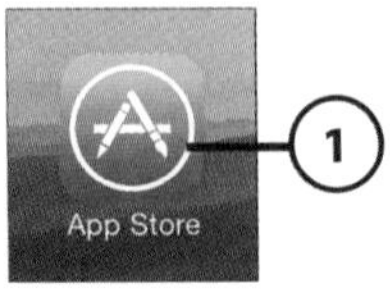

App Store
1

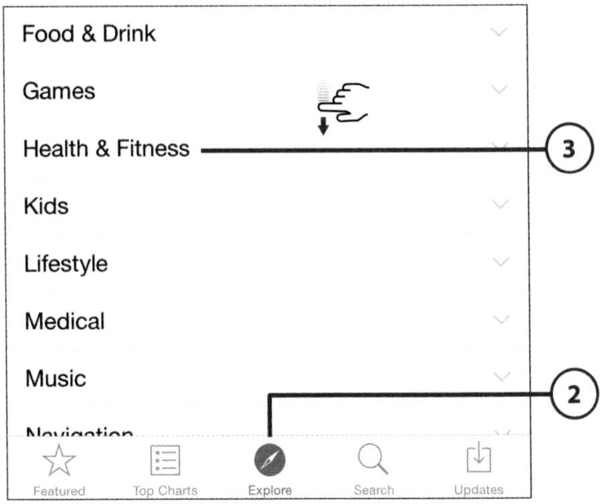

Food & Drink
Games
Health & Fitness
3
Kids
Lifestyle
Medical
Music
Navigation
2
Featured
Top Charts
Explore
Search
Updates

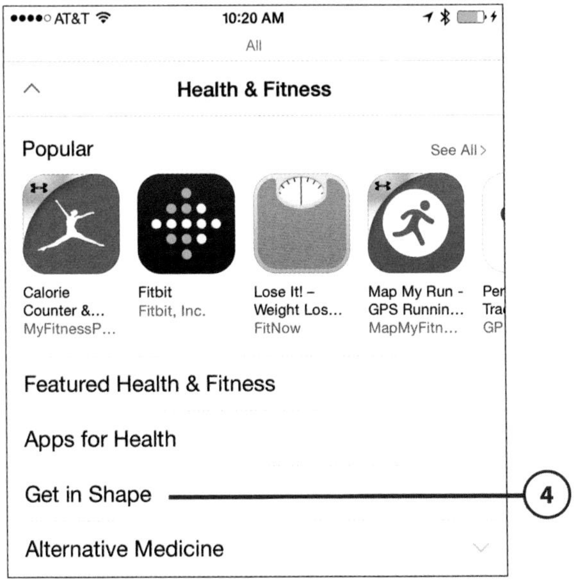

●●●●○ AT&T
10:20 AM
All
Health & Fitness
Popular
See All >
Calorie Counter &...
MyFitnessP...
Fitbit
Fitbit, Inc.
Lose It! – Weight Los...
FitNow
Map My Run - GPS Runnin...
MapMyFitn...
Per
Tra
GP
Featured Health & Fitness
Apps for Health
Get in Shape
4
Alternative Medicine

5. Tap an app to go to the description page and read more about the product. You can purchase or get the app for free via the description page. Before you can download anything from the App Store, you must first sign in to your Apple account.

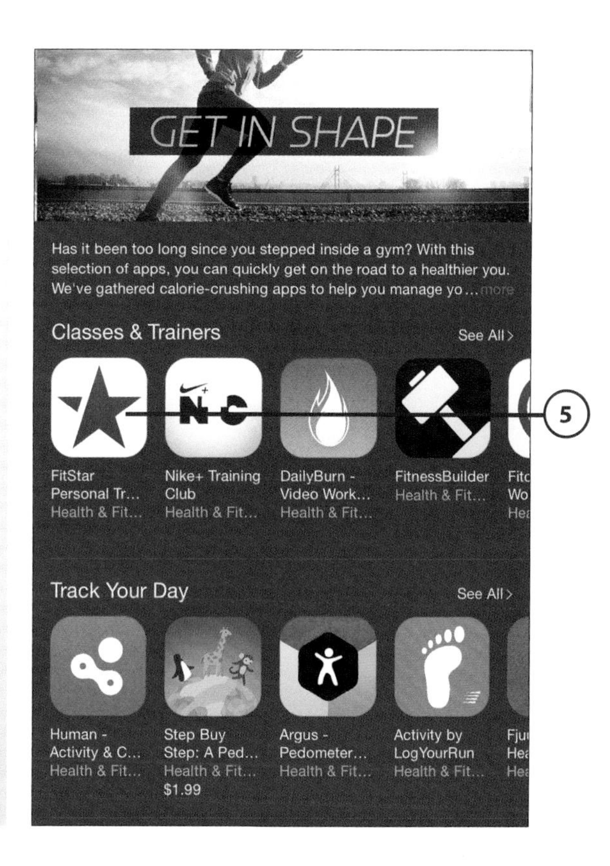

Use the Apple Watch App

This option is for those who have already landed in the Apple ecosphere or are planning to get an Apple iPhone. The Apple Watch app makes it easy for you to browse content that you can download to your Apple Watch. You can access the Apple Watch on your iPhone's main screen.

1. Tap the Apple Watch icon on the screen. The settings for configuring your Apple watch appear.

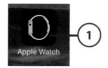

2. Tap Featured. All the featured apps for your Apple watch appear in categories.
3. Swipe down the screen using your finger, and locate the Healthy Living category.
4. Swipe from right to left with your finger to view the available apps. If you know the specific name of the app you are looking for, you can tap the Search option at the bottom of the screen.
5. Tap an app to go to the description page and read more about the product. You can purchase or get the app for free on the description page. Before you can download anything from the App Store, you must first sign in to your Apple account.

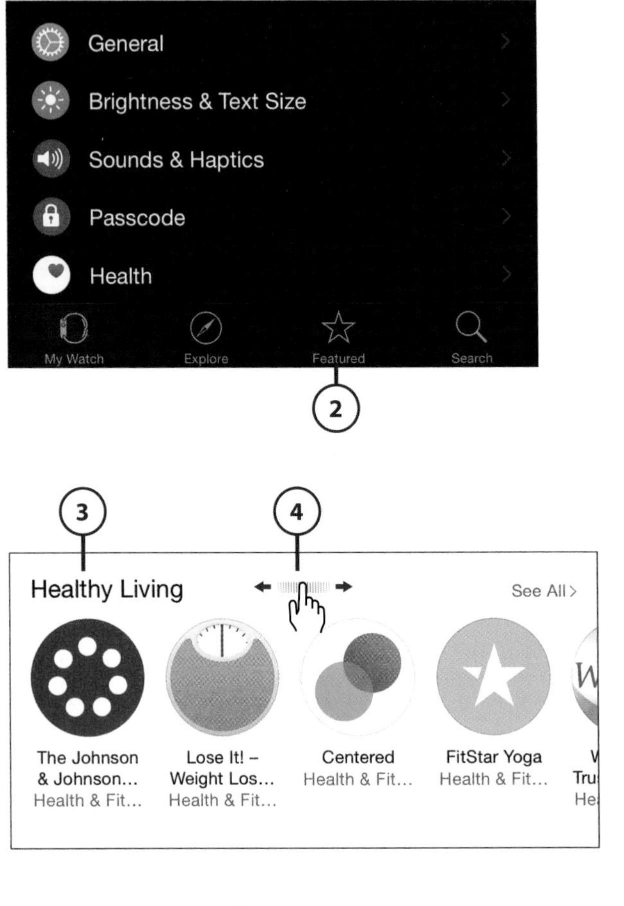

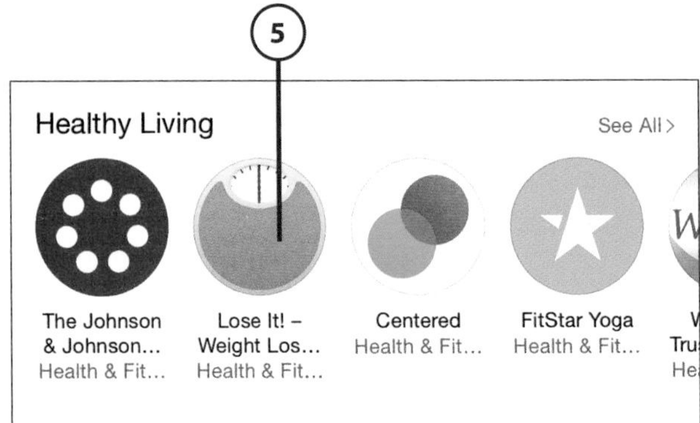

Visit a Fitness Tracker's Website

Many fitness trackers come with a dedicated phone app to be used as a portal to browse apps for that particular device. For example, the Pebble line of watches has the Pebble App Store where you can peruse its Health & Fitness section. Whichever tracker you choose, go to its company's website to learn more about the apps available for that device. After you know the name of the app you are looking for, you can find most of these apps in the Google Play Store and Apple App Store. You can also subscribe to blogs for the fitness tracker, or follow the brand on Twitter or Facebook to keep up-to-date with new apps and features.

Exploring Web-Based Solutions

Web-based and mobile services have grown into a viable option for bringing health care into your home and providing some extra transparency. A friend's recommendation of a doctor is a great way to get you started in your search, but now apps and web-based resources can help you find doctors and peruse anonymous reviews, such as on Angie's List. Online services have moved well beyond just being able to book an appointment; you can actually participate in a doctor's visit on your computer, as with Doctor On Demand and Teledoc. This can save you the hassle of calling in to a doctor's office for an appointment and having to wait weeks before an opening. Of course, not every health situation can be properly treated this way. A doctor online can help you make that determination. Resources such as Co-Patient, Good RX, and WeRx also enable you to compare prices at different pharmacies to avoid paying exorbitant fees for medication. You can find additional resources for helping your family prepare if something should happen to you, including Checklist for My Family and Everplans. This book lists only a few of the web-based services that you can and should vet for yourself. Read what other people are saying online about these services. Does the service provide real value? Do people like the service?

>>>Go Further

HARDWARE NEEDED FOR WEB-BASED SERVICES

To take full advantage of all the Web-based resources in this book, you will need a computer. Some of the options covered in this book also include apps, so a smartphone or a tablet would help you take full advantage. Your computer must also have a camera: internal or external. Internal cameras are located at he top of your monitor, right in the middle. You also need a microphone. Chances are if your computer has an internal camera, it also has a built-in microphone. Internal microphones are usually just a small, single hole, and might be marked with the word *MIC*. Most tablets and smartphones are equipped with front-facing cameras so that you can, for example, video visit with a doctor online.

Taking a Look at What Wearables Can Do for You

Wearable technology is the new frontier of mobile devices. By the time you read this book, there will be new devices to discover. More and more manufacturers are tapping into this new trend. This section helps you separate hype from practicality, and provides, in tandem with the other sections of this book, a better understanding of how fitness trackers and smartwatches can help you live a healthier lifestyle and manage many health conditions.

One distinction needs to be made before we go further. The term *wearable* usually encompasses fitness trackers, smartwatches, and even smart eyeglasses. This book does not cover smart eyeglasses because their practicality has yet to be determined, but it does cover some products, such as medical bracelets, pendants, and dedicated pedometers, that might not traditionally fall into the mainstream tech definition of wearable. These added products are included so you can choose the most effective and practical resource for your lifestyle.

If you have a pacemaker or other implanted electronic device, consult your doctor before using any wearable products.

Decide Between Fitness Trackers

The first step in picking the best device for your lifestyle is to understand the difference between a fitness tracker and a smartwatch. If you can track your activity and monitor your heart rate on a smartwatch, does that make it a fitness tracker? If you can tell time on your fitness tracker, does that make it a smartwatch? It all boils down to purpose.

Fitness trackers almost exclusively do what the name implies: track and evaluate how much physical activity you're exerting. This book includes "running watches" and "swimming watches" in the fitness-tracking category as well. On the other hand, *smartwatches* include many features outside of health and fitness that you might or might not have a use for. The upcoming section, "Do You Really Need a Smartwatch?," provides more information on those features. The following discussion provides some guidance on buying a fitness tracker.

What Fitness Goals Do You Want to Achieve?

Choose a fitness tracker that fits not only your current needs, but also what goals you hope to accomplish in the future. At their very core, most fitness trackers can show you how many steps you've taken and how many calories you've burned. If you are new to exercise and are looking to become more active, fitness trackers such as the Withings Activité Pop and the Fitbit are wonderful multipurpose devices. Withings and Fitbit offer a range of activity levels to choose from.

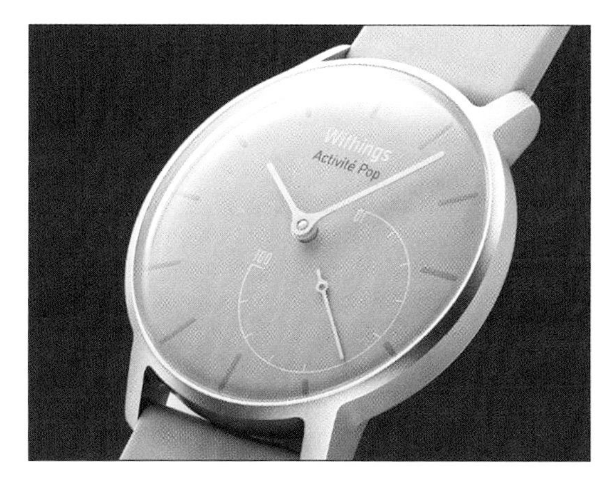

© 2009-2016 Withings SA

Withings Activité Pop

If you walk every day, but you want to work up to a 5K, 10K, or beyond, choose a fitness tracker whose strength is tracking running performance. This usually means having a GPS and a running mode. This could include the Garmin Forerunner 220 or the Fitbit Surge. If you love to swim, get a fitness tracker that is designed for it, such as the Moov Now Multi-Sport Wearable Coach or Swimovate PoolMate HR. If you perform a variety of activities, both Garmin and TomTom make many products that track elevation, pace, biking, intervals, and more.

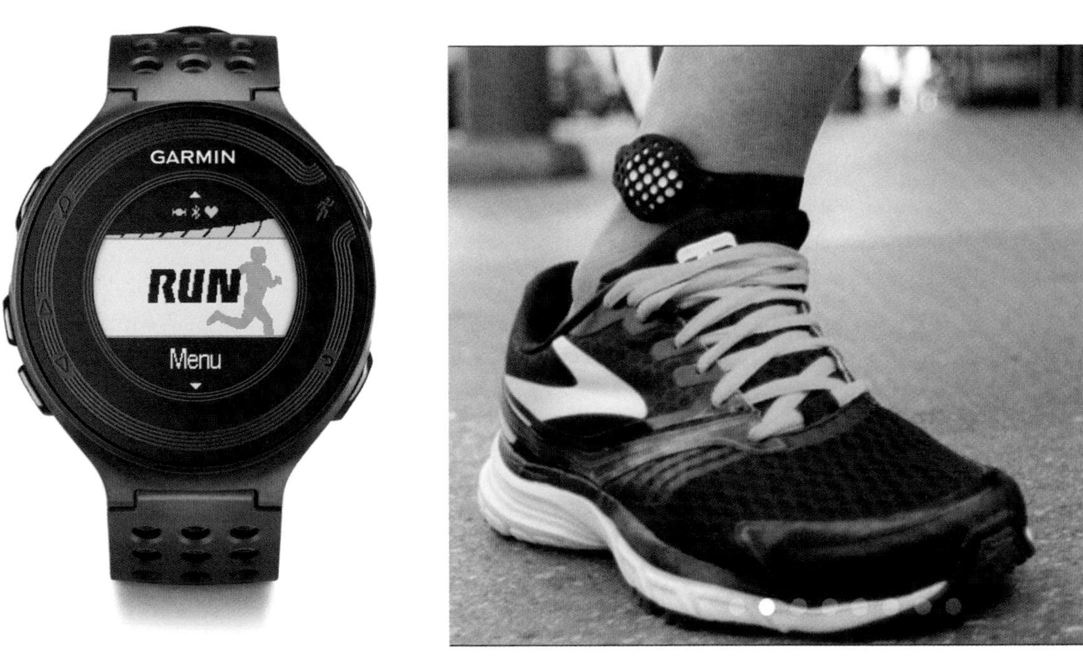

© 2009-2016 Withings SA
Garmin Forerunner 220

© 2015 Moov, Inc
Moov Now Multi-Sport Wearable Coach

Water Resistance

If you have not purchased a watch that can be used for tracking swimming performance, you should at least know a device's water resistance level. Can you shower with it on? Splash resistance typically implies being sweat-resistant, as do the words *fitness* and *activity*. Water-resistant can mean safe for showering but not for swimming. Waterproof implies the device is safe for swimming. Make sure whichever tracker you choose is right for your needs.

It's Not All Good

Varying Results in Tracking Accuracy

Accuracy in readings can vary among the many activity trackers. Some activity trackers might do a better job at calculating the correct distance travelled or steps taken. Some activity trackers with heart rate monitors prove less accurate in monitoring heart rate if you have dark skin. Fortunately, manufacturers are receiving a lot of feedback and are working out the issues. Do your research before purchasing a product. Read product reviews and join online community discussions to help determine which devices perform best for your needs.

What Design Fits Your Needs?

Aesthetics aside and diving straight into practicality, some fitness trackers are made to be worn in various locations on the body. Most of the fitness trackers are designed for wearing around the wrist. Some clip on to clothing. The Misfit Flash and the Jawbone UP MOVE are designed for both options. The Moov Now Multi-Sport Wearable Coach enables you to wear the sensor around your ankle or intertwined in the laces on your shoes. Depending on which activities you perform, you might prefer one location over another. You can wear a fitness tracker all day long or just when you need it. Some of the running watches have big faces that you might find too gaudy to wear all day. If you do choose to wear one all day, you might find you don't interact with it much. However, when you do use your watch, you want the interaction to be intuitive. This is where the display is important.

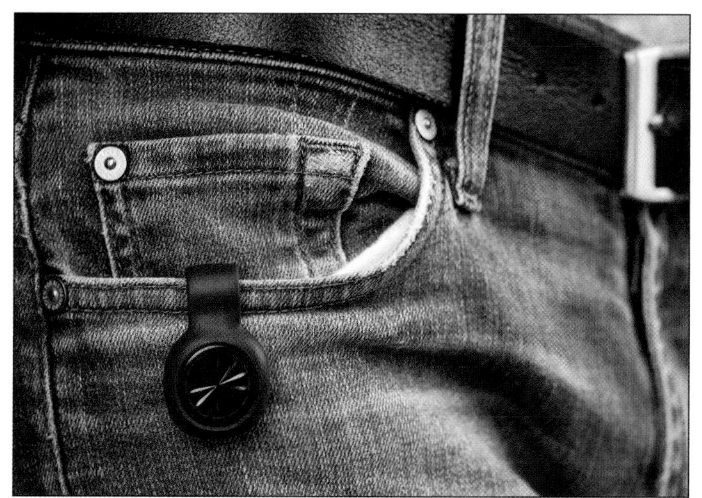

Jawbone UP MOVE

Some fitness trackers, such as an entry-level Fitbit devices, take a minimalist approach and use LED lights to show information, whereas others offer an attractive analog interface, such as Withing's Activité Pop. Some devices might have a touch screen that you tap or swipe to view information. Larger faced devices enable more information to be shown onscreen.

Which Features Do You Need or Want?

As stated earlier, most fitness trackers can count steps. The sleep monitoring feature that can help you form healthier sleep patterns is also quickly catching on, as found on the Activité Pop and the Microsoft Band. If you want to know how many flights of stairs you climbed, or the intensity of your physical activity, look for a fitness tracker that includes an altimeter, which measures altitude, as well as an accelerometer, which measures speed.

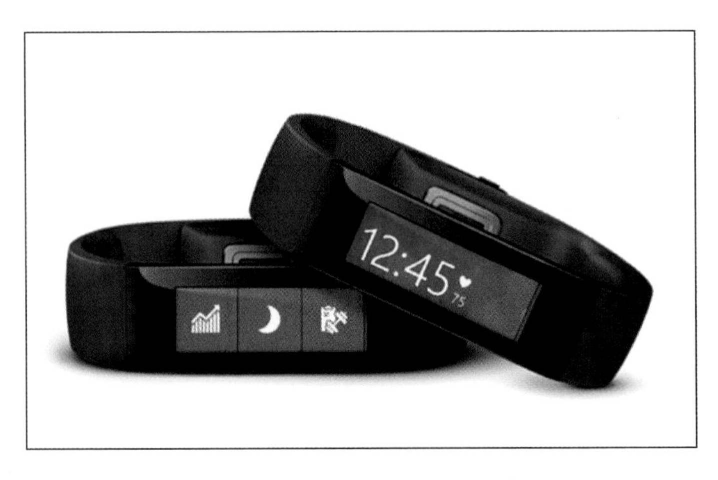

Microsoft Band

Heart rate monitoring and GPS capability are feature sets of higher-end fitness trackers. Some fitness trackers, such as the Basis Peak and the Microsoft Band, can monitor your heart rate without the chest strap, via sensors on the back of the tracker that are pressed against the skin. Some bands can use the chest strap as well. GPS capability is great for runners, cyclists, hikers, swimmers, and anyone who wants to monitor their speed, distance, and route.

What Apps Are Available for the Device?

Most fitness trackers have companion apps that you install on your phone. Some also have dedicated websites. You synchronize your fitness tracker to the app or website to store and review your activity data. These apps and websites also offer some additional features such as food logging, calorie counting, and other nutritional information for a healthier diet. Some trackers even allow you to use apps made by other companies, such as Lose It!, to track and sync data.

When vetting a fitness tracker, make sure its companion app or website is easy to read. Is the information presented in an intuitive, easy-to-understand presentation? If a fitness tracker uses a website, go to the website and take a look for yourself to see whether it works for you.

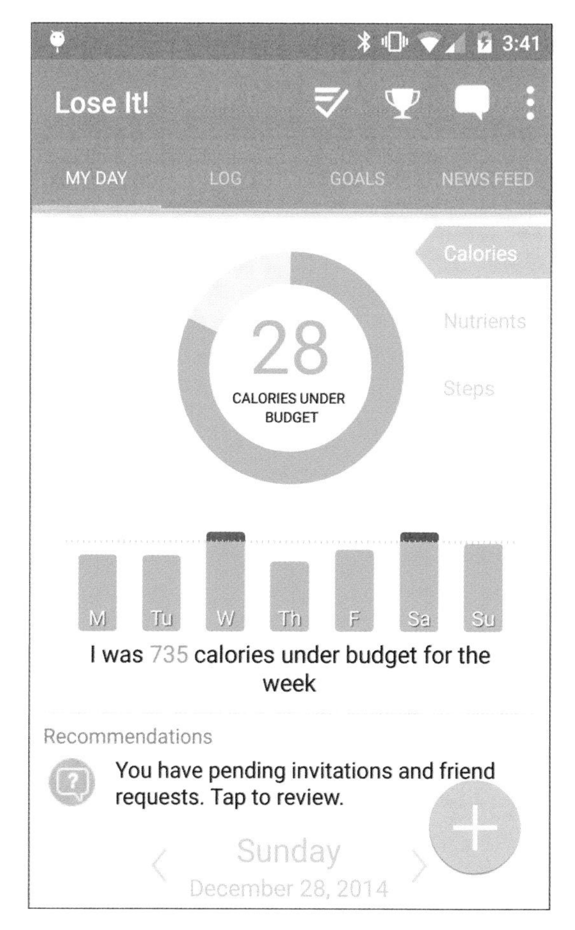

The Lose It! App

Is the Device Compatible with Your Phone?

Most fitness trackers are designed to sync with Android and Apple (iOS) Phones. Windows Phone–compatible devices are rare. If you are interested in a specific activity tracker, first see whether it's compatible with your current phone. It will usually state this on the box, product website, or Amazon. This information alone could lead you to a specific line of devices.

What's the Price?

Fitness trackers typically range between $50 and $420 dollars. This is when it is important to once again ask, "What is it that you want to achieve? What do you need to be the healthiest version of you?" If you want to count steps and calories, then you can save a lot of money and go with a baseline fitness tracker. If you want to improve your time in the annual 5K race, a higher-end tracker that provides detailed information on pace and stride will serve you better. As your fitness goals change or progress, you might need a fitness watch. Overall, as with most products, the more you pay, the more features and options are available. Not to pigeon-hole any of these devices into a superficial category, but here is a brief categorization of a few fitness tracker features and associated cost that might help you decide on a device that's right for you.

- **Introductory:** An introductory fitness tracker under $50 (USD) is a good place to start if you are looking to lead a more active lifestyle and get your body moving. Fitness trackers at this level, such as the Jawbone UP MOVE and the Misfit Flash, enable you to track steps and calories, and monitor sleep activity. You can wear the Jawbone UP MOVE around the wrist or on a belt clip, and the Misfit Flash includes a clasp and sport band so that you can wear it on your waist, wrist, sleeve, shoes, pocket, lapel, or even shirt. Each is compatible with Android and Apple (iOS) devices and a variety of apps.

If You're New to Working Out

Always consult a physician before beginning any exercise program.

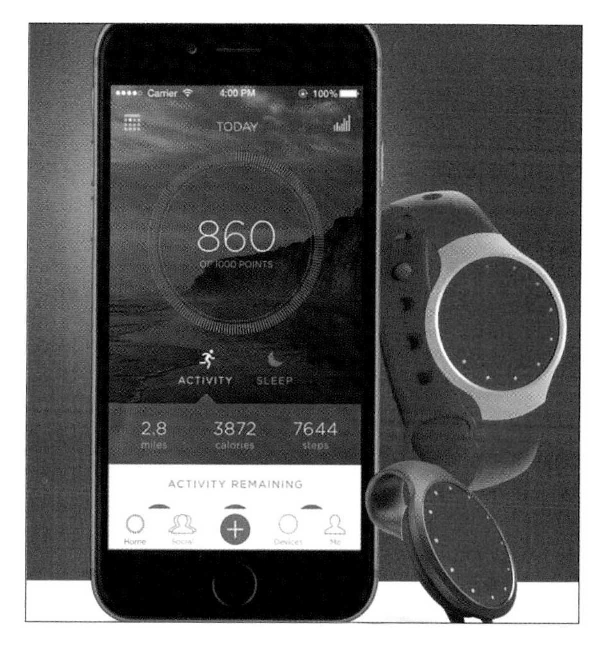

Misfit Flash

- **Intermediate:** An intermediate fitness tracker, from $50–$100, is for the individual for whom exercise and the gym have become a regular pastime. The Moov Now can track your running, cycling, walking, guided workouts, swimming, boxing, and sleeping activity. It even talks to you as you work out. The Fitbit Flex can track steps, distance, calories burned, and active minutes. It also enables you to monitor how well you sleep and even has a silent alarm to wake you. Both devices are water-resistant. They are compatible with Android and Apple (iOS) devices so you can use their accompanying apps to collect data on your activities. The Fitbit Flex is even compatible with Windows Phones. Due to the rate at which these technologies expand, do still make sure that your particular phone is supported.
- **Midrange:** Most fitness trackers fall under the midrange category, costing about $100–$200. This is a great range to grow into if you currently fall into the introductory or intermediate category, and it is a range in which a competitive athlete can find a solid device. Heart monitoring capability is prevalent in this category, as well as GPS-enabled devices. The Microsoft Band can track your heart rate, steps, calories burned, and sleep quality.

You can also receive email previews and calendar alerts when you need to stay connected to the outside world. The Fitbit ChargeHR can track your heart rate, calories burned, floors climbed, and active minutes. The Fitbit app also lets you see your progress and analyze trends with intuitive charts and graphs. You can log workouts, use a monthly exercise calendar, and use the MobileRun app to track run stats, map routes, and keep a food log. Both devices are compatible with the leading Android and Windows devices and Apple (iOS devices).

- **High-End:** The high-end trackers, $200 and up, carry some of the widest range of feature sets for fitness buffs and some of the most highly specialized. You can find trackers that feature an altimeter, barometer, and compass, like with the Suunto Ambit3 Peak. The Suunto Movescount app lets you plan your own route by offering maps, and you can even set up notifications for seeing calls and text messages. The TomTom Runner Cardio helps you run in your optimal heart rate zone with its built-in heart rate monitor. If you're a triathlete, like my mother-in-law, take a look at the TomTom Multisport Cardio, which also tracks cycling and swimming. The TomTom My Sports app can collect all of your activity data for a detailed report. The Suunto Ambit3 Peak and both TomTom Cardio devices are compatible with Android and Apple (iOS devices).

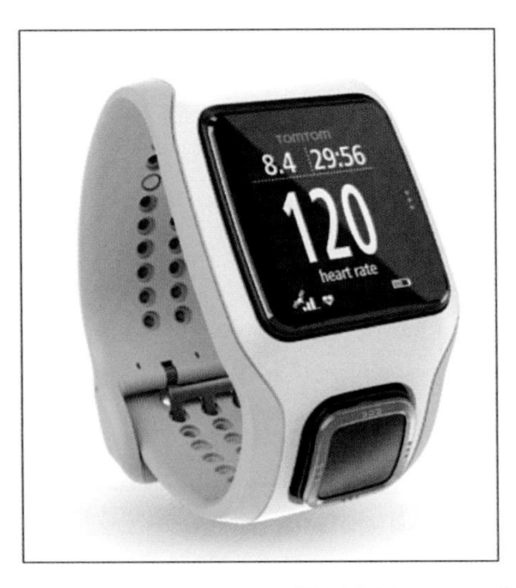

TomTom Runner Cardio

Determine Your Need for a Smartwatch

Some confusion tends to surround what makes a smartwatch different from a fitness tracker. As stated earlier, first and foremost, fitness trackers almost exclusively track and evaluate how much physical activity you're exerting. Smartwatches have fitness tracking capabilities, but go far beyond this and incorporate many of the same functions as your cell phone. Notifications and apps are the biggest difference between activity trackers and smartwatches. Email and text messages sent to your phone can be viewed on your smartwatch, along with incoming call notifications and calendar event notifications. You can even browse through photo galleries located on your phone from your smartwatch. If you have an Android or Apple phone, you can also access the Google Now or Siri virtual assistants using voice commands.

Like fitness trackers, more and more of the popular smartwatches— including Android Wear—are starting to work on both Android and Apple (iOS) systems. With that being said, as of this writing, Android smartwatches still work best on Android devices, and the Apple Watch works exclusively with Apple products. For the time being, you're better off choosing a platform. One of the exceptions is the highly popular Pebble line of smartwatches that work nicely on both Android and Apple (iOS) phones.

Many of the points used to decide on an activity tracker can also be used to make an informed decision about purchasing a smartwatch. Again, it all boils down to purpose and practicality.

What Are Your Priorities?

Do you make time to perform calorie-burning activities and need something that can quickly and easily relay your email, text messages, and calendar events? A smartwatch might be right for you. If you would like to glance at a message or swipe across your watch screen to answer a call or review your calendar, then a smartwatch can give you this and much more. Because the smartwatch shares many of your phone's features, you'll find yourself picking up your phone less frequently during the day. If you don't want to be bothered by all these notifications while you're out for a run or walk, you can easily turn them off. Think of a smartwatch as an accessory to your smartphone.

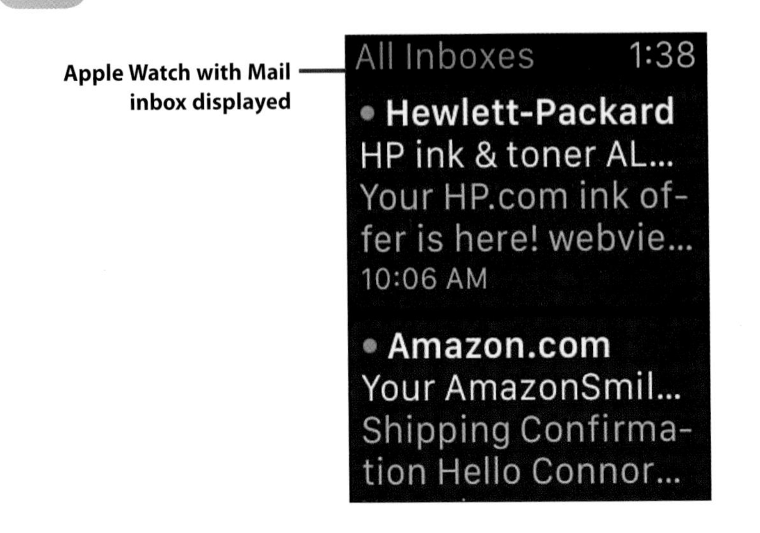

Apple Watch with Mail inbox displayed

Is the Watch Compatible with Your Phone?

The most popular smartwatches land in four categories: Android Wear, Apple Watch, Samsung Gear, and watches produced by other manufacturers (including Pebble and Sony) that are compatible with Android and Apple phones.

As of the writing of this book, the latest line of Android smartwatches is compatible with Android 4.3 Jelly Bean or higher. The newer Android Wear watches are now compatible with iPhones running iOS 8.2 or higher. The Apple Watch is compatible with the iPhone 5 models (5, 5C, or 5S) and up, running iOS 8.2 or later. The Pebble line of smartwatches works with Android devices running 4.1 (Jelly Bean) and above, and with iOS 6 or higher.

Confirming Your Phone's Operating System

If you already own an Android or Apple phone and need a refresher in how to check which operating system you are running, review the previous "Explore Android Devices" and "Consider an Apple iPhone" sections.

What Are the Health and Fitness Possibilities?

The smartwatches' strength rests in the wealth of health and fitness apps available for them. The most popular fitness apps are made for Android and

Apple smartwatches, and many health and fitness apps are making their way to the Pebble App store.

Because Android and Apple have their own line of phones, they come with their own fitness apps for their phones. After you sync your device to your phone, you can begin taking advantage of these apps. Some apps enable you to track your everyday activities, receive coaching to achieve your daily goals, and choose from a variety of fitness plans. With the Pebble line of smartwatches, you can download activity tracking apps such as Fitocracy, Jawbone, Misfit, and RunKeeper. You can go to the Google Play Store and Apple App Store and add many, many more health and fitness apps depending on your own personal needs.

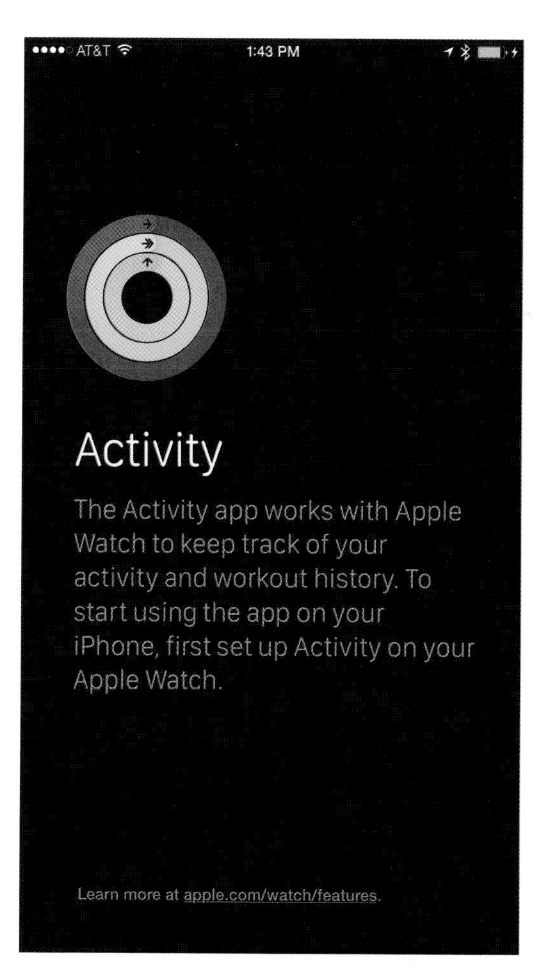

Apple Activity app

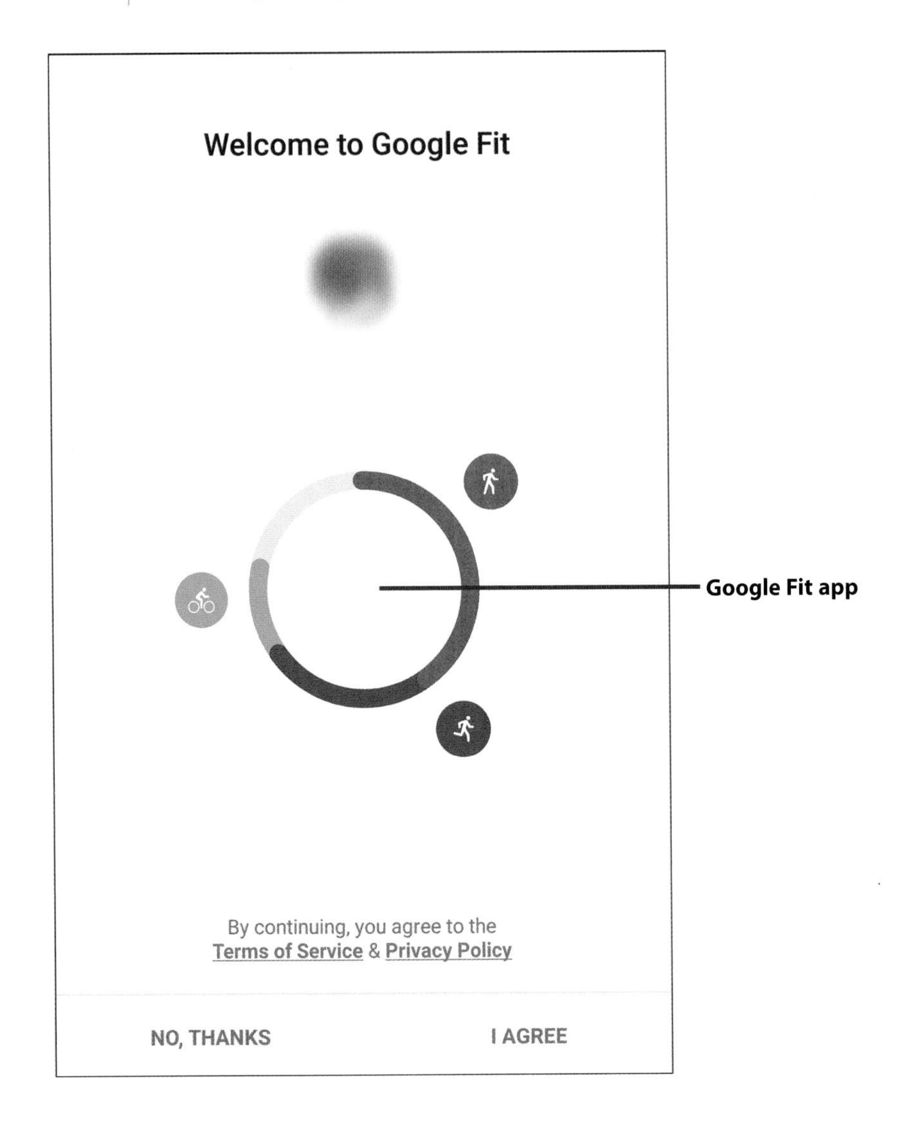

Each watch also comes with its own personalized health and fitness functions right out of the box that provide personalized insight into your performance while running, walking, cycling, hiking, and other activities.

What Design Fits Your Needs?

In the conversation of smartwatches, aesthetics ranks up there with screen navigability. This is because many people buy a smartwatch to replace their current watch and plan to wear it all day, so they are more concerned with the design of this watch than those who might only wear their fitness tracker during activities. The Android Wear, Apple Watch, Pebble line, and Samsung Gear are the most popular smartwatches. Let's look at some specifics to help you choose.

- **Android:** Currently, Android Wear offers the widest variety of watch designs on the market. This collection offers stainless steel, large, round displays as well as the square form you find in most smartwatches. The Android Wear collection is comprised of phones made by a variety of manufacturers including Motorola, LG, and even Samsung. Each Android Wear model comes with standard fitness apps, but you can expand their health facility through the Google Play Store. Because there is no analog face, you can easily switch between digital watch faces. Google has also just started adding functions to the watch face itself that can allow you to tap or swipe for super-easy access to some of your favorite apps and fitness-tracking information. There are also a variety of bands to choose from. Currently, the most popular devices in the Android Wear line are the Asus Zen Watch, LG Watch Urbane, and the Moto 360.

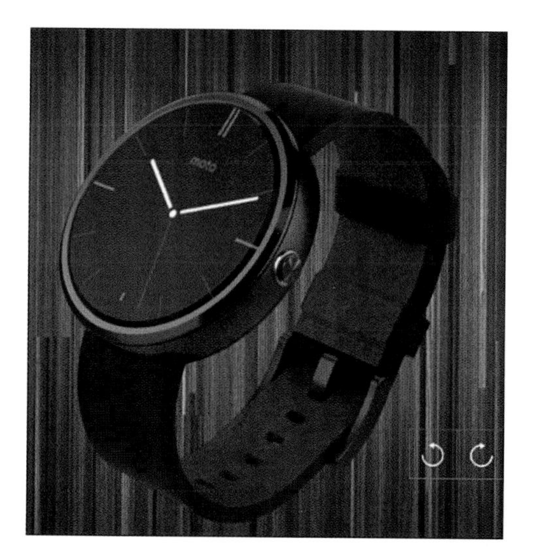

Moto 360 by Motorola

- **Apple:** The Apple watches come in three collections: Watch Sport, Watch, and Watch Edition. All have the same features, including the ability to switch watch faces/themes, and are available as either a 38mm or 42mm watch. The differences lie in the materials used to make the watches. The Watch Sport has an aluminum case, and its flexible fluoroelastomer band comes in various colors. The Watch collection currently has a stainless steel body, with various styles of metal or leather bands, or you can use the sport band. The Watch Edition comes in a gold casing with various styles of bands, including the sport band if you choose.

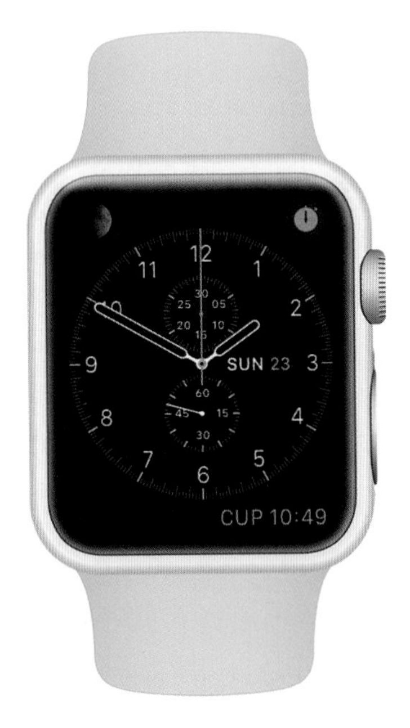

Apple Watch Sport

- **Pebble:** The Pebble line of smartwatches consists of the Pebble Time (the newest of the collection), Time Steel, Pebble Watch, and Steel. Each is made of stainless steel in a curved ergonomic design. This line has fitness-tracking functions that you can expand on by adding new apps. You can change watch faces and choose between steel, leather, and silicone watchbands. One distinctive characteristic of the Pebble watches compared to most smartwatches is their Electronic Paper Display (EPD), sometimes referred to as E-Paper. This simply means that screen content replicates the look of ink on paper.

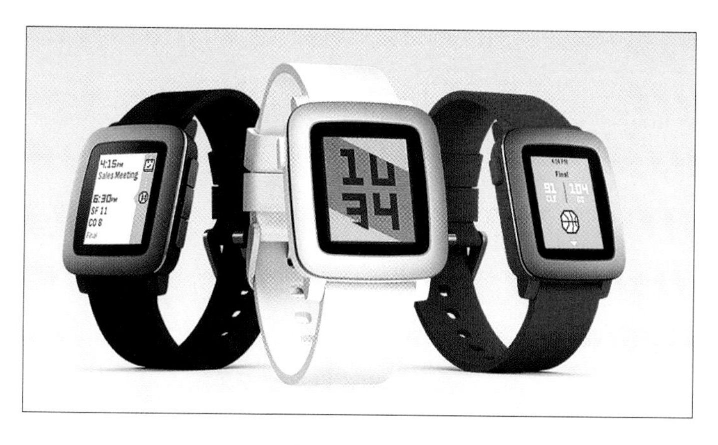

Pebble Time

- **Samsung:** Currently the Samsung Gear line includes six models: Gear Fit, Gear 2, Gear 2 Neo, Gear Live, Gear S, and Gear S2. The Gear Fit is more akin to a fitness tracker than a smartwatch, although it does allow you to receive notifications for calls, emails, and calendar events, and it displays the time. All the Gear models are equipped with health and fitness apps. Each has a large display and is available in various band colors. The Gear Fit and the Gear S are the models with curved screens, but the entire Gear line allows you to switch watch faces/themes for a different look. All have a metallic body, although the Gear 2 Neo is equipped to be more durable and lightweight than the other models. The Gear S2 is Samsung's newest watch to date, complete with a newly designed round body. It comes in two designs, standard and classic, and with a selection of different materials, including stainless steel. The list of compatible devices continues to grow, so continue to check back with the Samsung website.

Some Gear Live and Gear S Standout Features

The Gear Live is the only device in the smartwatch lineup that can be used on both Samsung and non-Samsung Android phones. With that being said, currently, it's no longer being sold on the Google Store online. You can still find it on Amazon, used. Currently, the Gear S and Gear S2 are designed to work independently from your phone. It's a cellular network-connected phone that enables you to make calls and check emails, texts, and more when your phone isn't nearby.

What's the Price?

Smartwatches typically start around $150 and can reach the astronomical price of $17,000 dollars. This is a good time to think again about your lifestyle; what your fitness goals are; and whether you would benefit from the productivity, communication, and entertainment features along with the health and fitness capabilities. Could a dedicated fitness tracker meet your needs?

Android Wear smartwatches can cost anywhere between $140 and $349.

The Apple Watch Sport can be purchased from $349 to $399. The Apple Watch costs between $549 and $1,099. The Apple Watch Edition collection can be purchased from a whopping $10,000 to $17,000.

You can get a Samsung Gear watch from $99 to $199. Currently, you can get the Samsung Gear S for $199.99 with contract at AT&T. Check your cellular carrier for any deals on the Gear S.

The Pebble line of smartwatches runs from $99 to $249.

Now that you have learned many of the features of smartwatches and fitness trackers, hopefully price comparisons can help you make a more informed decision on what is the best option for you.

Consider the Need for a Medical ID

One of the lowest tech health precautions you could take might just be the very thing that saves your life. A Medical ID or ICE ID (In Case of Emergency) is an easily accessible record of your medical conditions, drug and food allergies, prescribed medicines, and emergency contacts. These IDs can be worn as a form of jewelry, but in case of an emergency—when you are unable to advocate for yourself—first responders will have a snapshot of your medical history that can aid them in your immediate treatment. You learn about some options for wearable medical IDs in Chapter 8, "Being Prepared for an Emergency."

You can also create a medical ID on your Android or Apple phone instead of wearing it in the form of a bracelet or pendant. You learn how to set up a medical ID on your phone in Chapter 8. After you see how it works on your phone, you can determine which option would likely be the most effective for you to get the correct medical attention you would need.

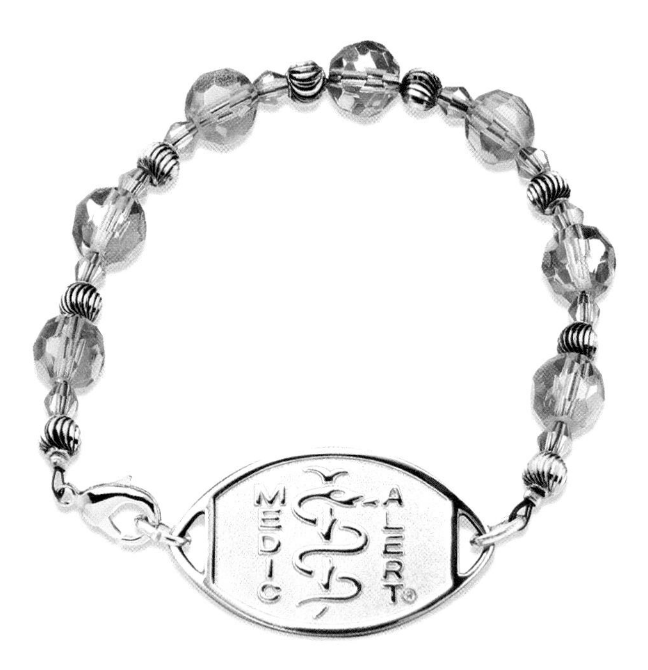

MedicAlert bracelet

Ask your doctor whether she or he recommends that you have a medical ID. If you or someone you care about has been diagnosed with a chronic condition, you should consider a medical ID. A variety of conditions for which you might be wise to get a medical ID include the following:

- Alzheimer's
- Asthma and COPD
- Autism
- Celiac disease
- Cerebral palsy
- Dementia
- Diabetes
- Epilepsy
- Food and drug allergies
- Gastric bypass surgery
- Physical disabilities
- Heart patients with pacemakers, arrhythmia, mitral valve prolapse, or heart stents

Medical IDs are also helpful if you are a caregiver—not only when you need to advocate for someone under your care, but also if you yourself become unable to advocate for those under your care.

Choose a Pedometer to Track Your Activity

A dedicated pedometer is a very straightforward device used to record the number of step-like movements you take, including walking, running, stair climbing, cross-country skiing, and even everyday chores. It then calculates an estimate of the distance traveled on foot. Smartphones also have this ability via health and fitness apps, with varying degrees of accuracy, as well as activity trackers. If you like to keep things simple, consider a dedicated pedometer. You can clip it on to your waistband, shoe, or pocket, and just go. Here are some points to consider when choosing a pedometer.

- **Accuracy:** Most pedometers are accurate in recording basic steps. The Garmin Foot Pod tests 98% accurate for speed and distance. If you are an avid hiker, consider a fitness tracker with an altimeter.
- **Ease of use:** Although most pedometers are just clip-and-go, some have more features, such as recording calories burned, that require more setup. For the most part, you just reset the counter back to zero before each day's activity and go. Some activity trackers might provide a more precise reading, but be prepared for a little more setup and perhaps having to search through a few more menus if you choose a tracker over a pedometer.
- **Features:** If your needs are simply to quantify your daily activity, just about any pedometer can do this. Pedometers store your daily activity for a few days, and then dispose of the old data to collect new data. The Omron HJ 321 Tri-Axis Pedometer has a seven-day memory that calculates steps and calories burned. If your goal is to track your data over time and to analyze long-term trends, you need a device that can upload to a computer or smartphone. The Fitbit Zip calculates steps and calories burned, and can be set up to sync automatically to a Mac (OS X 10.6 and up) or PC (Windows Vista and up), as well as leading Android, Apple (iOS), and Windows devices.

- **Price:** Low-end pedometers can cost as little as $2 online. You can find many for under $15. The problem with these low-end devices is that they simply aren't accurate and they physically wear out faster.

  Mid-range pedometers cost between $15 and $35. Many top-rated devices in this range provide accurate readings but are still susceptible to wearing out more quickly than their higher-end counterparts.

  High-end pedometers cost up to $60. Higher than $60, high-end pedometers start to enter into fitness tracker territory. The high-end range pedometers offer precise step counters, distance measurements, and burned calorie calculators. For the options over $60, you might be venturing into paying premium prices for features you personally don't need.

Exploring Technology for Your Household

Chapter 8 explores digital health technology you can use in your home for a higher quality of living and an independent lifestyle. It presents many options for how technology can help you monitor your health, diet, exercise, and sleep, and be prepared for emergencies. Here are some very practical solutions for your home.

Smart Bathroom Scales

Smart scales are a great way to help you stay on track, whether your goal is to maintain your weight, gain weight, lose a few pounds, or lose many pounds. Smart bathroom scales do a lot more than just show you your weight; they can calculate BMI (Body Mass Index), lean mass, and body fat percentage. Three such devices are:

- Fitbit Aria Wi-Fi smart scale
- Weight Gurus Bluetooth Smartscale + body composition
- Withings WS-50 Smart Body Analyzer

All three scales are capable of recognizing multiple users and can connect to the user's individual, compatible, Android and Apple (iOS) devices. The Fitbit Aria is capable of connecting with Fitbit trackers and the Fitbit app. Each scale produces charts that display weight stats and progress as charts and graphs and syncs stats wirelessly. (The Aria and the Withings Smart Body Analyzer sync via Wi-Fi network, and the Withings scale can also sync using Bluetooth. The Weight Gurus scale syncs via Bluetooth.)

Talking Measuring Cups and Food Scales

Regardless of your weight goals, food portion control can play an important role. Speaks Volumz Talking 3-cup measuring cup makes measuring ingredients easier. Instead of having to eye each measurement, the cup speaks measurements in English. You can measure in cups, ounces, milliliters, and grams. This can be a great kitchen companion for anyone, especially for people who are blind or have low vision. The Vox 3000TS Talking Kitchen Scale can help you accurately weigh even larger portions of food.

Medicine Adherence

Taking your medicine at the right time, at the right dose, on a consistent basis can be critical. It can be crucial in determining your quality of life, and in some circumstances, can make the difference between life and death. Apps and devices like the CleverCap® can help make sure that you adhere to your prescribed dosage by providing audible and visual reminders. Reminders can also be sent by text, calls, email, and/or alerts to your phone, depending on which product you choose. The CleverCap® adds an extra level of adherence and dispenses the right dosage at the right time. The CleverCap® also generates feedback reports so that you and your caregiver can analyze whether you are taking your medicine as prescribed. Each product does this in its own way, and you will get to see which works best for you later in the book.

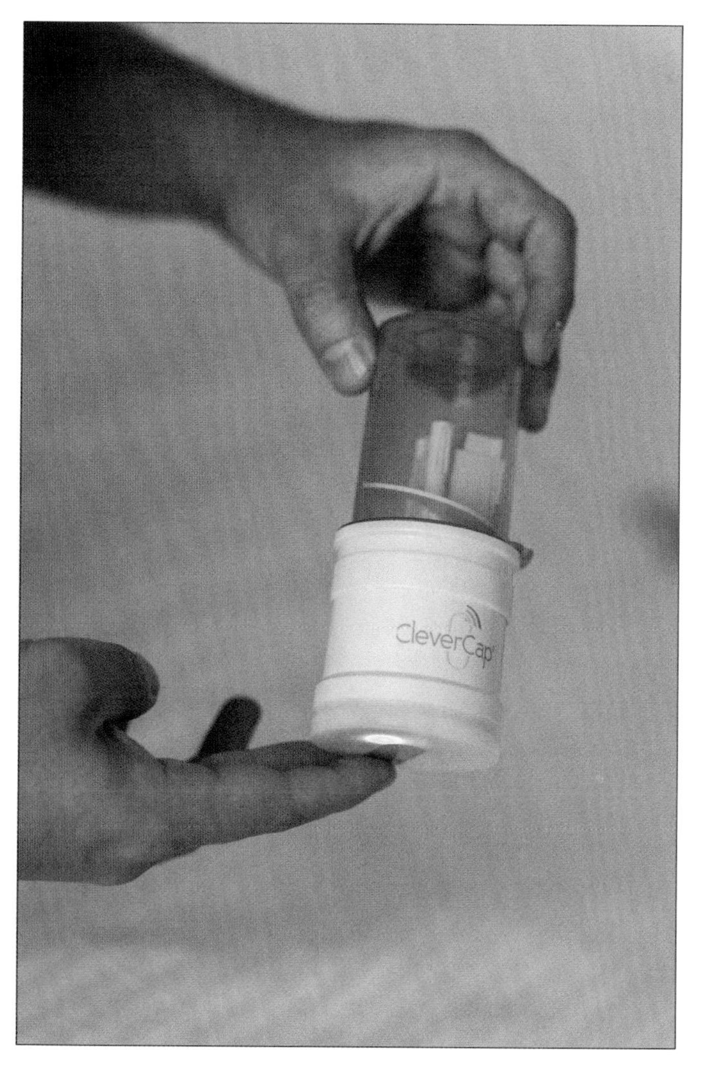

© 2015 CleverCap

The CleverCap®

Reminder Rosie is another product that can help you remember to take your medications. It is an advanced voice-controlled system that can remind you to take your medication throughout the day. Rosie can be operated almost completely by voice. Record up to 25 reminders for any time or any date. We dive deeper into the CleverCap®, Reminder Rosie, and much more in Chapter 5, "Staying on Top of Your Medicine."

Anti-Scalding Devices

Automatic temperature control faucets and showerheads can help prevent burning yourself. If you accidentally turn the hot water faucet too far, instead of the water becoming too hot and scalding you, these devices ensure that the water stays at a safe temperature. After the device is installed, if the water temperature becomes too hot, the device automatically shuts off the water flow. These devices can even help regulate water temperature if you are in the shower and someone flushes the toilet. Everyone can benefit from these devices, but check out the Alzheimer's Store for some anti-scalding devices: http://www.alzstore.com/water-temperature-control-devices-p/0200.htm.

Turn On Lights Remotely

You can turn on your lights in a number of ways without having to first fumble through the dark for a light switch. Many of them let you use your smartphone as a remote control to access software that can "flip" the switch. This is a valid method, but a few low-tech options might be quicker and easier. The sound-activated light switch, the Clapper, has been around for a long time; it's been tried and tested, and it's easy to use. Depending on the number of times you clap your hands, the light turns on or off. The Feit Automatic Sensor LED Night Light is another convenient option.

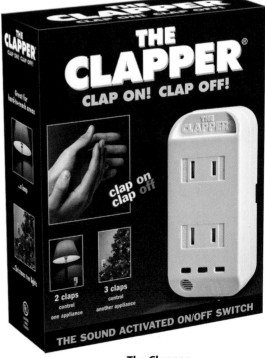

The Clapper

Clapper® is a registered trademark of Joseph Enterprises, Inc. in the United States and other countries. Clapper trademark and image are used with permission.

Medical Alert Services

A home medical alert system can be a wonderful thing. It can enable you or a caregiver to respond to a health emergency while you live a comfortable, independent life. A personal medical alert system can be a simple push-button worn around the neck or wrist, or a base station, which enables access to 24/7 emergency assistance. When you're on the go, some systems can connect with your smartphone. A sophisticated system might include sensors that can be placed around the home so that a caregiver can tell whether someone has gotten out of bed on time and is eating properly or taking her medicine. Some of the systems you learn about in this book go much further than just detecting falls but can also allow caregivers to monitor vitals and activity online and through apps. Certain systems even include online community features, offering more ways for you to stay in contact with family and friends.

In Chapter 8, you get a chance to take a closer look at the grandCARE monitoring system, Life Alert, and the Lively Medical Alert System. All are effective, subscription-based services with their own unique features for you to choose from.

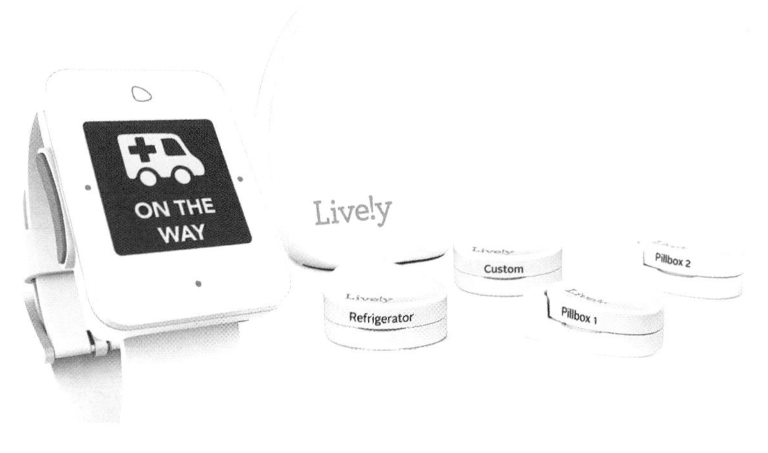

Lively Medical Alert System

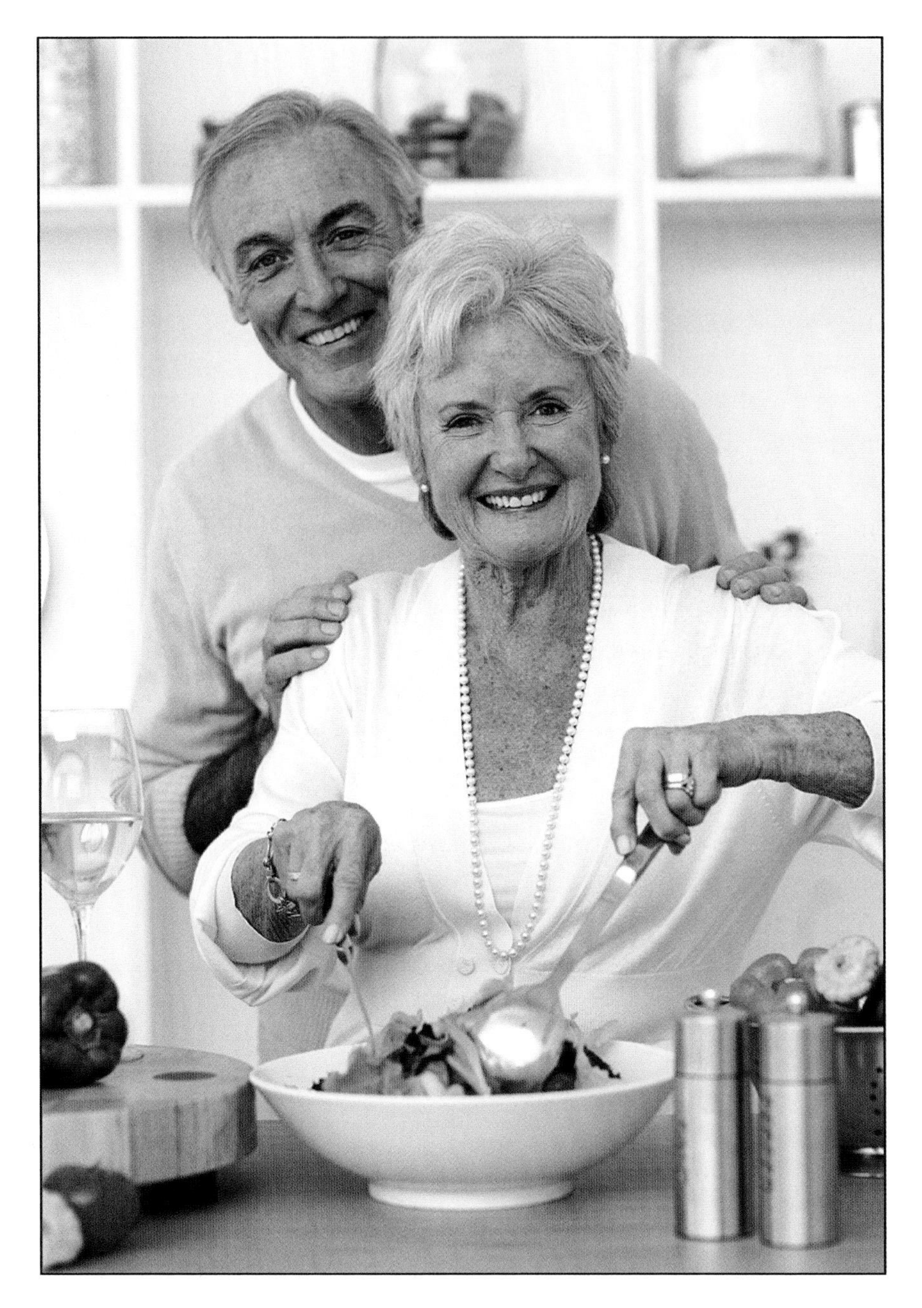

Credit: © WavebreakMediaMicro/fotolio.com

Use smart weight scales, intelligent water bottles, nutrition apps, food scales, and grocery delivery services to help obtain and maintain a healthy body.

In this chapter, you learn about devices that help you track your weight and body composition. You learn about devices that weigh food portions or monitor fluid intake, and apps that help you choose healthier food options. You also discover some food delivery services that help make grocery shopping easier.

2

- → Knowing Your Body Measurements
- → Watching Your Weight
- → Watching Your Food Portions
- → Tracking Your Daily Hydration
- → Making Better Food Choices
- → Getting Groceries Delivered to Your Door
- → Exploring Diet-Specific Delivery Resources with Recipes

Maintaining a Healthy, Balanced Diet

The quality and quantity of food you put into your body is an important factor in living a healthy lifestyle, regardless of your weight goals. The word *diet* has almost become synonymous with weight loss. However, whether you are looking to maintain your current weight, lose a few pounds, or work toward profound weight loss, the fuel you put in your body plays an important role in the quality of your life. In this chapter, you are introduced to digital resources that help you accomplish your goals. They not only help to educate you on the quality of the foods you eat, but also provide greater insight into your body composition—body measurements beyond just the metric of weight. You explore how to monitor your weight on an app with information acquired from a scale.

You see how to measure food portions so you'll know exactly how much you're eating. You learn the value of apps that help you make better nutritional choices and can journal what you eat. You even learn of devices that ensure you reach your daily fluid intake. Toward the end of the chapter, you are provided many options for having your food delivered straight to your door, including diet-specific foods such as vegetarian, heart healthy, and gluten-free grocery lists.

Knowing Your Body Measurements

There is more than just one way to measure your health and fitness. Knowing your body mass index (BMI) and body fat percentages are great ways for you to gain further insight into your body composition, beyond just monitoring weight. The reason for this is that the ratio between fat and muscle changes as you become more fit. The bodies of two people who are the same height and weight can look drastically different if they are on opposite ends of the spectrum when it comes to body fat versus lean body mass. This is where smart weight scales come in handy. Some can help you track both. Before we jump in to the hardware, here are some things you should know about BMI and body fat percentage—and ways to measure them.

Calculate Body Mass Index (BMI)

Calculating BMI is a way to estimate whether a person is at a healthy weight for his or her height. It's an easy way for a person to determine whether a person is normal weight, underweight, overweight, or obese. It is not a perfect indicator; more on that in just a moment. The CDC (Centers for Disease Control and Prevention) formula for calculating BMI using pounds is BMI=(weight in pounds x 703)/Height in inches^2. Fortunately, there are devices (some of which we'll cover shortly) and many apps that can do this calculation and provide weight categories you might fit into. These apps include the Fitter Fitness Calculator for the iPhone and the BMI Calculator by Splend Apps for Android phones.

Although BMI is used to screen for weight categories that could lead to chronic conditions, it provides an educated guess at best as to the fatness or overall health of an individual. BMI does not take into consideration how much muscle a person might have. For example, a person who does a lot of weight training and is very muscular might have a BMI that places him or her into the obese category. This is where fat percentages come into play.

Track Your Body Fat Percentage

The formula for calculating body fat percentages is a bit more complex than the formula for calculating BMI. However, it can be broken down into Body Fat Percentage = Fat Mass/Body Weight. The ability to track your lean mass and body fat percentages helps you determine whether you are losing fat and building muscle. Fortunately, smart scales and apps can calculate body fat percentages and help you track this data. The Fitter Fitness Calculator for the iPhone and the Body Fat Calculator app by Voiche Apps for Android phones can do the calculations and track your progress.

Watching Your Weight

Bathroom scales have become a whole lot smarter. Not only do they show your weight, but they can also calculate your body fat percentage, BMI, and lean mass. Access to lean mass and body fat percentages help you determine whether you are losing fat and building muscle. Some scales are equipped to track data from multiple individuals and can even determine who you are as soon as you step on them. The information collected by these scales can also be accessed through websites and apps where you can view your progress in the form of charts and graphs. Some smart scales work in tandem with compatible fitness trackers to help you achieve your goals.

It's Not All Good

Do Not Use a Smart Scale if You Have a Pacemaker or Other Internal Medical Device

Due to the technology used by these smart scales to analyze body mass, which involves sending a small electrical signal through the body (Bio-impedance Analysis), people who have pacemakers or other internal medical devices should not use these devices before consulting their doctor.

Measure Weight with the Fitbit Aria Wi-Fi Smart Scale

The Fitbit Aria Wi-Fi Smart Scale tracks weight, BMI, lean mass, and body fat percentage. The Aria can track up to eight users. As soon as you step on the scale, the Fitbit Aria identifies you. The scale wirelessly transmits your stats, using your home Wi-Fi network, to your Fitbit account, where it can be privately viewed on the online Dashboard or the Fitbit app. From these two locations you can access charts and graphs so that you can view long-term trends in your progress and make meaningful adjustments to your diet or exercise regimen. The Fitbit Aria Wi-Fi Smart Scale works with Fitbit Trackers so that you can set goals and use calorie coaching. The scale's measurement range is from 20 to 350 pounds.

In addition to a Wi-Fi network, you need to visit www.fitbit.com/scale/setup/start to set up your Aria using a Mac or Windows computer or mobile device.

You can purchase the Fitbit Aria Wi-Fi Smart Scale on fitbit.com and amazon.com, in addition to other sites, or at your local electronics store.

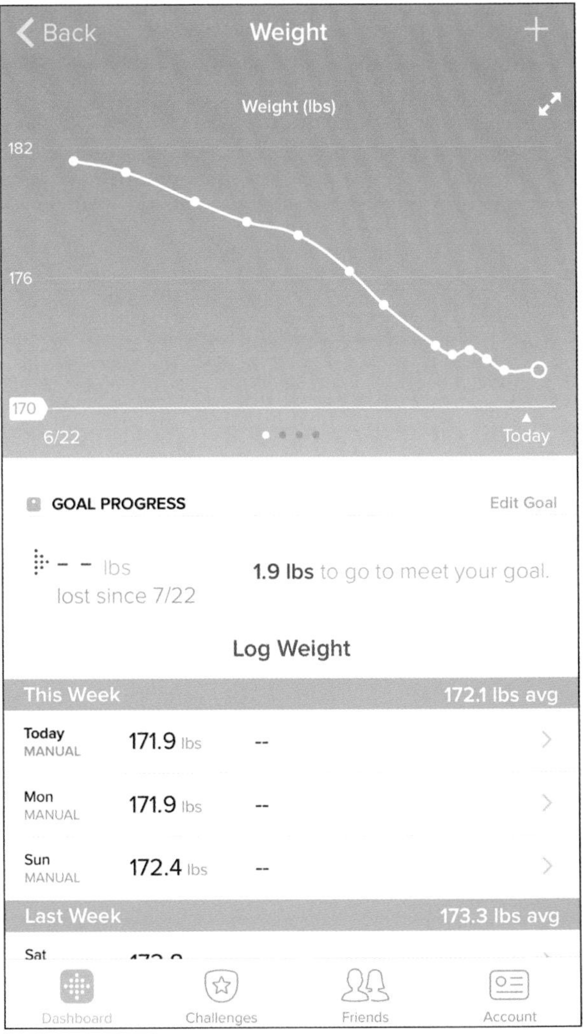

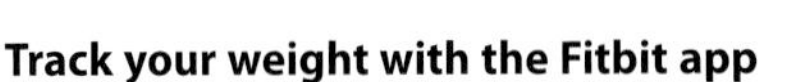
Track your weight with the Fitbit app

Monitor Weight with the Weight Gurus Bluetooth Smart Body Fat Scale

The Weight Gurus Bluetooth Smart Connected Body Fat Scale is another option for accurate measurements. The scale has a 400-pound capacity. This device calculates BMI and other health indicators including lean mass, body fat, water weight, and bone mass. This smart scale supports up to eight users and can automatically detect a specific user as soon as he steps on the scale. Bluetooth technology is used to sync your measurements to your smartphone. Be sure to visit the Greater Goods page on amazon.com to see whether your device is on the compatibility list. The Greater Goods app for Android and iOS charts your progress, enabling you to identify trends so you can make the necessary adjustments to your diet and workouts to reach your goals. You can purchase this scale by visiting greatergoods.com, bedbathandbeyond.com, amazon.com, or by searching the Internet. You can download the apps on the Google Play Store and the App Store.

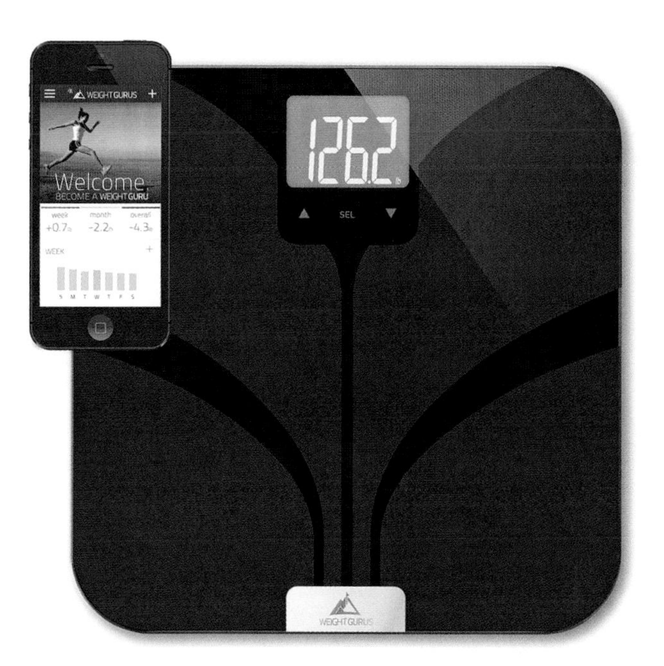

The Weight Gurus Bluetooth Smart Connected Body Fat Scale and Greater Goods app

Track Your Weight with the Withings WS-50 Smart Body Analyzer

Withings WS-50 Smart Body Analyzer not only tracks your weight, BMI, and body fat, but it can also measure your pulse through your feet so that you can set goals to lower your standing heart rate (a good indicator of heart strength). If you work out vigorously, this scale also lets you switch to "Athlete mode" so it can more accurately calculate the fat mass measurement. The Withings WS-50 Smart Body Analyzer also has the ability to track environmental metrics such as carbon dioxide concentration and indoor temperature to let you know when it is time to clear the air, and it even provides the daily weather. This scale can accommodate up to eight different users and automatically recognizes each user after he or she steps onto the scale. If two people are of a similar weight, it will prompt you to lean either left or right to choose the right person.

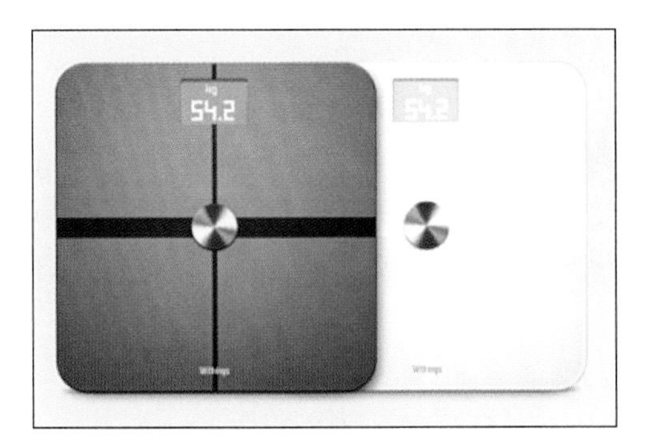

© 2009-2016 Withings SA

Withings WS-50 Smart Body Analyzer

You pair the Withings Smart Body Analyzer to your Android or iOS device using Bluetooth. Then download the Health Mate app from the Google Play Store or the App Store. The app walks you through setting up an account, connecting to your Wi-Fi network, and configuring measurement units. After you're set up, just step on the scale and let it go to work. With the Health Mate app, you can keep your progress history on hand. You can also track your health using the web-based interface. If you are not familiar with some of the readings, Withings does a good job providing helpful information so you can understand the data being tracked.

Visit withings.com to learn more and to purchase the device. You can also search for the device on the Internet.

Watching Your Food Portions

If you regularly eat out in restaurants, it's hard to ignore the fact that food portion sizes have grown larger and larger over the years. This trend can also influence you when you're preparing meals at home, giving you a skewed perspective of what an actual serving size really looks like. Knowing the proper serving size helps you know the calories, fat, sodium, and other nutritional values of the food that you put in your body. Resources like digital food scales and measuring cups that talk can help you take control of portion sizes and help build a healthier you. If you don't already practice this, there will be a learning curve; you'll have to start reading packages and learning what constitutes a recommended serving size instead of just eyeballing. You just might learn that the plate of pasta you enjoy at your favorite Italian restaurant in fact might be an entire package of pasta! The tools to watch your food portions are really quite simple. Consider the following products as examples to get you started. There are many, many more to choose from.

Weigh Food Portions with Digital Scales

Knowing your food portions when you're preparing meals has never been easier. Digital kitchen scales have been around for a long time and are hardly high tech, but sometimes simple and low tech is all you need. Enjoy the foods you love, but eat less. A digital food scale provides more precise measurements of portions when preparing food. Consider one of these scales.

The Ozeri Pronto Digital Multifunction Kitchen and Food Scale is a popular product that lets you accurately weigh up to 11 pounds in graduations of 0.05 ounces (1 gram). The weighing platform is large to accommodate large bowls and food items. It comes with a tare feature, which allows the scale to subtract the weight of the bowl or plate so you can get an accurate measurement. You'll need to place the empty container on the scale first, and then press the Tare button to zero out the scale before you add the food. You can change the unit of measurement with just a press of a button. The widescreen LCD displays results in grams, ounces, pounds, and kilograms. Visit ozeri.com and choose For the Kitchen at the bottom of the screen to view more scales by Ozeri. Go to amazon.com and search for Ozeri Pronto Digital Multifunction Kitchen and Food Scale to purchase the item.

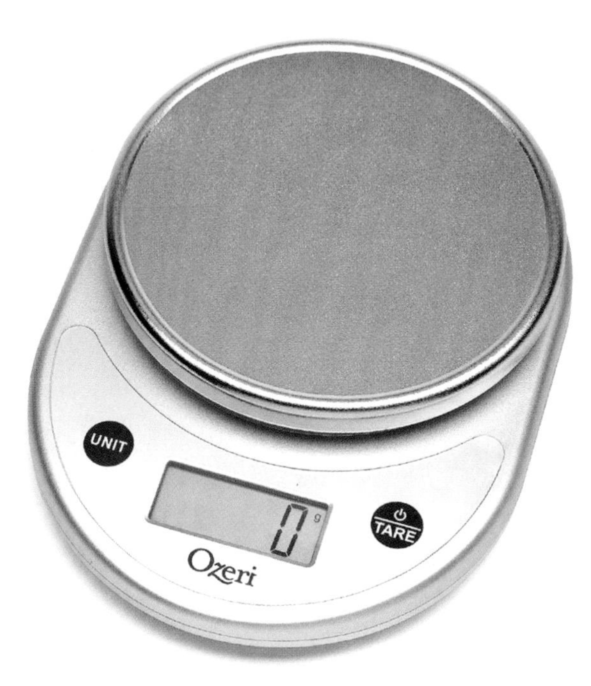

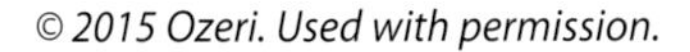

The Ozeri Pronto Digital Multifunction Kitchen and Food Scale

The DecoBros Digital Multifunction Kitchen and Food Scale is another popular option with precise 0.1oz accuracy. It has a capacity of 11 pounds and also has a Tare function, sometimes labeled "Zero," which subtracts any extra weight on the scale (such as a container) before you add the food. You can switch between units of measurement by pressing the Mode button. Visit amazon.com to purchase the DecoBros Digital Multifunction Kitchen and Food Scale.

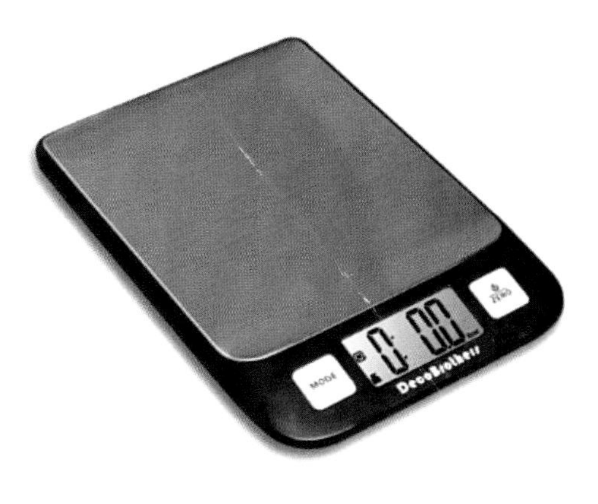

The DecoBros Digital Multifunction Kitchen and Food Scale

Work with Talking Measuring Cups

If you're looking to measure cooking and baking ingredients accurately, the Speak Volumz Talking 3-Cup Measuring Cup might be just what you are looking for. The cup actually speaks the measurements and can be a wonderful accessory in the kitchen for anyone, but especially for those who have low vision or who are blind. The unit consists of a cup, a base that it sits in, and a lid. The cup measures weight and volume up to 3 cups, 24 ounces, 690 milliliters, and 720 grams. It even performs conversions for water, oil, milk, flour, and sugar. The cup also has a tare function so you can add ingredients without emptying the cup. It's also dishwasher and microwaveable safe. As of this writing, the cup speaks measurements only in English. The Speak Volumz cup has easy pushbutton controls that are quickly accessible from the front. The buttons are embossed as such:

V: Volume; measures in cups or milliliters

W: Weight; measures in ounces or grams

S: Density; switch between water, oil, milk, flour, and sugar

T: Tare; on/off

The dimensions of the product are 6.5" × 4.75" × 6" high.

Just press the T button to hear "Scale ready," and then press the S for the density you want. Pour, and after you finish, the cup speaks the measurement. The cup has a spout that makes the contents easy to pour.

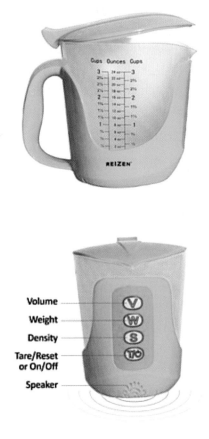

The Speak Volumz Talking 3-Cup Measuring Cup

Tracking Your Daily Hydration

Proper hydration is important for everyone. You'll want to pay special attention to your hydration needs when you exercise. Medications such as drugs for blood pressure and other cardiac conditions can also contribute to dehydration. And as you age, dehydration becomes more of a concern. Your sense of thirst can lessen, and your body isn't able to conserve water as well. Water bottles are available that can help you monitor water consumption and meet your daily hydration goals. One water bottle you'll read about is intelligent enough to calculate the water you need to consume for various activities and reminds you to hydrate. Proper hydration varies by individual and is based on a variety of factors, including gender, age, weight, environment, and activity level. Before you begin any hydration program, consult your doctor.

Monitor Fluid Intake with HydraCoach

HydraCoach is a smart device that helps keep you properly hydrated. This intelligent water bottle holds up to 22 ounces of fluid and calculates, monitors, and reminds the user to consume enough fluid for his or her individual needs. HydraCoach tracks your fluid consumption in real time, as well as paces you throughout the day using a time tracker. You can customize your fluid intake regimens. Along with tracking the average amount of fluid you consume per hour, this device shows you in percentages how you are progressing toward your hydration goal.

HydraCoach is a BPA-free bottle and comes with a pre-installed CR2032 3 Volt Lithium battery that lasts approximately 6 months under normal conditions. When it's time to change the battery, a Low Battery icon appears in the upper-right corner of the display. Learn more and purchase HydraCoach by visiting hydracoach.com and amazon.com.

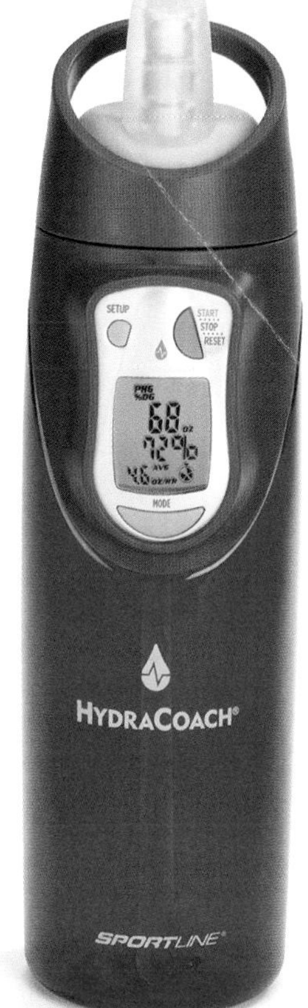

The HydraCoach water bottle

The HydraCoach Personal Hydration Calculator can use your weight to automatically calculate a recommended daily hydration goal. Follow these steps to have the HydraCoach automatically calculate a daily, Personal Hydration Goal. To activate the bottle, you first manually remove the battery insulation tab and reinstall the battery.

1. Screw off the lid and then lift the bezel to access the back of the computer.
2. Unscrew the screw, and then open the door.

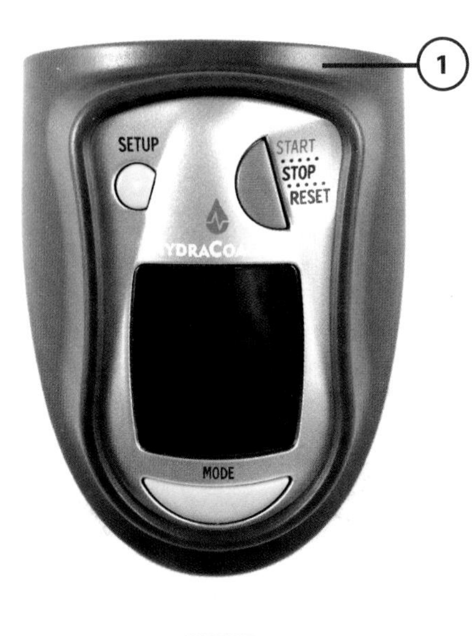

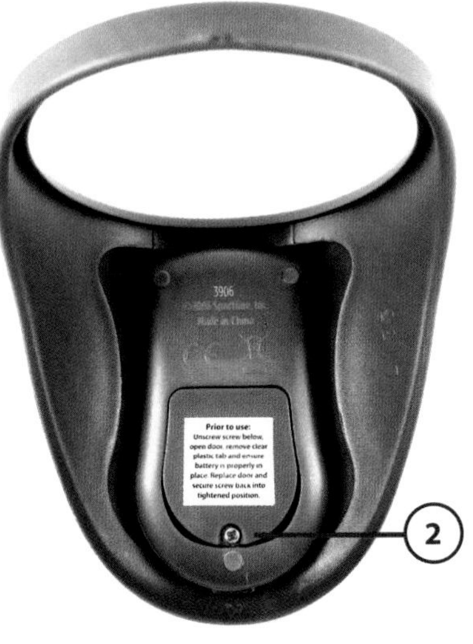

Another Way to Enter Initial Setup Mode

You don't need to remove the battery each time you want to enter Initial Set Up Mode. Press the Setup and the Start/Stop/Reset buttons simultaneously to enter Initial Setup Mode from now on.

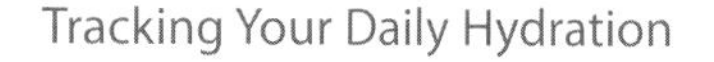

(3) Remove the clear plastic tab. As you raise the tab, the battery comes out. Place the battery back into the slot and screw the back onto the computer. SEL now displays on the computer screen. You are now in the Initial Setup Mode.

(4) Place the lid and bezel back onto the bottle.

(5) Press the Mode button to toggle through units and advance digits. The default unit of measure is OZ (Ounces). You can hold down the button to quickly advance through the options. The highlighted option blinks.

(6) Press the Setup button to select OZ. Setup advances to the next screen—Units Of weight.

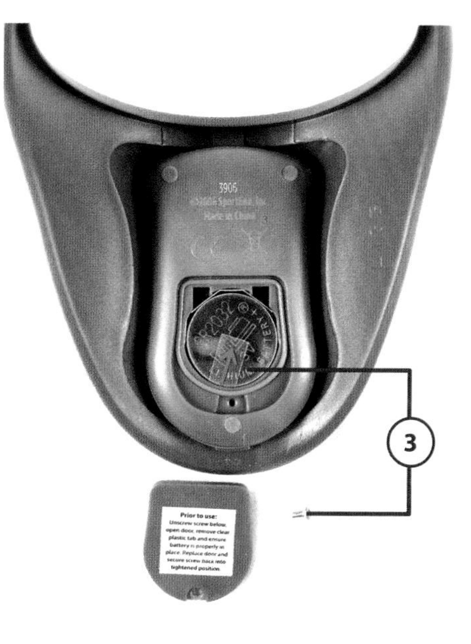

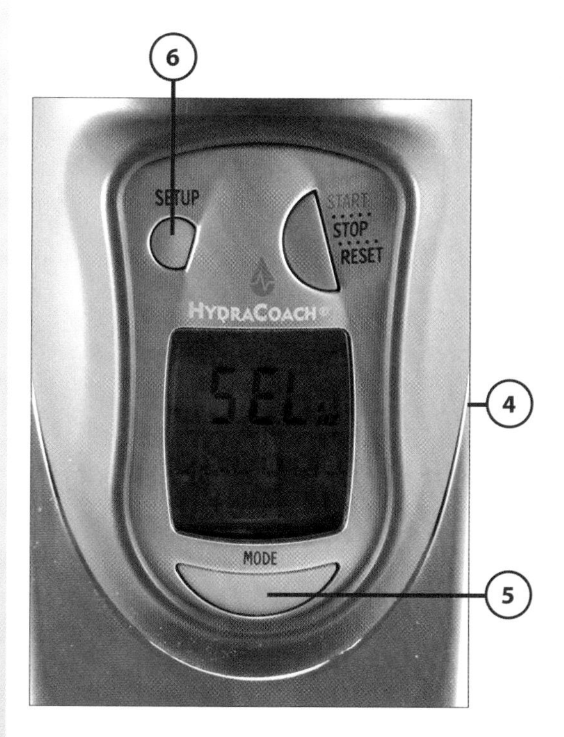

7. Highlight LB (Pounds) or KG (Kilograms) as the default unit of weight by pressing the Mode button. The default unit of weight is LB.
8. Press the Setup button to select LB and progress to the next screen.
9. Enter your current weight one digit at a time using the Mode button. You can move between digits using the Setup button after you input the proper digit.
10. Press Setup after you enter the final digit for your weight. HydraCoach uses your weight to calculate a daily Personal Hydration Goal (PHG).
11. View your calculated daily Personal Hydration Goal (PHG) onscreen. You can adjust this value up or down to meet your personal requirements.
12. Accept the goal by pressing the Setup button. The Clock Format screen displays.

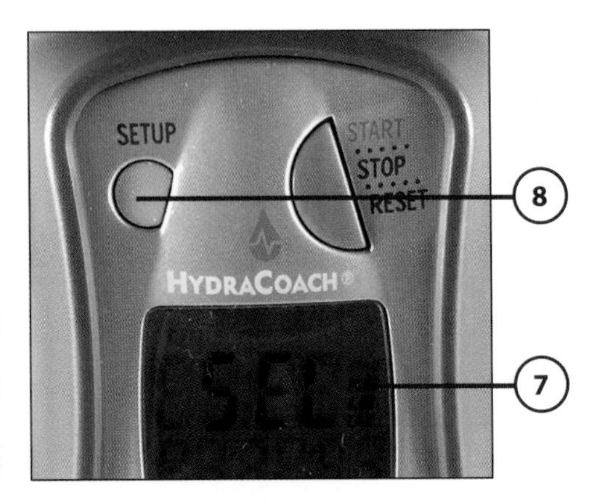

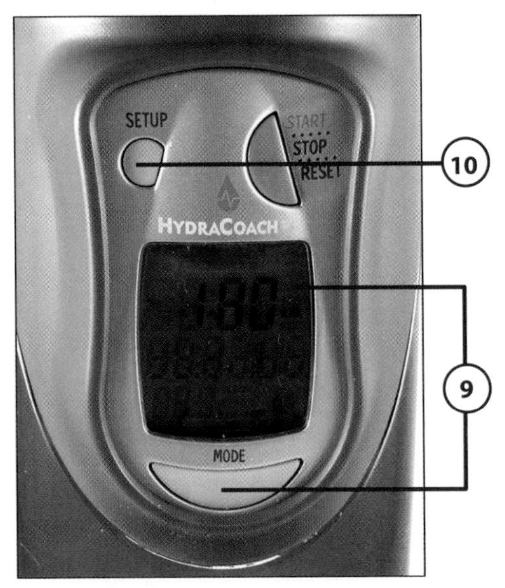

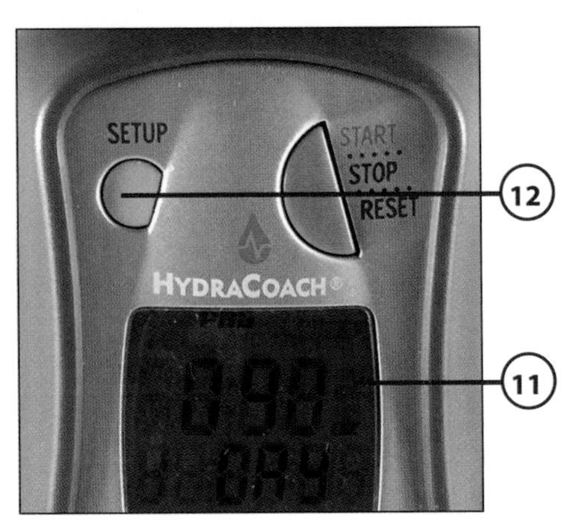

(13) Select a 12- or 24-hour clock format using the Mode button. The default format is 24 hours.

(14) Press the Setup button to accept the chosen clock format and proceed to the current time screen.

(15) Enter the current time in hours and minutes.

(16) Press the Setup button to proceed to the Current Date.

(17) Enter the current, day, month, and year, and then press Setup to accept it.

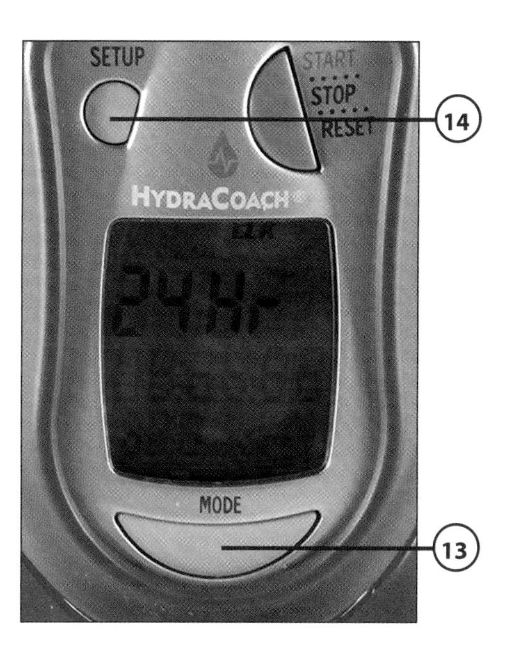

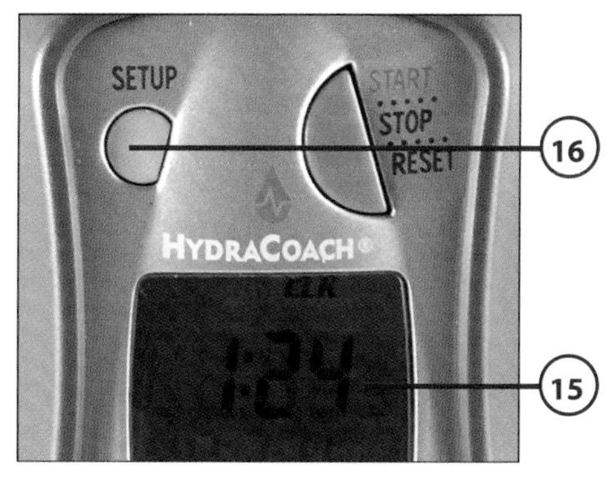

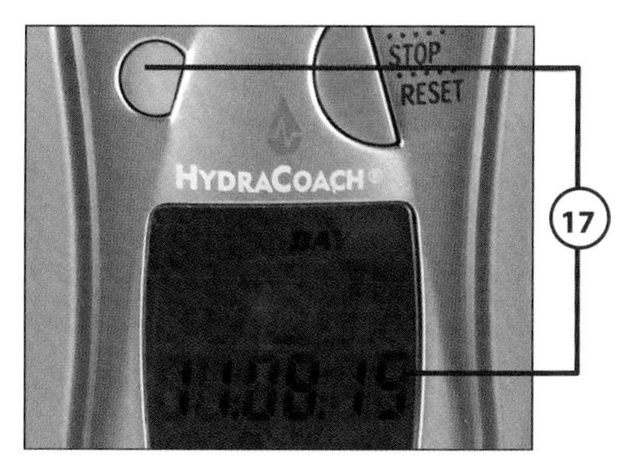

(18) Press Start. Your HydraCoach is now ready for use.

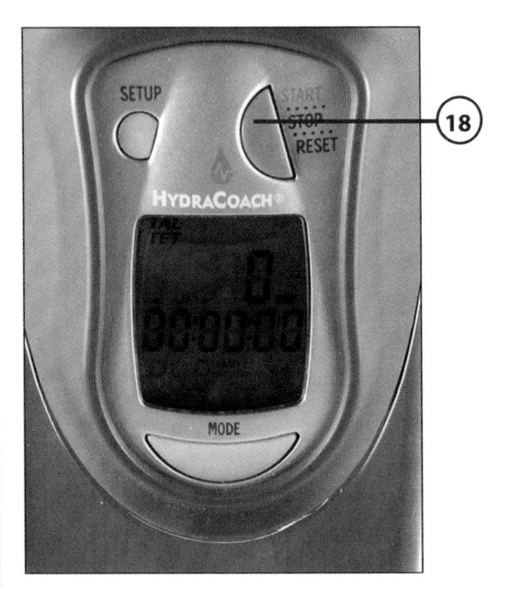

>>>Go Further

TIPS FOR USING HYDRACOACH

Drinking from the HydraCoach might be different than water bottles you are used to and is a two-step process. Place your mouth on the mouthpiece and use your teeth to bite down on the indents to open the slit. Suck in the water like you would with a straw to draw the water into your mouth. Keep the bottle oriented in a vertical position for accurate reading. Be sure to refill the bottle when the water line reaches the Refill mark located toward the bottom of the bottle and only fill with water. It's okay to put ice into the bottle, but don't store the bottle in the refrigerator. The HydraCoach disassembles into seven main components. The bottle portion can be placed in the dishwasher. The computer display may be polished with a soft cloth or a slightly damp cloth if necessary. Do not place it in the dishwasher.

Online and Mobile Tracking in the Works

As of this writing, a future version of this bottle is under development that will allow your hydration data to be tracked on a computer, smartphone, and tablet.

Monitor Fluid Intake with the Thermos® Connected Hydration Bottle with Smart Lid

Another solid option for achieving your daily hydration goals is the Thermos® Connected Hydration Bottle with Smart Lid. Thermos has been in the business of making durable bottles for a long time. Thermos offers a 24oz, BPA-free, connected water bottle that monitors your intake and temperature of your water, and communicates that data to compatible devices. The Thermos Smart Lid app lets you set your daily hydration goals using the baseline average or create a custom goal for your desired intake. You also have the option of using the integrated hydration calculator to set goals based on your personal data. This bottle also works with Fitbit®. By connecting your Fitbit account with the Thermos Smart Lid app, your profile information links for easy setup, and then you can instantly see your hydration stats sync each time a bottle of water is finished. Visit thermos.com to learn more. You can also purchase the bottle from retailers and download the Thermos Smart Lid app from applicable online stores.

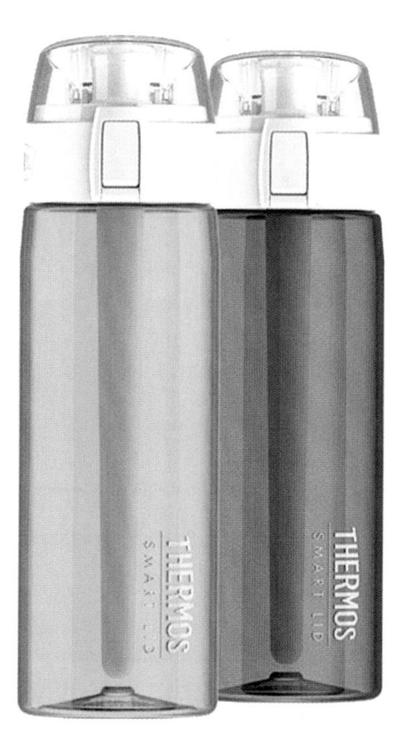

The Thermos® Connected Hydration Bottle with Smart Lid

The Activity Dashboard in the Thermos Smart Lid app shows you the current liquid level in the bottle, water temperature, and how much progress you're making toward your hydration goal. The app tracks your daily, weekly, and monthly hydration progress with charts and graphs. It also advises you on your daily average consumption. To stay on track, turn on goal reminders and create custom reminders to keep you on pace throughout the day. The app also makes it easy for you to share information with family, friends, and a caregiver by connecting with Facebook, Twitter, Instagram, and Pinterest.

Getting started with the Thermos® Connected Hydration Bottle is pretty straightforward. Follow these steps to track your water intake with the Thermos Smart Lid app.

1. Connect the Micro USB cord into the socket located on the lid and let it charge for at least 3 hours. After your Smart Lid is charged, it always stays on and is ready to connect to your mobile device.

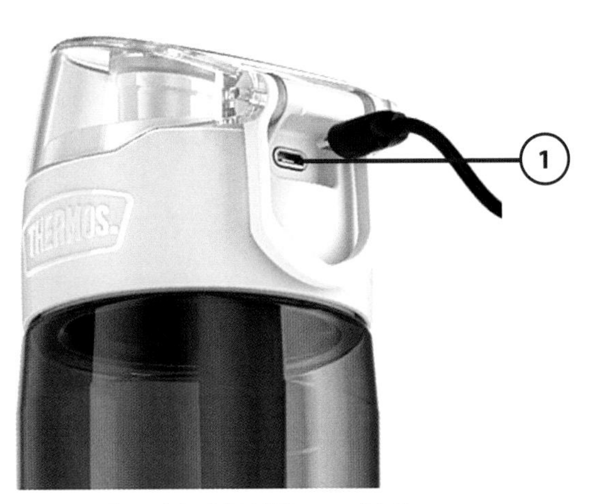

Copyright © 2015 Thermos L.L.C.

Battery Life

The Smart Lid has up to 12 days of battery life.

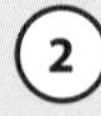
2. Download the Thermos Smart Lid app from the App Store.

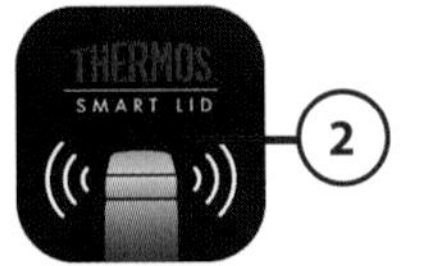

Device Compatibility

Be sure to visit www.thermos.com/smartlid.aspx to see whether your device is compatible.

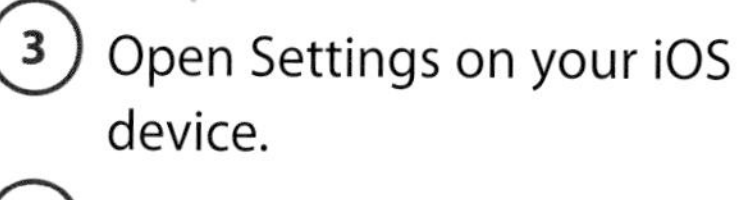

3. Open Settings on your iOS device.

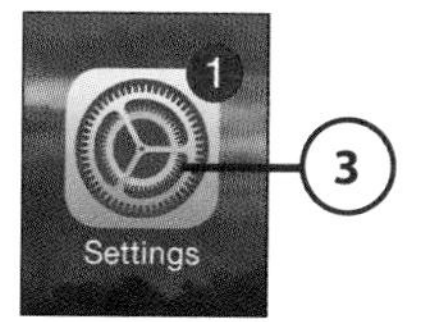

4. Tap Bluetooth. Make sure Bluetooth is in the On position and that the lid is within 75 feet of your mobile device, and then tap the SP400 Smart Lid under My Devices to connect.
5. Go to your device's home screen and open the Thermos Smart Lid app. A message asks for permission for the app to send you notifications.
6. Tap OK. A message asking your permission to receive alerts appears.
7. Tap OK. This Alert message might appear twice. Tap OK for each instance.

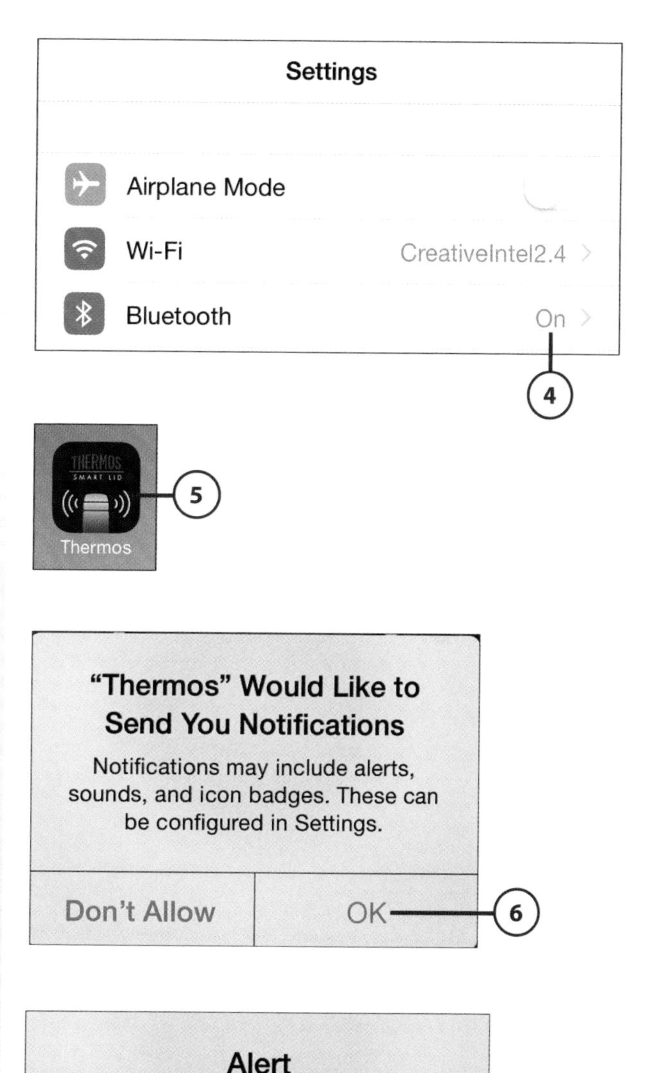

8. Tap Get Started.
9. Tap Use Fitbit Profile if you have a Fitbit account and want your hydration stats to be synced automatically to your Fitbit app each time you finish a bottle of water. The information in your Fitbit account will be used to create your Thermos Smart Lid app profile. If you don't have a Fitbit account, proceed to the next step.
10. Tap Create My Own Profile Account. This option was used for this example.

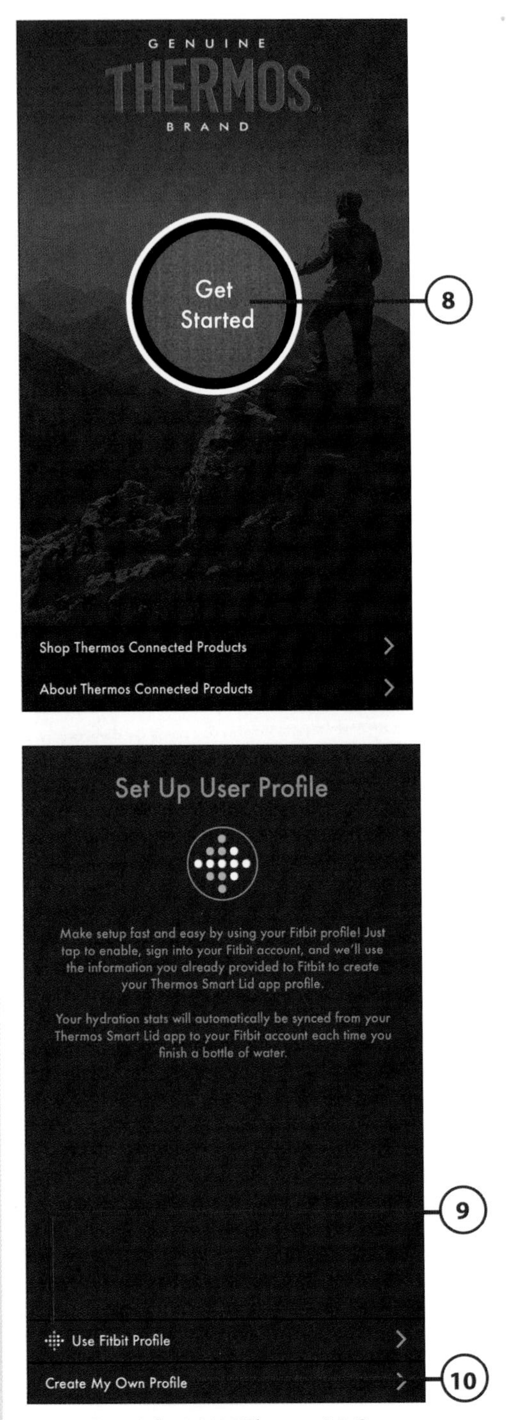

11. Tap Edit.
12. Tap to enter your profile name, and then tap Next.
13. Tap Add A Photo to take a photo or choose one from your photo library, and then tap Next. Thermos might ask you whether it's okay to access your photo library. Tap OK if this happens, and then select the photo you want to use. You can skip this step by tapping Skip This Step at the bottom of the screen.

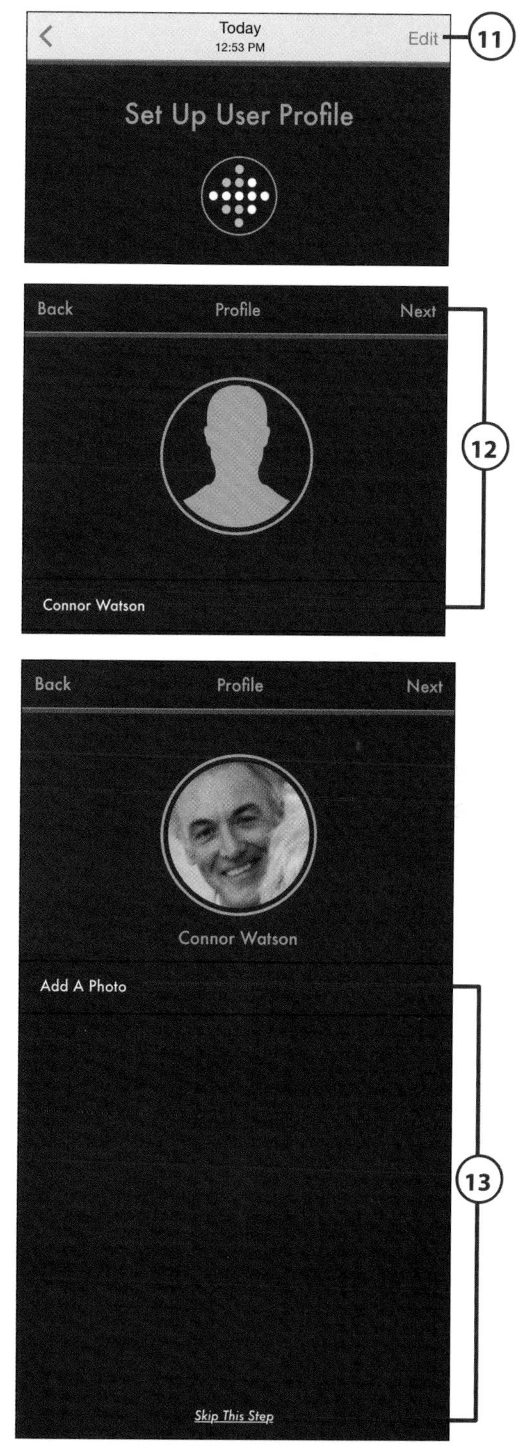

Copyright © 2015 Thermos L.L.C.

(14) Tap to enter your email if you want to receive updates, notices, and promotions from Thermos. You can skip this step by tapping Skip This Step at the bottom of the screen.

(15) Wake up your Smart Lid by using the provided charger to plug the device into a power source, and then tap Next.

(16) The app searches for your Smart Lid. If it's able to find the device, it will ask you to pair the device. After you choose Pair and pair the devices, you are ready to set hydration goals.

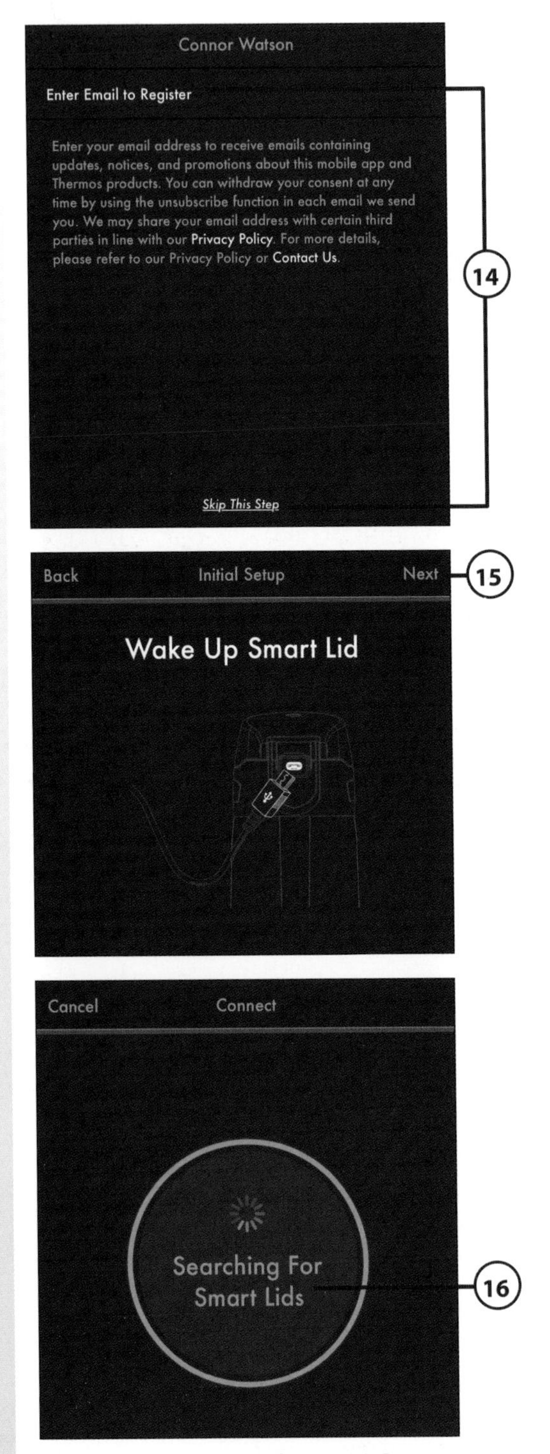

(17) Tap Setup My Suggested Goal or Continue With General Baseline Goal. This example shows the latter goal chosen. The general baseline is 64oz of water.

(18) Drink from your hydration bottle; the device automatically tracks your intake. If you have synced with your Fitbit account, you'll see your hydration stats in the Fitbit app once you have finished a bottle of water.

(19) Tap the main menu (three horizontal bars) to access the Dashboard, monitor your activity, manage reminders, and edit your profile.

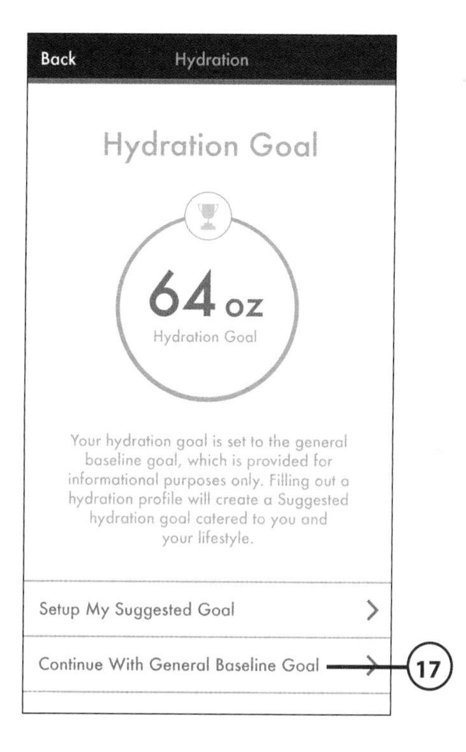

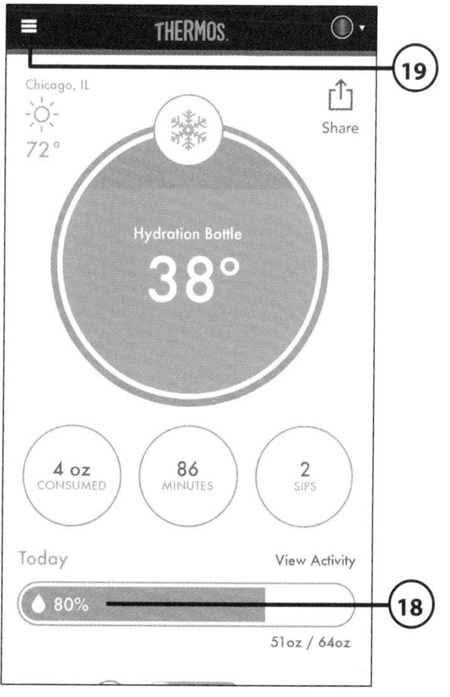

Making Better Food Choices

Changing the quality and quantity of your food can have a profound effect on your health. Your choice to eat smarter doesn't have to be driven by body weight, although it can certainly help you lose or gain weight if that's your goal. Making better food choices can just simply make you feel better, have more energy, and improve your emotional health. A number of apps are out there that put plenty of nutritional information at your fingertips, so you can track the amount of calories, fat, and sodium you are consuming, and much more. It used to be that when you ate out at your favorite restaurants you had very little knowledge about the nutritional value of the food you ate. Apps such as Calorie Counter, Fooducate, Lose It!, and MyFitnessPal have built-in food databases containing foods from many popular restaurants, so you can make educated choices when you dine out. These apps let you scan barcodes to add new foods. The Fooducate app can even offer healthier alternatives to some foods you crave and help you tailor specialized diets, including gluten free.

When you start monitoring the nutritional values of your food, you might find that one of your favorite meals contains an entire day's recommended daily caloric intake! Consider the following apps so you know what you're putting into your body, and keep a food journal. You can even receive customized daily caloric budgets to help you achieve your weight loss goals.

Track Calorie Consumption with the MyFitnessPal App

- MyFitnessPal lets you set a target goal weight, asks you how active you are, and then calculates the maximum number of calories a day that you should eat. It also tells you how much weight you can expect to lose each week and gives you milestone dates for when you can expect to lose a specific number of pounds. This app has a database of more than 5 million foods. It is highly likely that what you eat is already in the database, so you might not have to manually enter information for most foods. The database makes it easy for you to simply choose your food items and edit portion amounts. MyFitnessPal automatically adds the nutritional value for that meal, and then subtracts each meal's calories from your daily calorie budget. If you don't see your meal in the database, MyFitnessPal recognizes more than 4 million barcodes, so you can scan barcodes using your phone's camera and manually enter food into the app. The app also remembers foods that you have eaten for breakfast, lunch, and dinner so you don't have to go looking for them again.

MyFitnessPal is a solid choice for connecting with other apps and devices. The app automatically inputs data from more than 50 apps and fitness trackers to provide a comprehensive picture of your calorie and fitness progress. Apps and devices include Fitbit, Jawbone UP, Garmin MapMyFitness, Runkeeper, Withings, and more. MyFitnessPal is available for Android and Apple (iOS) devices.

Follow these steps to track your calorie consumption using MyFitnessPal. The following examples are shown on an iPhone.

1. Download the app from the App Store, and then tap the MyFitnessPal icon on the Home screen.
2. Tap Sign Up.

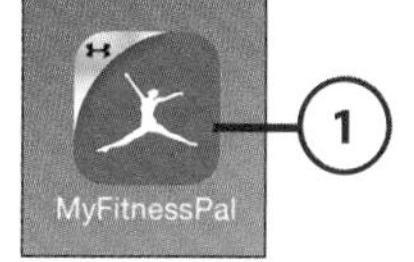

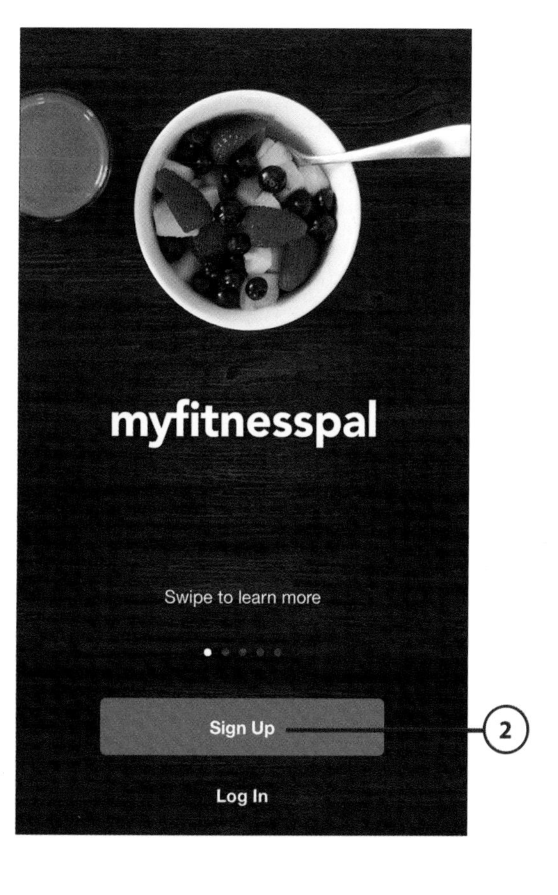

Social Media Privacy Issues

Keep in mind that logging in via Facebook can pose privacy issues by giving the app access to your social media data. Consider signing up using an email account instead.

3. Tap Sign Up with Email. If you already have a Facebook account, you can sign up with that account information.
4. Tap the option that best describes your goal. Lose Weight was chosen for this example.
5. Tap in the box to enter the amount of weight you want to lose. You can edit this number later.
6. Tap the arrow to proceed to the next screen. Follow the prompts as MyFitnessPal gathers more information about you, so it can calculate a custom plan to help you achieve your weight loss goal. Tap the arrow to proceed to the next screen when it is required. When you have finished entering all of your information, your daily net calorie goal is displayed.

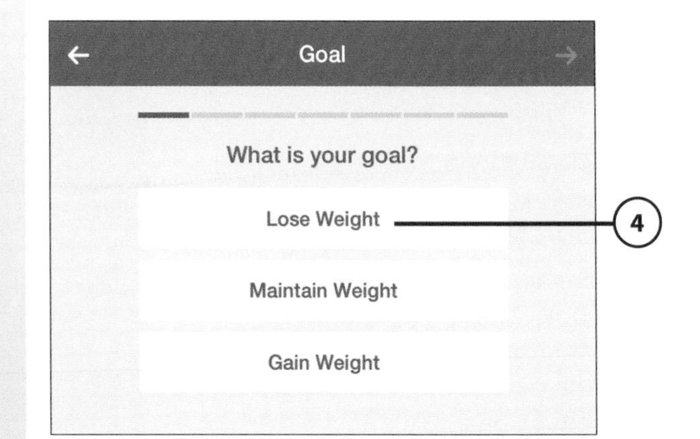

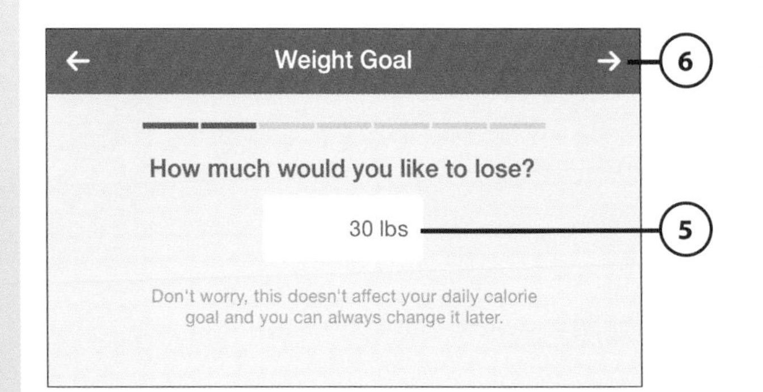

Upgrade to Premium?

As you're filling out your personal information so that MyFitnessPal can calculate your daily net calorie goal, you will be asked whether you want to upgrade the app to the paid Premium version. You can download the app and use some features for free, but Premium unlocks more features for the app including customer support, dietician-approved recipes, and a nutrient dashboard.

The nutrient dashboard provides deeper insight into what is in the foods you eat. If you want to eat more protein and fewer carbs, the nutrient dashboard provides the information you need. You can choose the information you want to see including Macronutrients: carbs, fats, protein, calories; Heart Healthy: fat, sodium, cholesterol, calories; and Carb-Conscious and nutrient breakdowns.

7. Tap a meal to add a food entry.
8. Tap in the field to type the food you are about to eat or that you ate. It's better to track your meals as you have them to help ensure the information is correct. You can also tap the barcode icon to scan the food you are about to eat, if it is not in the database.
9. Tap Search. A list of all the foods that closely match your search in the database appear.

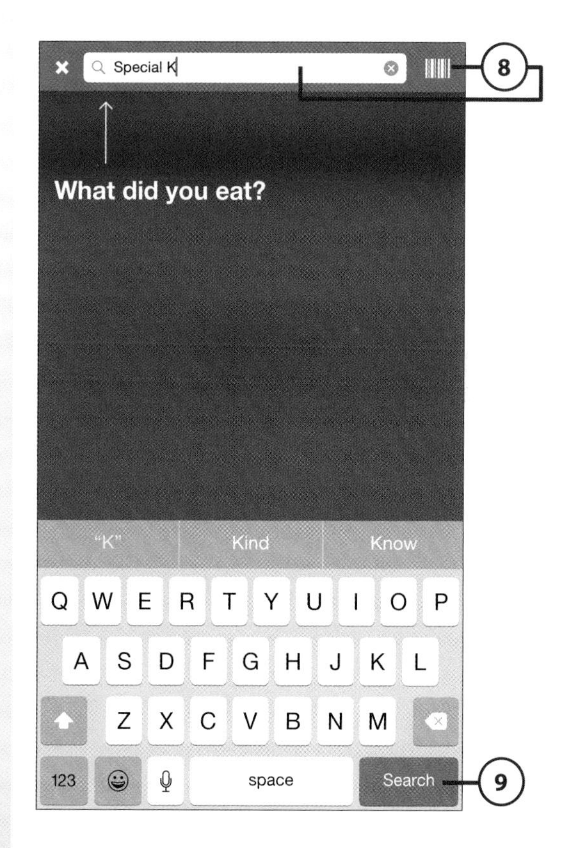

10. Tap the correct search result.
11. Adjust the serving size by tapping in each field, and then tap the check mark in the upper-right corner of the screen.
12. Tap OK, I'm All Done to end the tutorial. The food has been added and your food diary opens.

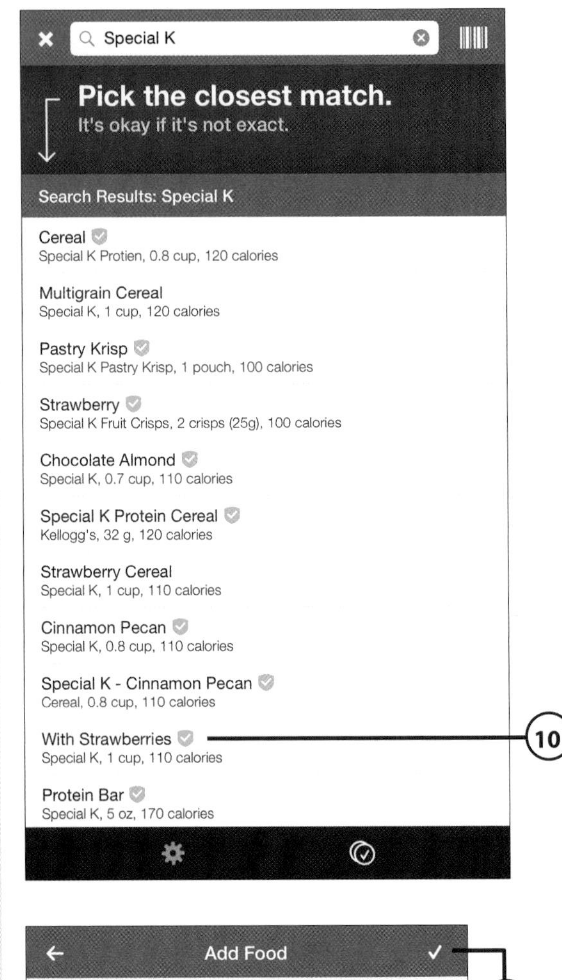

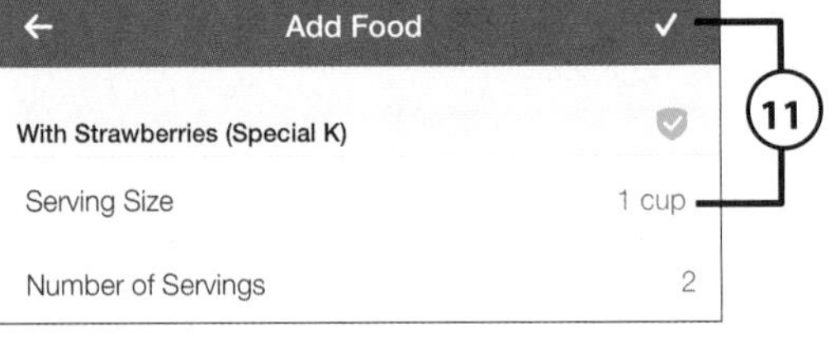

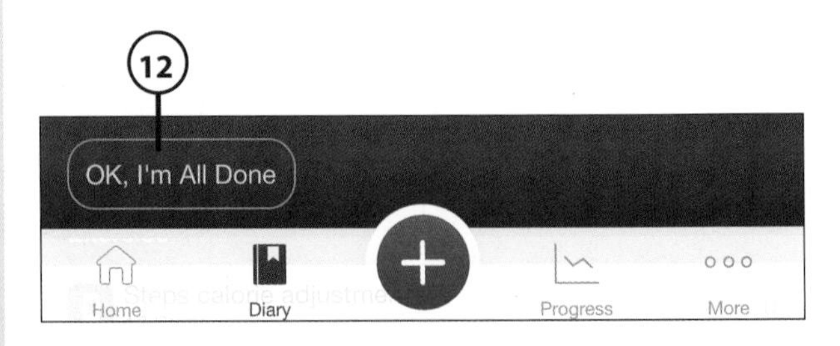

13. View the calories you have remaining. MyFitnessPal even gives you some added information on the food you just ate. For example, "This food has lots of Vitamin C."
14. Tap a plus icon in any food category to add a food for each meal.
15. Tap the large plus icon at the bottom of the screen to add notes pertaining to Status, enter water intake information, make a food entry, add exercise information, and enter a new weight.

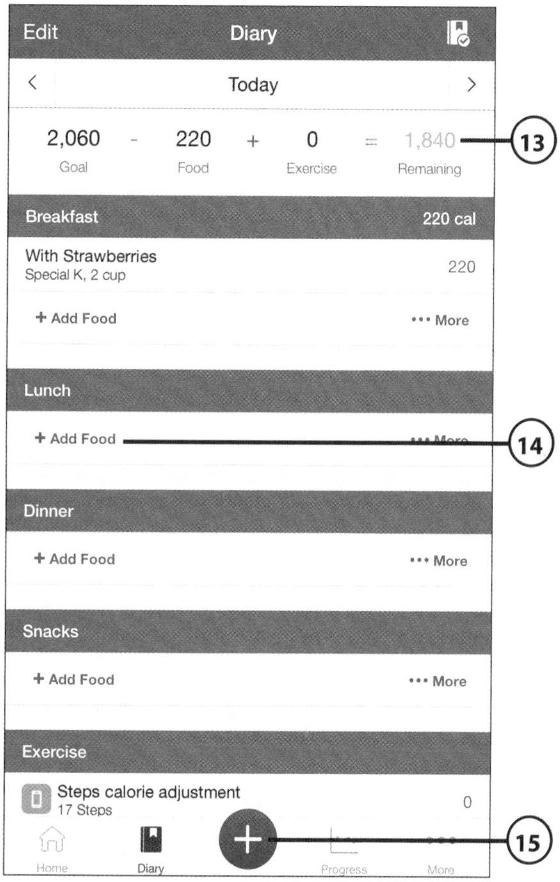

Learn What's Really in Your Food with the Fooducate App

Fooducate calculates a daily calorie budget and journals your food and it helps you lose weight by showing you how to eat right. As the name suggests, think of Fooducate as an educational app that helps you track the quality of calories, not just the quantity. Track exercise and food, including your recipes. This app helps you lose weight by providing suggestions for healthy alternatives for food that you already eat and by grading foods by nutritional value from A (Great) to D (Avoid). More than 250,000 unique products are graded. Fooducate gives you access to a huge food database where you can view calories per serving and additives and preservatives that you might not be aware of in the foods you eat. You can download and use some features of the app for free, but if you upgrade to paid Premium services within the app, you can tailor your diet even further by choosing a low-carb diet, paleo diet, gluten-free diet, and more. This app also helps you stay motivated by having community features that let you share your progress with others. Fooducate is available for both Android and Apple devices.

Fooducate is a healthy diet partner that might be the one app you need to get yourself in better shape by eating better. Follow these steps to use Fooducate to learn what's really in your food and start making better choices. The follow examples are shown on an Android phone.

1. Download the app, and then tap the Fooducate app icon on the home screen. The Welcome screen opens.
2. Tap Next.
3. Tap Sign up. If you already have an account, tap Log in. You can also log in using an existing Google+ or Facebook account.

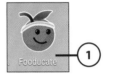

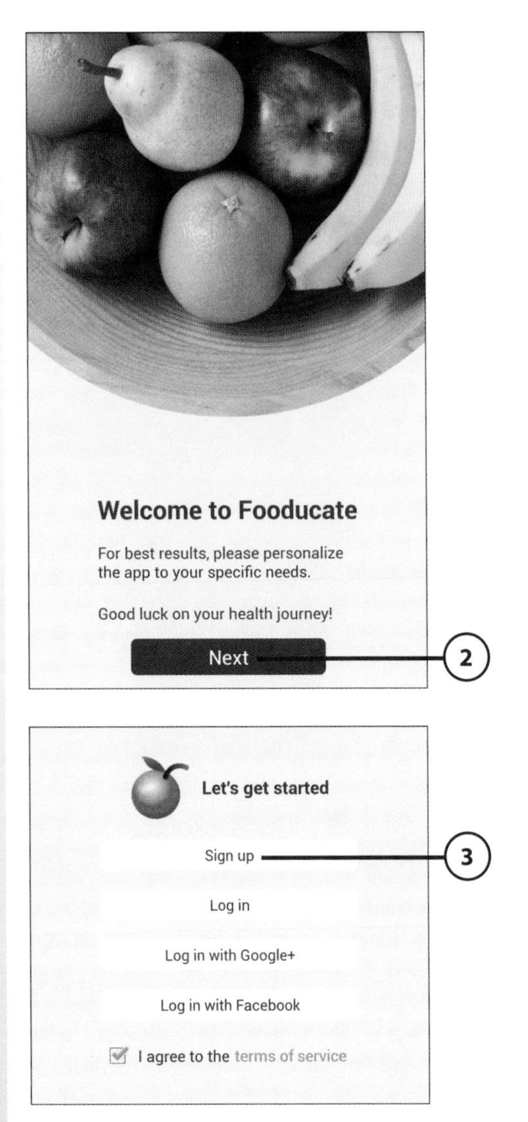

Social Media Privacy Issues

Keep in mind that logging in via Google+ or Facebook can pose privacy issues by giving the app access to your social media data. Consider signing up using an email account instead.

4. Enter an Email address, new password, and your Zip code, which is optional but improves recommendations.
5. Tap Signup. A message appears asking you to confirm your email.
6. Tap Confirm.
7. Tap Take a Selfie to add a profile picture by taking a picture of yourself using the front camera of your smartphone or choose a picture from the photo gallery on your phone.
8. Write something about yourself in the Something About Me field; it can be your favorite food or your goal weight, and so on. Tap Next.

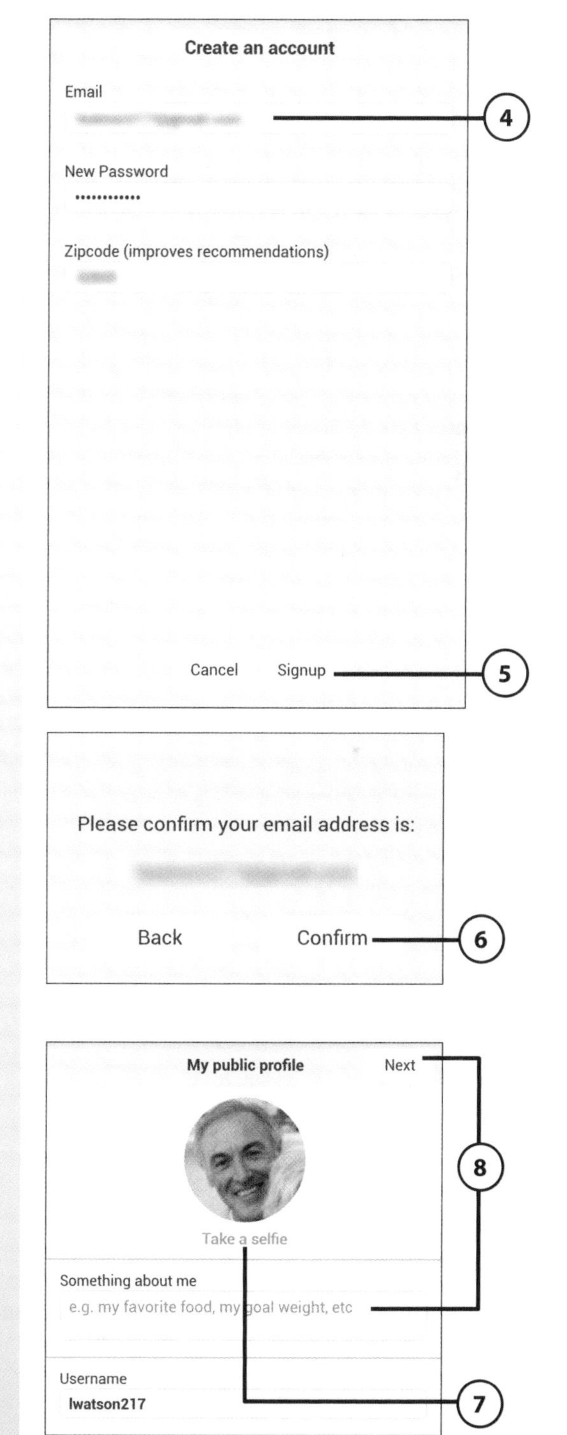

9. Fill in your personal information, and then tap Next.
10. Fill in your goals. You can see that Fooducate goes beyond giving you a daily calorie intake. It also gives you a food points score and gives you the option for recommended daily max added sugar allowance.
11. Tap Next. The next page is for further tailoring your diet if you have upgraded to Premium.
12. Tap one of the options to the On position if you want to upgrade to premium and further tailor your diet.
13. Tap Done. Your "personalized weight loss toolbox" opens, providing options to navigate the app. More options may be available when viewing this screen on the Apple (iOS) version.

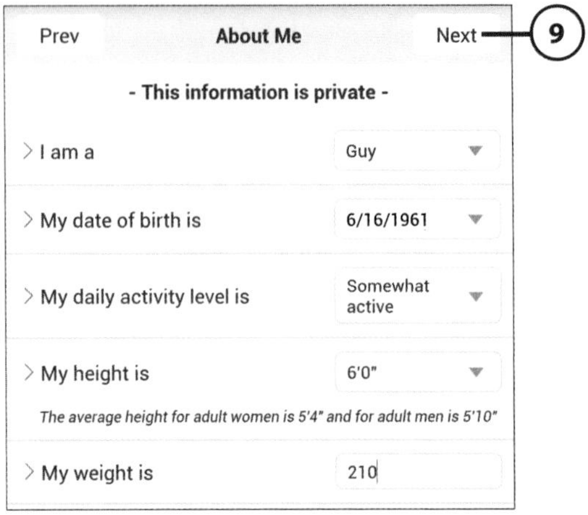

Prev | About Me | Next — 9

- This information is private -

I am a: Guy

My date of birth is: 6/16/1961

My daily activity level is: Somewhat active

My height is: 6'0"

The average height for adult women is 5'4" and for adult men is 5'10"

My weight is: 210

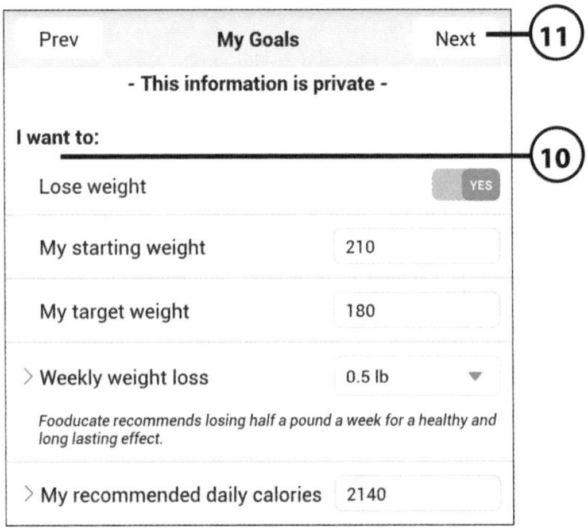

Prev | My Goals | Next — 11

- This information is private -

I want to: — 10

Lose weight: YES

My starting weight: 210

My target weight: 180

Weekly weight loss: 0.5 lb

Fooducate recommends losing half a pound a week for a healthy and long lasting effect.

My recommended daily calories: 2140

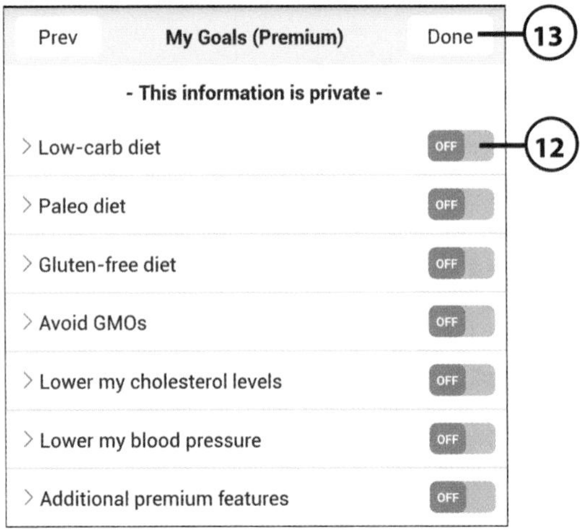

Prev | My Goals (Premium) | Done — 13

- This information is private -

Low-carb diet: OFF — 12

Paleo diet: OFF

Gluten-free diet: OFF

Avoid GMOs: OFF

Lower my cholesterol levels: OFF

Lower my blood pressure: OFF

Additional premium features: OFF

14. Tap Food Finder. The screen automatically opens up to a camera view so that you can scan a barcode. You can also type in a search for a food.
15. Type a search for a food, and then tap the Search button. A list of foods appears along with their nutritional grade.

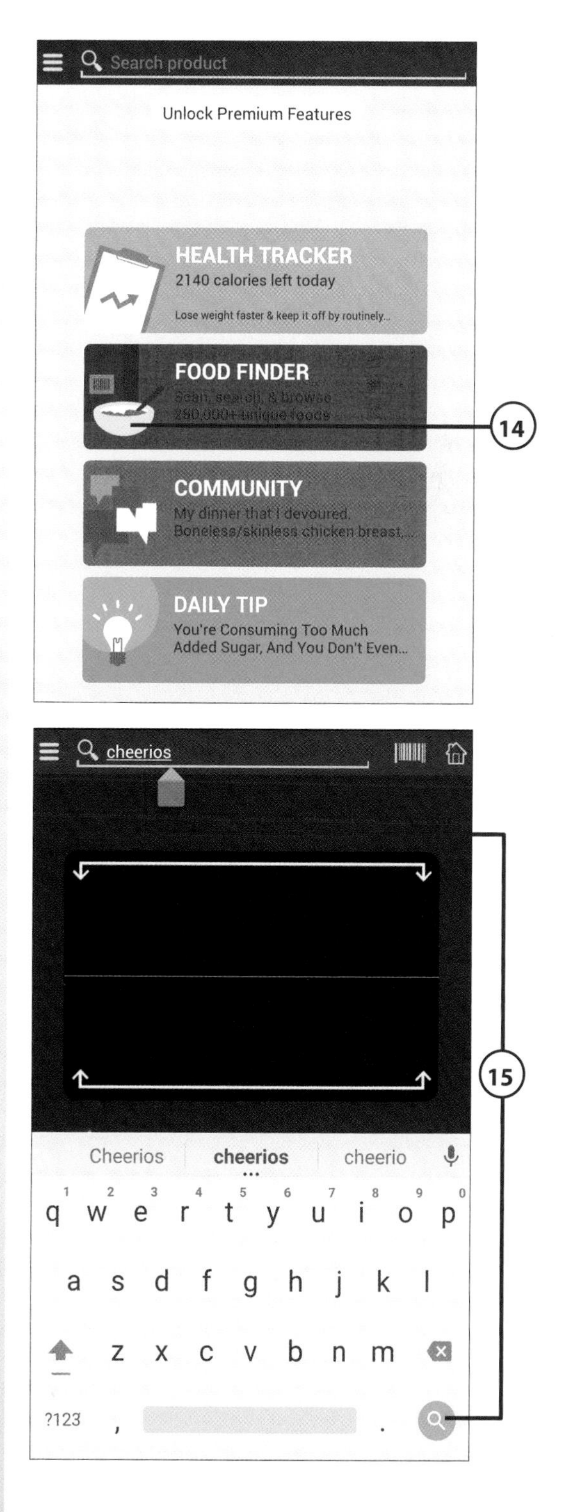

16. Tap on the product you want to know more about.
17. View the grade and the calories per serving. Toward the bottom of the stage you view other users' comments about this product and type your own comments. You can tap Explanations at the top of the screen to see how the product received this grade.

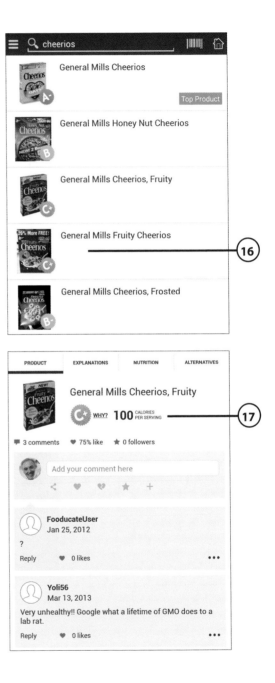

(18) Tap Nutrition to view all the nutritional information about this food. You can see how the nutritional information of this food fares to keep you on track for the daily goals you have set. Healthy nutritional values that keep you on track are marked with a green check mark to the far right; those that don't are marked with a red exclamation point. Other unhealthy attributes including "controversial artificial colors," "highly processed," and "low fiber" also receive red marks.

(19) Tap Alternatives to see what other healthier options are out there for this particular food. For this example, a product with an average nutritional grade was chosen. Healthier alternatives are shown for you to make better choices when shopping.

PRODUCT EXPLANATIONS NUTRITION ALTERNATIVES (18)

100 Calories per serving 20 120100

about average — Products in this category have on average 178 calories.

Serving size: **1 oz(s) - 27 g**

	Amount per serving	My daily value	
Calories	100cal	5%	
Calories from Fat	10Kcal	2%	
Total Fat	1g	1%	
Saturated Fat	0g	0%	✓
Trans Fat	0g	0%	
Cholesterol	0mg	0%	✓
Sodium	135mg	9%	
Total Carbohydrate	23g	8%	
Dietary Fiber	2g	7%	
Sugars	9g	17%	
Added Sugars	9g	25%	!
Protein	1g	2%	

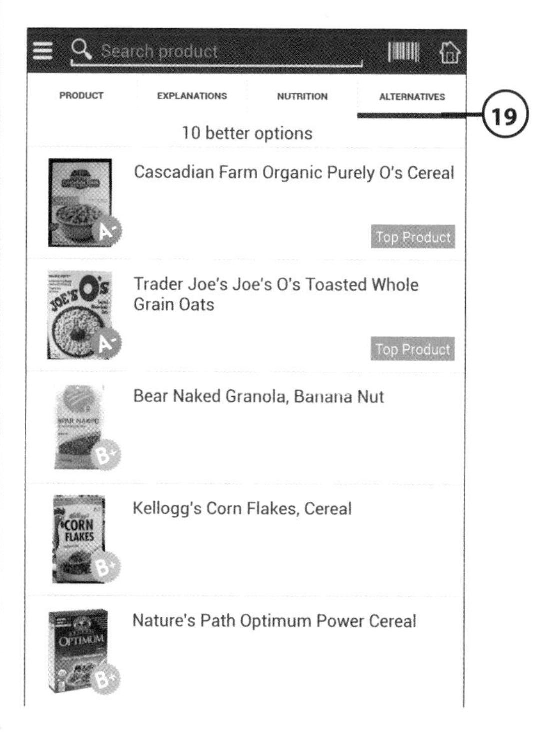

Lose Weight with the Lose It! App

Lose It! is an all-in-one resource for losing weight. It tracks your meals, exercise, and nutrition. Set your goal weight, and Lose It! puts together your daily calorie budget. This app has an extensive food and exercise database with more than a million entries, so you can easily find and journal the foods you eat without manually entering each meal. You can scan the barcode for food not found in the database so that they're easy to track in the future.

Lost It! is a free app, and you can use many of its features for free. If you pay to upgrade to Lose It! Premium, you can track steps and exercise calories; access exercise planning; track body fat; and track body measurements such as neck, hip, and waist. You can even track your hydration, and monitor your sleep. Without the Premium upgrade, Lose It! syncs with activity trackers including the Nike FuelBand, Fitbit One, and Jawbone UP. This app even works with wireless scales like the Withings Scale and Fitbit Aria. For motivation and support, Lose It! lets you connect with friends and family and connect to social apps such as Facebook and Twitter. Lose It! is available for both Android and Apple (iOS) devices.

It's very easy to get started with Lose It! Just enter a few details about yourself including your weight loss goals. Lose It! puts together a custom weight loss program. The following steps are shown on an iPhone.

Download the app from the App Store, and then tap the Lose It! app icon on the home screen. The Welcome screen opens.

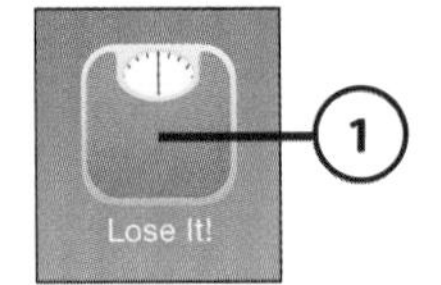

2. Tap Start Losing It! to answer a few questions about yourself.
3. Enter your current weight, and then tap Next.
4. Enter your goal weight, and then tap Next.
5. Tap to choose a Gender, and then tap Next.

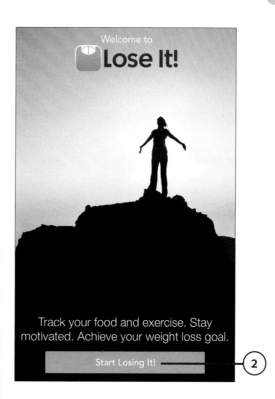

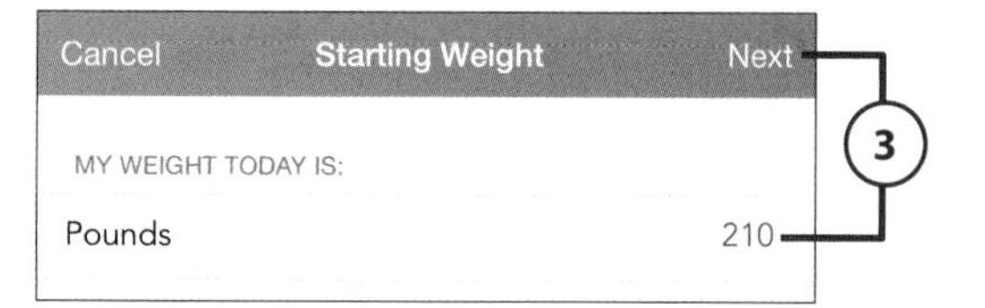

Starting Weight Goal Weight Next
MY GOAL WEIGHT IS:
Pounds 180
4

Previous Gender Next
Female
Male
5

6. Use the scroll wheels to enter your height, and then tap Next.
7. Use the scroll wheels to enter your birthday, and then tap Next.
8. Tap to designate your personalized weight plan. Depending on which plan you choose, the date you are expected to achieve your weight goal is shown at the bottom of the screen, along with your daily calorie budget.
9. Tap Next.

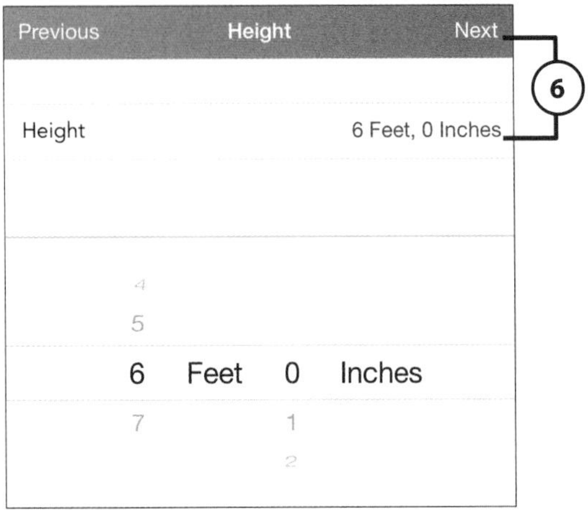

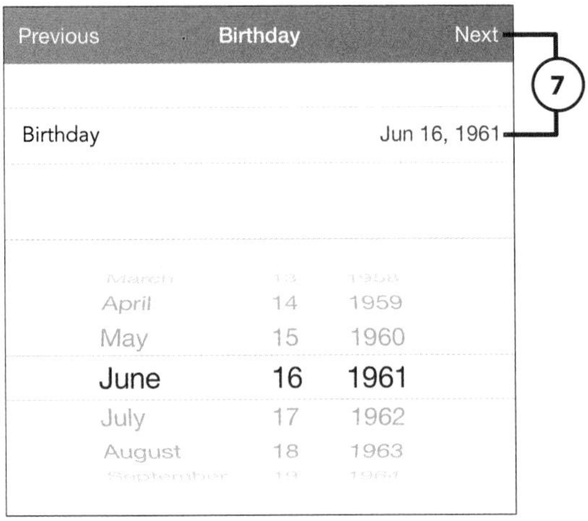

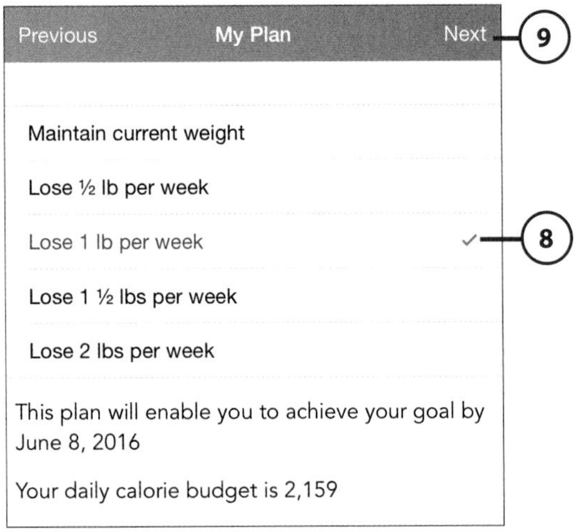

10. Enter your account credentials to create your Lose It! account, and then tap Next. A message appears asking for permission for the app to send you notifications.
11. Tap OK.
12. Tap the Add button that looks like a plus sign in the upper corner of the screen to add a food or exercise to your log. The Add to Log screen opens.

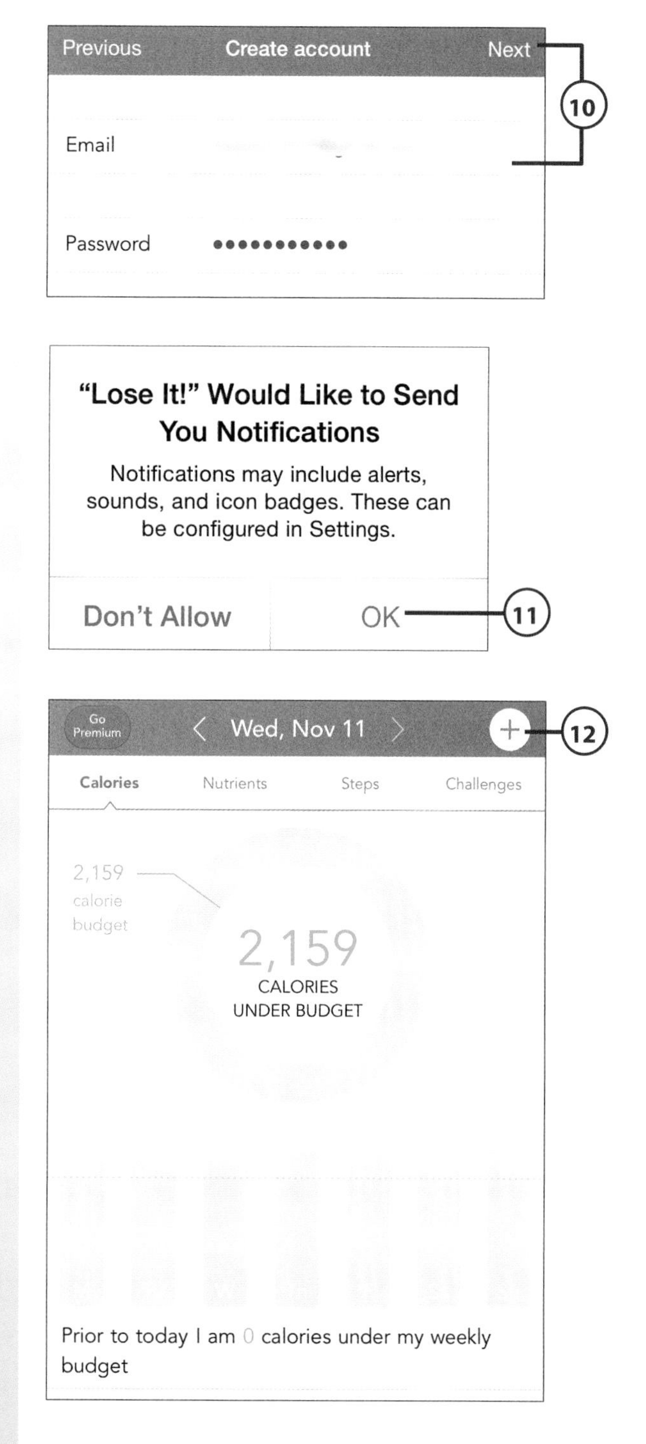

Adding Exercise

Note that you can also select exercise from the option on this screen. A wide range of exercises is arranged in alphabetical order including aerobics, Pilates, running, walking, water aerobics, and a whole lot more. You can tap an exercise to add the duration and calories burned. You can also create new exercises.

---

13. Tap the meal you want to log. Breakfast was chosen for this example. A message may appear asking whether it's okay for the app to access your location while you use this app. Access to your location enables Lose It! to determine nearby restaurants for faster logging.

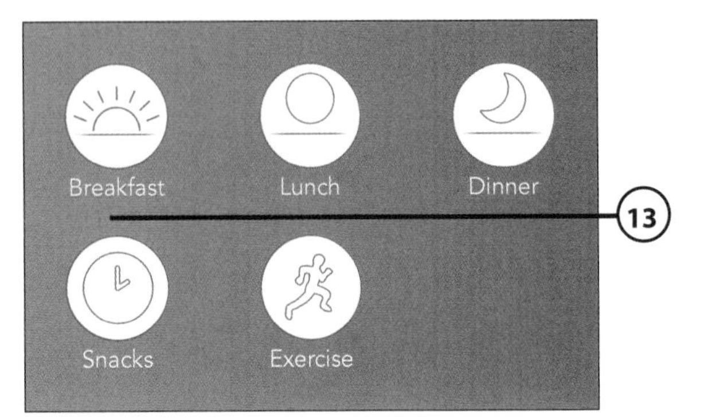

14. Tap Allow, but use your own discretion if you want to allow this location access. The page that allows you to search for a food opens.

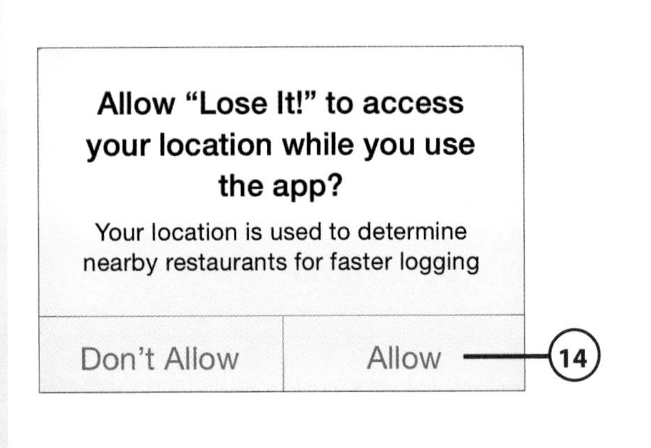

15. Tap in the search box and enter a search for the food you are about to eat or that you have eaten. To be accurate, try to log your food as you go. A list of possible search results appears beneath the search box.

16. Tap the correct search result to add it to your journal.

16 15
quaker oatmeal
Search My Foods Meals Recipes Brands
Oatmeal, Weight Control, Flavor Variety, Inst
Quaker Oatmeal – 160 cals per package
Oatmeal, Express, Brown Sugar, Golden, Inst
Quaker Oatmeal – 200 cals per package
Oatmeal, Express, Baked Apple, Inst
Quaker Oatmeal – 200 cals per package
Oatmeal
Quaker Oats – 150 cals per ½ cup
Oatmeal, Express, Cinnamon Roll, Inst
Quaker Oatmeal – 200 cals per package
Bar, Granola, Wholesome Favorites, Oatmeal...
Quaker Chewy – 111 cals per ounce

17. Use the scroll wheel to adjust the portion size for this food.
18. Tap Add to add it to your journal. Here, 320 calories of oatmeal for Breakfast has been added to the journal.
19. See that 320 calories have been subtracted from your calorie budget. You can tap the add button that looks like a plus sign for any category to add to your journal. Get the most out of Lose It! and tap Go Premium in the upper-left corner of the screen.

>>>Go Further

OTHER WAYS TO SEARCH FOR FOOD

On the Search for a Food page, there are multiple ways to search for food located under the Search box. Under Search, you have the option to type a search or scan a barcode for food not included in the database. Create New Food enables you to name a new food and manually enter all the nutritional information. The Add Calories Option lets you add calories to a given meal as well as optional nutrients, including fat, carbohydrates, and protein for a food. Lose It! saves past meals that you journal. Tap the My Foods menu option to quickly add a food that you have added previously. Tap the Meals option to add meals or combinations of foods you have journaled before. Tap Recipes to enter nutritional information for unique recipes you have made. Tap Brands to search the database for Supermarket Foods and Restaurant Foods.

Getting Groceries Delivered to Your Door

Grocery shopping can be time consuming, between travelling to the store, searching aisles, and possibly having to drive to a different store. Doing your grocery shopping online and having your food delivered can be convenient and time efficient. Not only do you not have to make the physical trip and do the leg work, but the online store is always open. Grocery shopping online also cuts down on impulse purchases, which many grocers are designed to maximize. Some online grocery services also provide easy-to-click coupons as you shop so you can save money. Then all you have to do is be there to receive your delivery.

There are many perks to grocery shopping online, but there are also a few potential drawbacks to consider. Some online grocery services charge a premium price for someone else to do the footwork, and some in-store discounts might not be available online. This might be reflected in the prices of food and delivery fees. Still, shopping online might be well worth it for you. So, when you further explore these services, take note of their prices (which aren't listed in this section, as they are subject to change before this book makes it to the shelves). Further, if you like to check the ripeness of produce by squeezing it or reach to the back of the shelf to get the freshest milk, you obviously can't do that online. When considering these services, keep in mind that there is usually a minimum order amount required.

With all the pros and cons in mind, let's take a look at some convenient options for getting groceries delivered to your door. Due to the regional variations in grocery chains, it's key that you follow the instructions as we continue, to see whether a given service is available in your area.

Explore Peapod Home Delivery

Peapod is an online grocery with delivery and includes the online grocery shopping for Giant and Stop & Shop. The process is easy. Sign up for an account, and then browse and search the aisles to add items to your virtual grocery cart. If you have a Giant card or Stop & Shop card, you can enter your card information to shop from a list of items you have previously purchased in the store. Book a time for home or workplace delivery, and Peapod does the heavy lifting for you. If you prefer, you can arrange an in-store pickup, and they load your trunk.

Use the following steps on your computer to get started. The service will update according to your Zip code to show Peapod, Peapod by Giant, or Peapod by Stop & Stop. Some options may vary based on your local stores. Peapod even has a mobile app available for both Android and Apple (iOS) devices. The following example is shown on a computer.

1. Go to peapod.com in your web browser.'

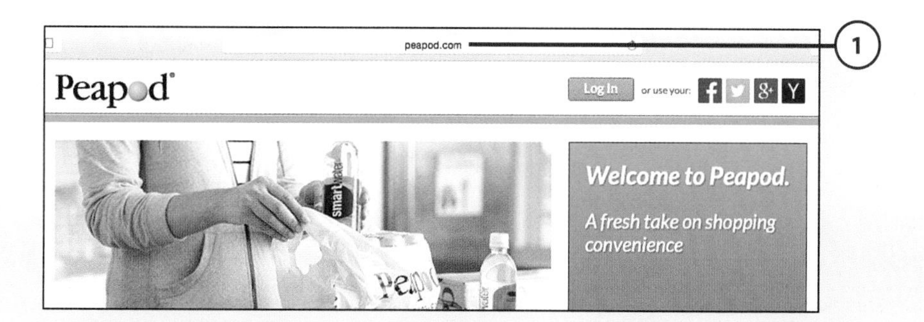

Social Media Privacy Issues

Keep in mind that logging in using a social media account can pose privacy issues by giving the app access to your social media data. Consider signing up using an alternative method.

2. Click View Service Areas to see whether Peapod delivers in your area.
3. Click New Customer to register an account.

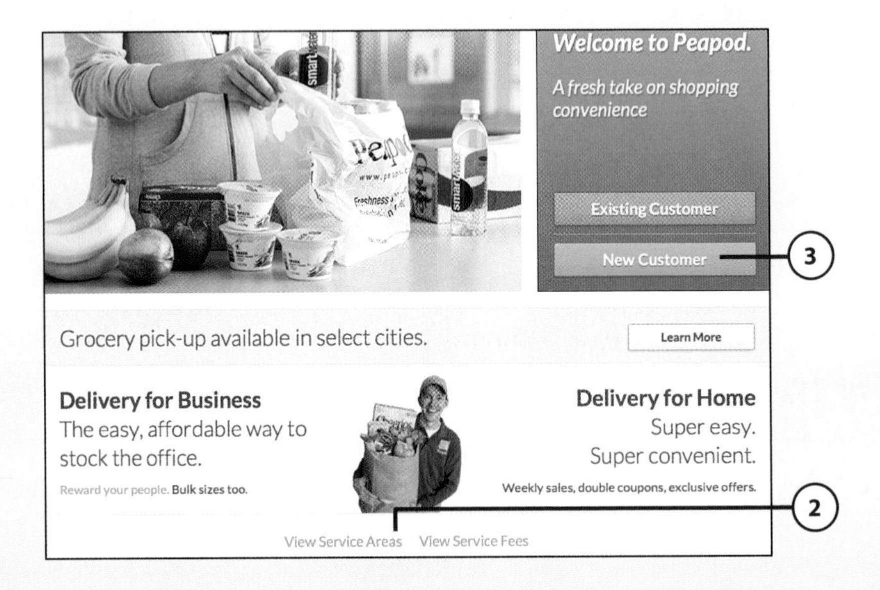

4. Enter your Zip code and type of address, and then click Start Shopping.
5. Sign in using one of your social networks or enter the username for your Stop & Shop (or Giant, as applicable) online account. If you don't have any of these, click No thanks, skip.

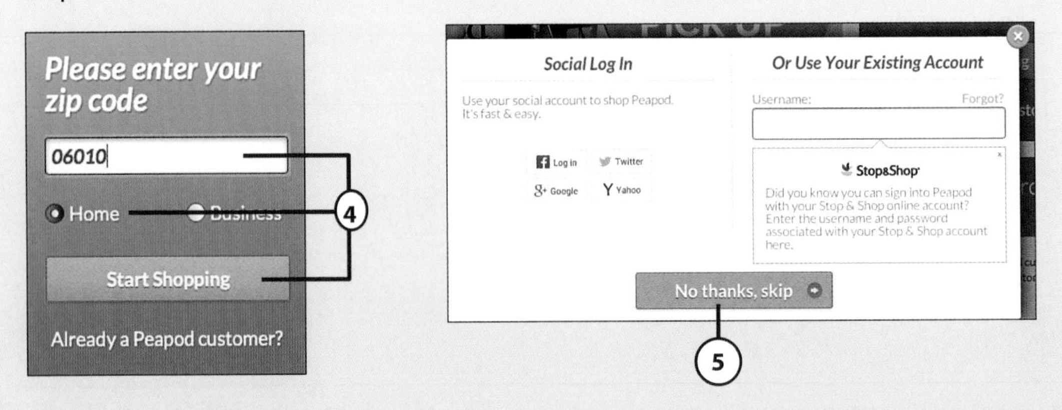

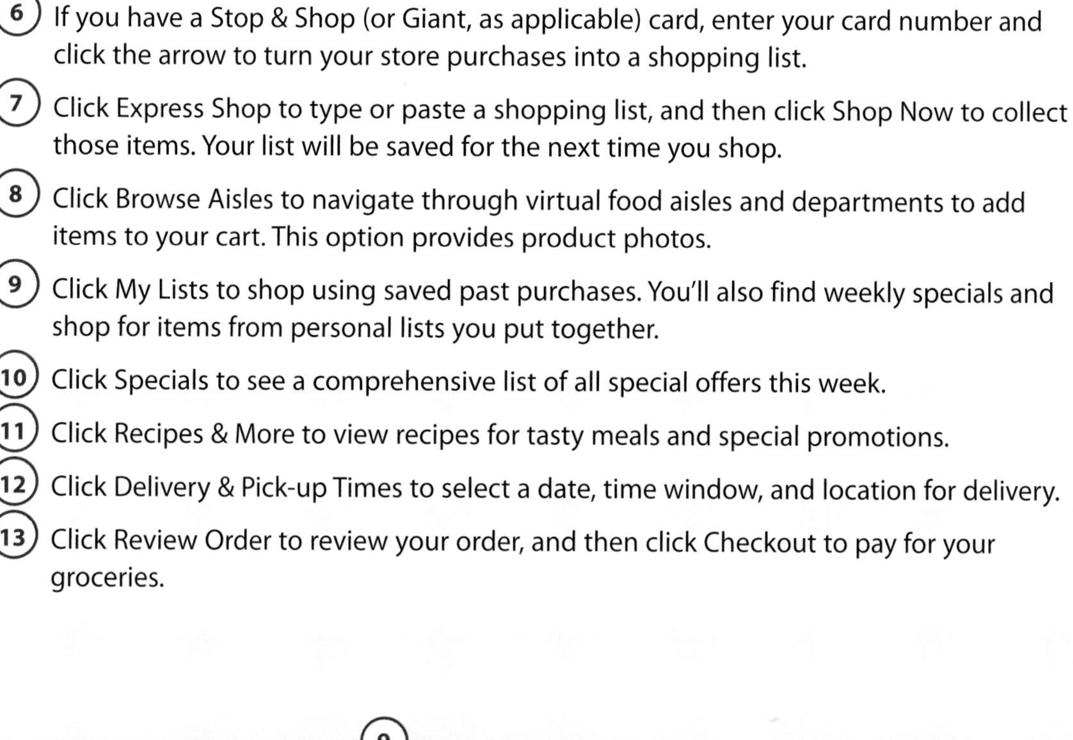

6. If you have a Stop & Shop (or Giant, as applicable) card, enter your card number and click the arrow to turn your store purchases into a shopping list.
7. Click Express Shop to type or paste a shopping list, and then click Shop Now to collect those items. Your list will be saved for the next time you shop.
8. Click Browse Aisles to navigate through virtual food aisles and departments to add items to your cart. This option provides product photos.
9. Click My Lists to shop using saved past purchases. You'll also find weekly specials and shop for items from personal lists you put together.
10. Click Specials to see a comprehensive list of all special offers this week.
11. Click Recipes & More to view recipes for tasty meals and special promotions.
12. Click Delivery & Pick-up Times to select a date, time window, and location for delivery.
13. Click Review Order to review your order, and then click Checkout to pay for your groceries.

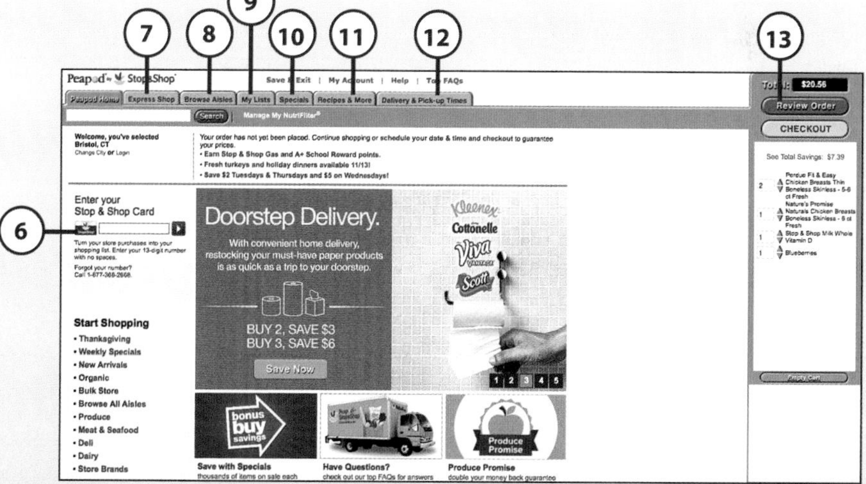

Use Schwan's Home Delivery Services

The Schwan Food Company delivers frozen foods and dairy products, including ice creams, entrees, meats, and desserts. There are three ways you can receive your groceries: delivery to your door, freezer bag drop-off (if you will not be home for several hours after drop-off), or mail order. If you do not live in an area serviced by Schwan's delivery trucks, mail order is the method for you. Schwan's currently offers discounts to AARP members for new Home Service customers. Schwan's also has an app for Android and Apple (iOS) mobile devices.

Follow these steps to use Schwan's Home Delivery Services. The following steps are performed on the Schwan's website via computer.

1. Go to schwans.com in your web browser.
2. Scroll down the page, enter your Zip code, and then click Submit to see the delivery options available in your area.
3. Scroll to the very bottom of the page and click Schwan's AARP Program to save money on your first order.

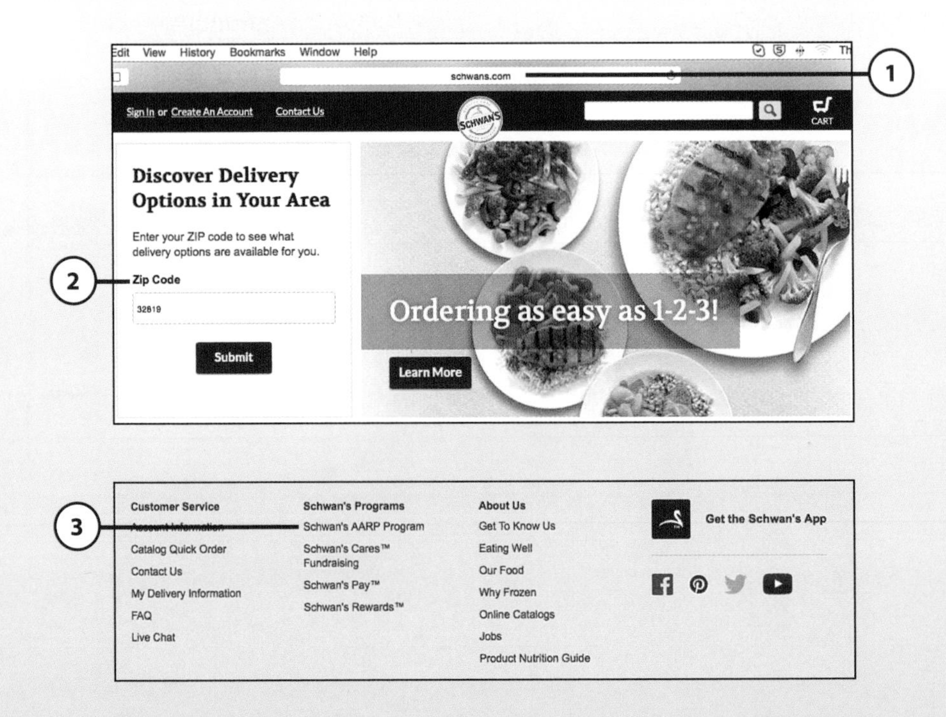

4. Scroll to the top of the page, and then click Create an Account to get started.
5. After you create an account, click a category to shop, and then click a subcategory.
6. Choose the quantity and then click Add to Cart for the items you want.
7. Click Cart to check out and specify delivery details. You can also use any coupon codes you may have.

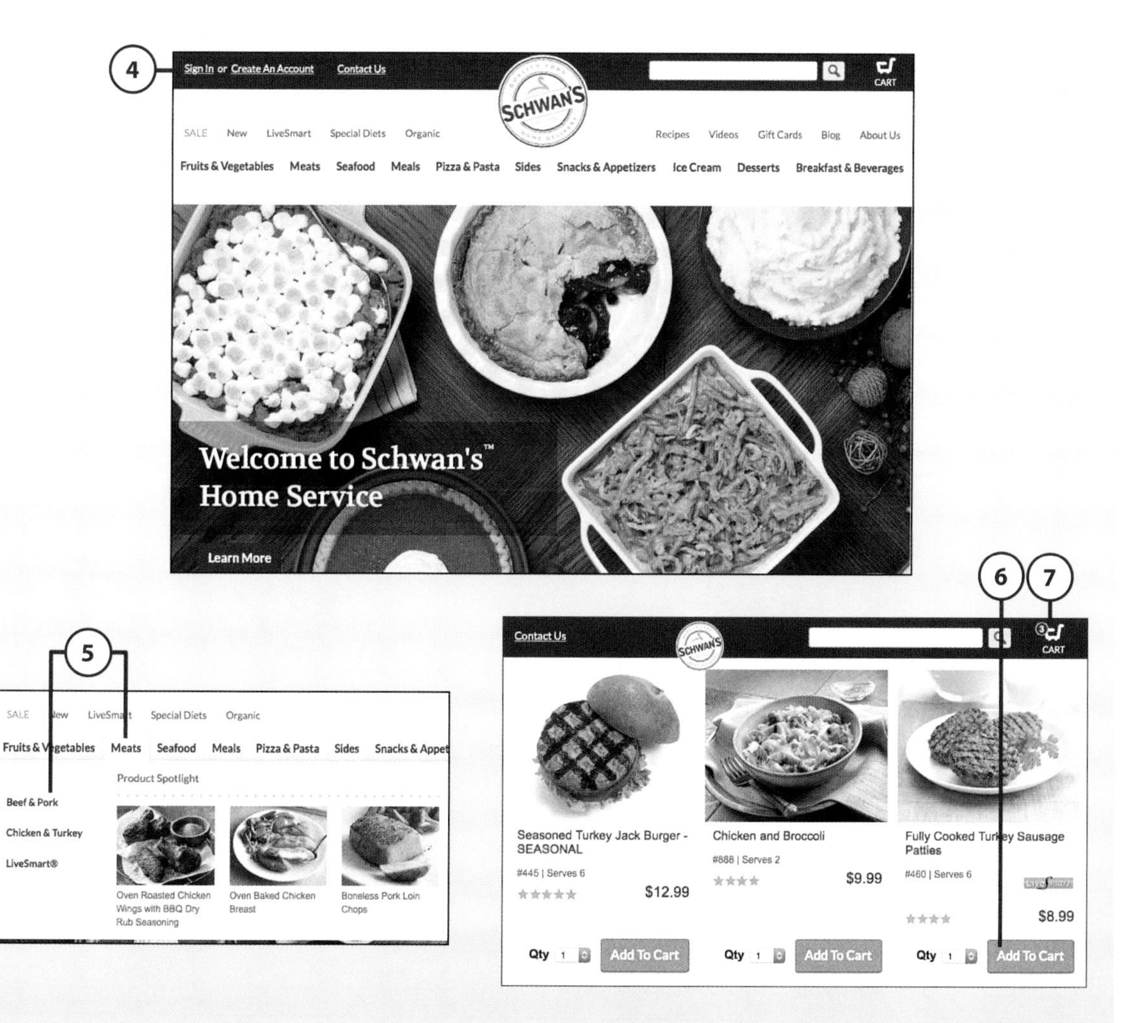

Order from AmazonFresh

Amazon is also in the business of delivering groceries with AmazonFresh. AmazonFresh delivers produce, dairy, meat, seafood, and more. You can also have other products from amazon.com delivered along with your food, so you can get fresh milk and a fitness tracker. AmazonFresh also lets you shop products from local shops and restaurants. As of this writing, AmazonFresh is available exclusively to Prime Fresh members. There is a 30-day free trial, but after that period you are billed for an annual membership. Find out more at fresh.amazon.com/welcome. You can download the AmazonFresh app for Android and Apple (iOS) devices. Use the following steps to get started ordering from AmazonFresh. These examples are shown on a computer.

1. Go to fresh.amazon.com/welcome in your web browser.
2. Enter your Zip code to see whether AmazonFresh delivers in your area, and then click Check. If AmazonFresh delivers in your area, you are taken to a local page.
3. Click the link to start your 30-day free trial.

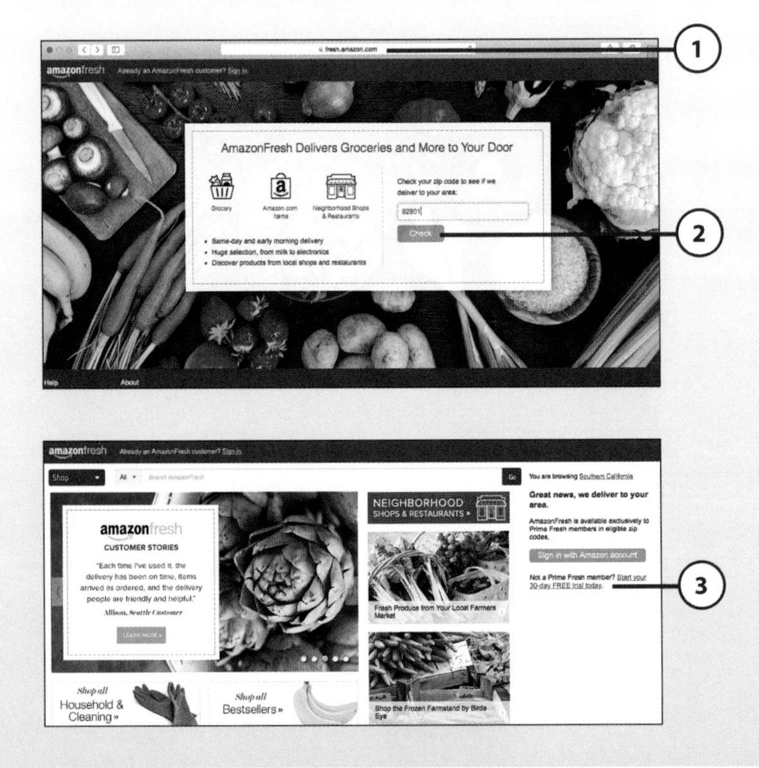

4. Scroll down to browse the categories of food, and then click a category.
5. Click a product to add it to your cart. After you have started your 30-day free trial, your cart will appear to the right. You can then choose to check out and specify delivery options.

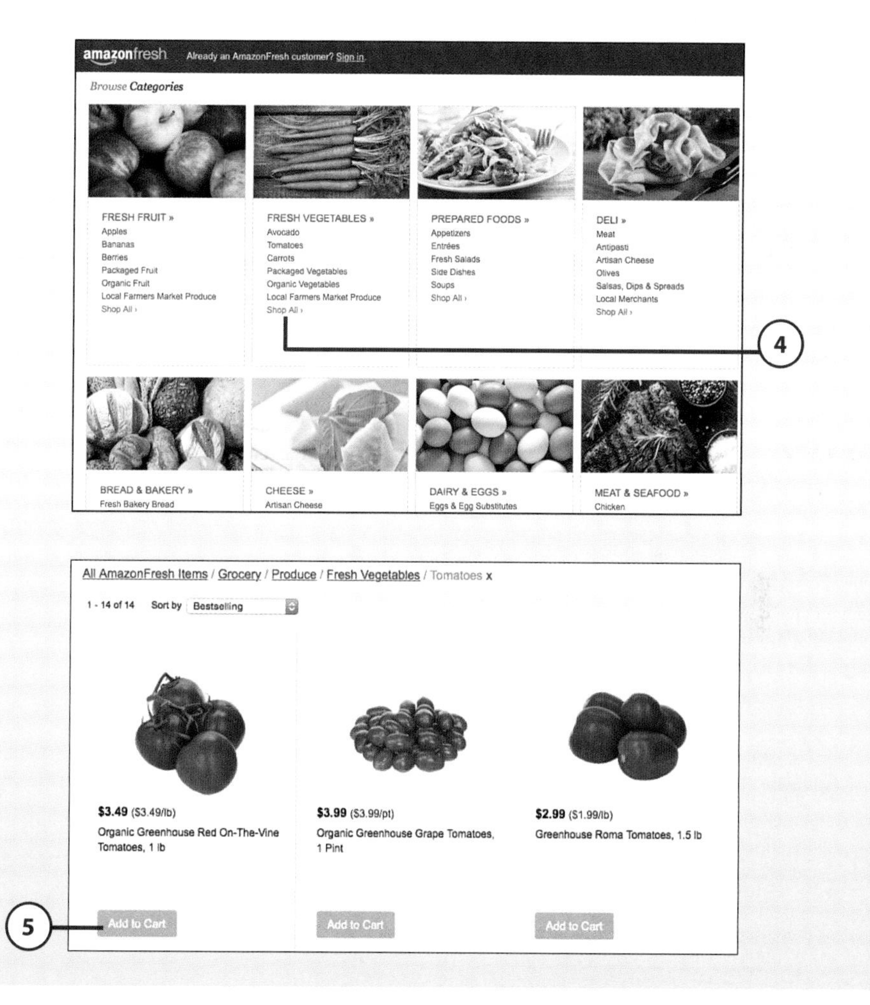

Consider Instacart Grocery Delivery

Instacart is a little different from the other services we've covered so far, because it's not a grocer. Instacart lets you grocery shop at stores with Instacart availability in your area, like BJ's Wholesale Club, Costco, Whole Foods Market, and Winn Dixie. Depending on your area, only the available stores will show after you create an account. In a few clicks you can create a grocery order of fresh fruit, vegetables, meat, seafood, and home essentials. Instacart Personal Shoppers pick and then deliver your order in as little as one hour. You can order from multiple stores at once, reorder deliveries, keep a shopping list, and set the delivery time that works best for you. Instacart also has a mobile app for Android and Apple (iOS) devices.

You can get started shopping with Instacart in just a few steps. The following examples are shown on a computer.

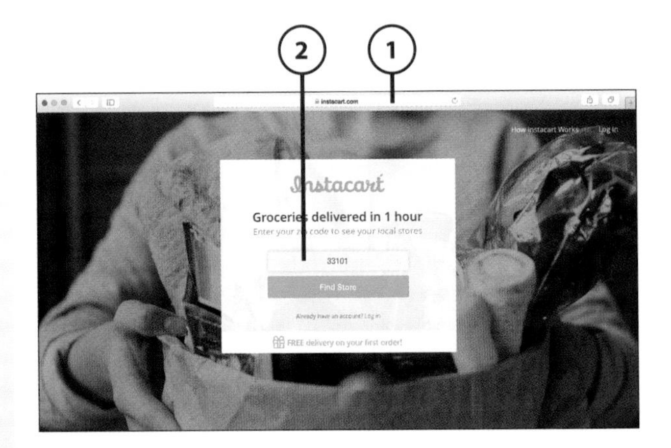

1. Go to instacart.com in your web browser.
2. Enter your Zip code, and then click Find Store to see whether Instacart services are available in your area. A dialog opens if the service is available.
3. Enter your full name, email, and a password to set up an account, and then click Shop Now. You can also set up an account using your existing Facebook account. The stores in your area available for Instacart appear.

Social Media Privacy Issues

Keep in mind that logging in via Facebook can pose privacy issues by giving the app access to your social media data. Consider signing up using an email account instead.

4. Tap a store. Winn Dixie is chosen in this example. The Winn Dixie online store page opens.
5. Hover your mouse pointer over an item that you want, and then click View. The item opens in a new screen. Depending on which web browser you use, such as Google Chrome, you might not see the View option while hovering. If you don't see View, just click the item.
6. Select the quantity for the product you want. After you select a new quantity, the item is automatically placed in the cart. If you want the default quantity, click Add to Cart. Under the Add to Cart button, you can save this item as a Favorite, or choose Add to List to add the item to a shopping list. These options will make your shopping experience go faster in the future. The item is placed in the cart.

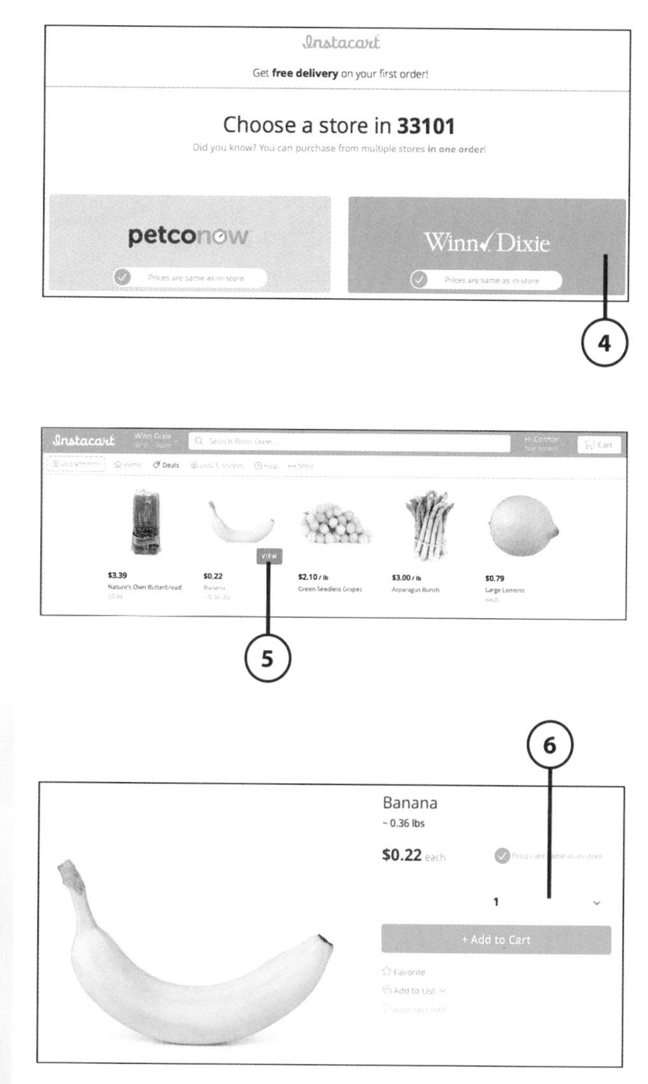

7. Click in the box, and then type to add any special instructions for the item. For example, "I want green bananas." Depending on the item, you might not be given the option to add special instructions.
8. Tap the X in the upper-right corner to close the item onscreen and return to the main screen.
9. When you have completed your shopping, click Cart to check out and specify delivery details. You are also making payment at this time.

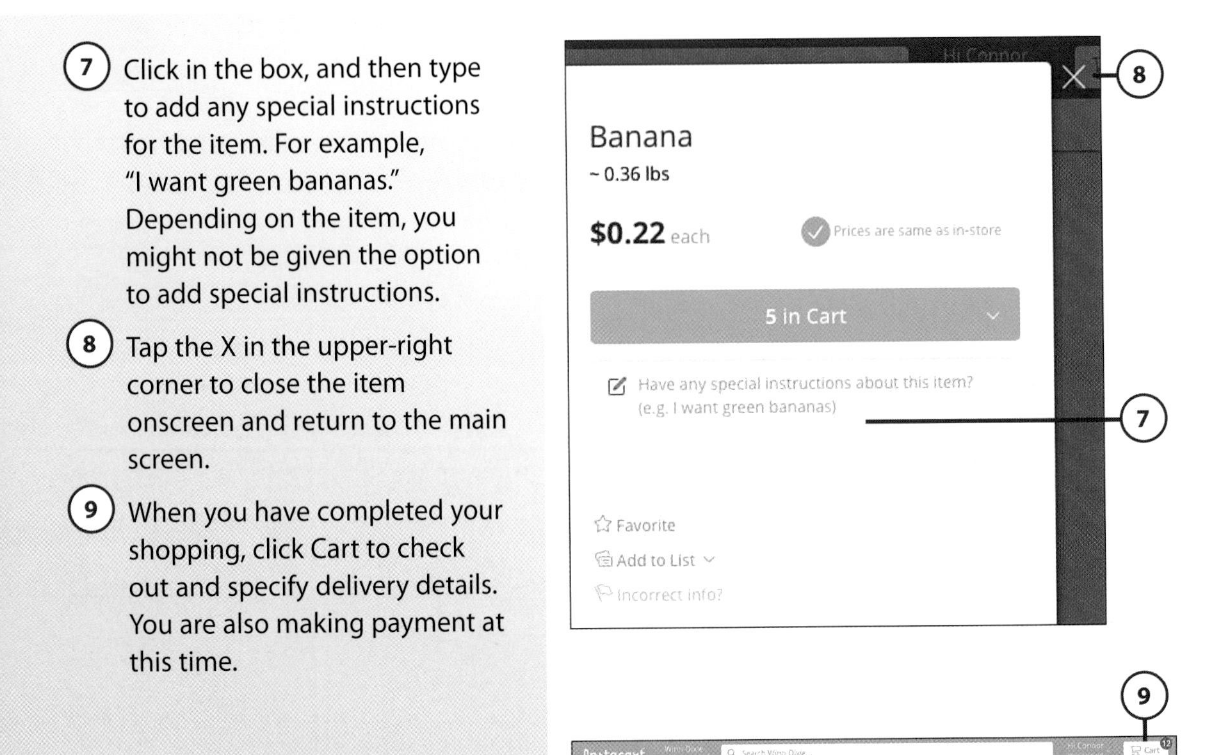

Exploring Diet-Specific Resources with Recipes

Some delivery services cater to individuals with specific dietary needs, including Kosher, vegetarian, gluten-free, and all-natural food diets. A couple of the delivery services that we've already talked about, Schwan's and Instacart, have such offerings. This section introduces you to some grocery delivery services that offer the diet-specific foods you might need and can deliver them to your door.

Explore All Natural, Gourmet Farm-to-Table Deliveries from Blue Ribbon Foods

Blue Ribbon Foods offers healthy food options with no steroids, no growth hormones, no preservatives, and no chemicals. It also doesn't add antibiotics, dyes, or coloring to its foods. If you're looking for an all-natural food alternative to your local grocery store, give Blue Ribbon Foods serious consideration for your meats, poultry, and seafood. You can also find Grade A natural and organic fancy vegetables and prepared items including lemon pepper chicken, chicken cordon bleu, lasagna, and pastas. On the Blue Ribbons Foods website, you'll also find some tasty recipes to prepare, including Slow Cooker Chicken and Rice, Mustard Shrimp, and Grilled Avocado. Visit blueribbonfoods.com and click on Our Service at the top of the screen to view delivery areas and see whether you qualify for a free sample.

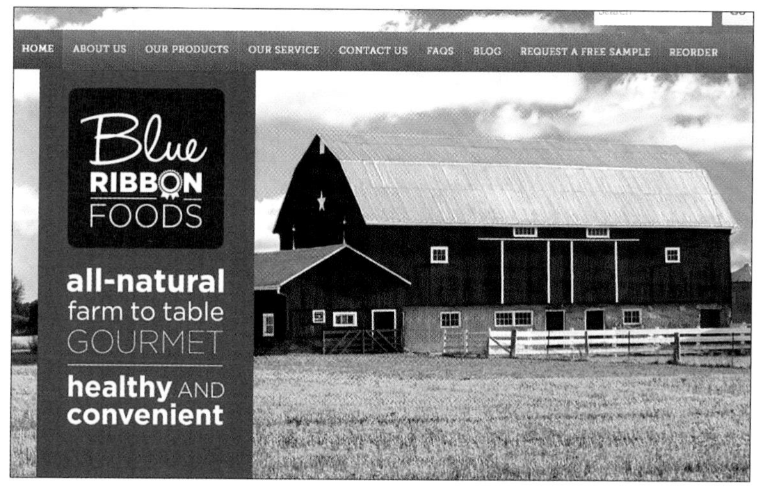

Go to blueribbonfoods.com to try this healthy option.

Receive Special Diet Deliveries from Schwan's Home Delivery

When we previously discussed Schwan's food delivery service, we only browsed the general foods that it offers. Schwans.com also has a section of its online ordering dedicated to Special Diets. In the Special Diets section you'll find hundreds of products, including Gluten Free, Vegetarian, No Sugar Added, Heart Healthy, Low Sodium, and Low Calorie foods. There are also hundreds of recipes that can help you add some variety to your meals, including Grilled Jalapeño Chicken Fajita Bites. You can find the Special Diets option located at the top of the screen at schwans.com. You should also check out the LiveSmart section of the website, also located at the top of the screen, to shop foods with moderate levels of fat, sodium, calories, and zero grams of trans fat. The LiveSmart section has hundreds of products and recipes for you to choose from, including Garlic Herb Shrimp and Grilled Chicken Breast with Avocado Lime Salsa.

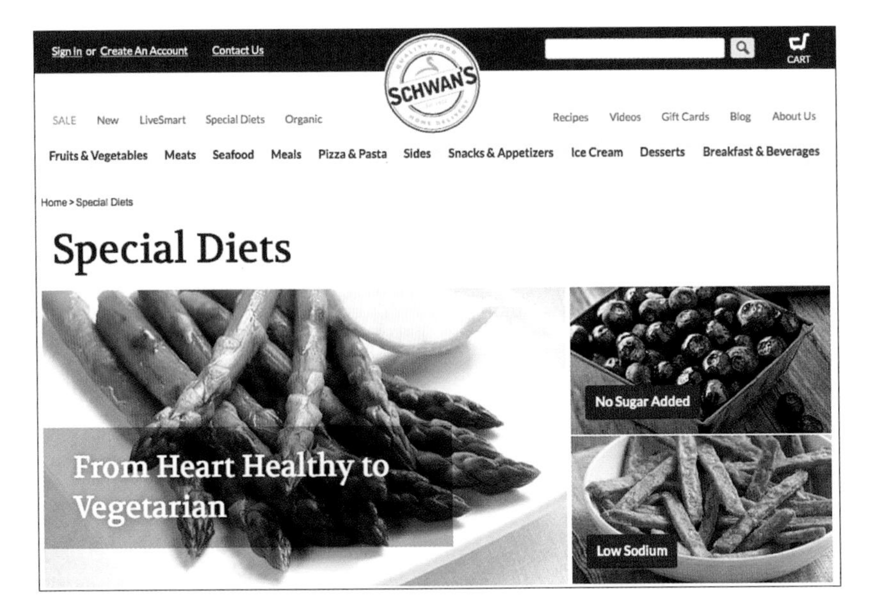

Make sure to check out the Special Diets section of Schwan's.

Consider Diet-Specific Grocery Delivery from Instacart

Because Instacart is strictly a delivery service, not a grocer, the stores offered in your delivery area dictate your choices for diet-specific foods. A Whole Foods Market will likely have more gluten-free options than a Winn Dixie, for example. If your store choices are limited in Instacart, don't throw in the towel just yet. Many grocers have diet-specific choices that you just have to look a little deeper to find. The following example uses Instacart to shop online at Winn Dixie. Under Lists & Recipes located at the very top of the screen, you can find links to Healthy foods and Ethnic Foods posted by users, which vary by store and Zip code. In this particular example featuring Winn Dixie, you can click on the Healthy category and find recipes including Roasted Beet Hummus, Thai Stir-fried Chicken with Cashew Nuts, and Vegan Berry Crumble Bars.

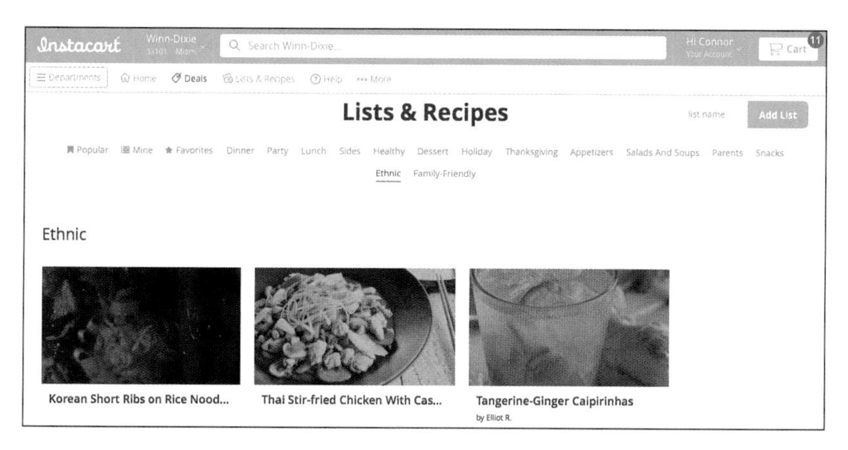

Make use of the Lists & Recipes section on Instacart to find diet-specific options, which may include Kosher, gluten-free, and other areas.

Eat Better by Planning Your Meals Using Edamam

Edamam lets you compare and select more than a million recipes across hundreds of websites using calorie, diet, and nutrition information. If you are looking for new recipes to add to your repertoire and/or have special diet or nutrition needs, the Edamam website or app for Android and Apple (iOS devices) can be a huge help. You can search recipes for free on the Edamam website, but some services are subscription-based, such as the Nutrition Wizard. The apps are free to download but have in-app purchases (services for which you have to pay). Here's how it works. Maybe you're looking for a new side dish to serve with dinner and you've just started cutting back on carbs. Enter a search for side dishes, filter the search for Low-Carb, and then Edamam searches the Web and provides you a bounty of recipes for low-carb side dishes. Filter the search using a calorie range, and Edamam goes to work presenting some wonderful recipes to choose from. All recipes have quality photos and a full nutritional profile so you can easily go through each result and do comparisons. All recipes have a complete ingredients list so you can take the Edamam mobile app on your phone to the store to shop for ingredients.

The Edamam website is very simple to use. Follow these steps (shown on a computer) to eat better and start planning your meals with Edamam.

1. Go to edamam.com in your web browser.
2. Click Sign Up so you can save your recipes.
3. Type in a search and click the Search icon. You can click Get Inspired at the bottom of the screen to see a random selection of tasty recipes, just to get you started. The Nutrition Wizard is a paid service that enables instant nutritional analysis of any recipe or ingredients list.
4. Click Calories and Diet. A menu of filter options appears.
5. Click the filter option(s) that you want. As soon as you click an option, a page of search results appears displaying calories and the number of ingredients. Depending on which web browser you use, you might have to click Done, located at the bottom-right corner, to see the search results. Notice that at the top of the results page you can edit the filter settings and the search.
6. Click a picture of a search result. A complete nutritional profile is displayed along with the ingredients.

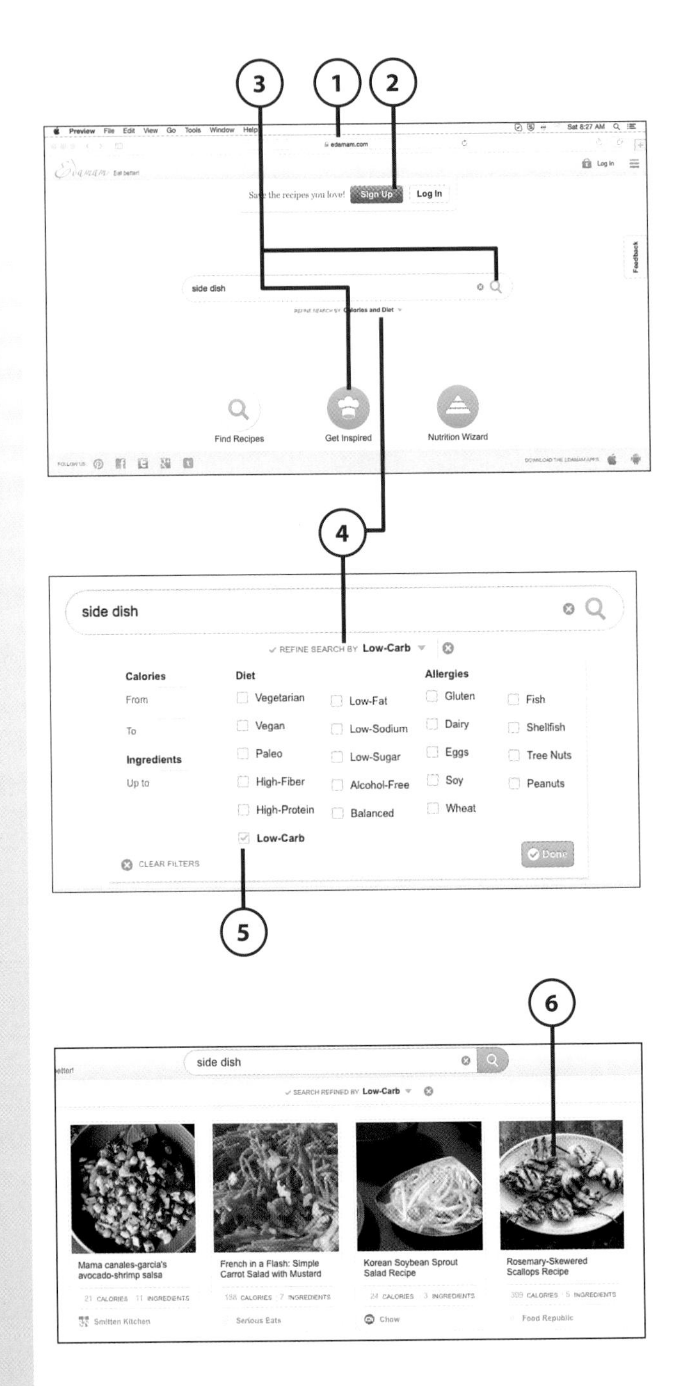

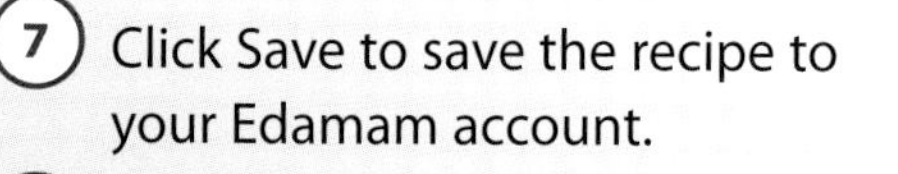

7. Click Save to save the recipe to your Edamam account.
8. Click See full recipe to view the full recipe.

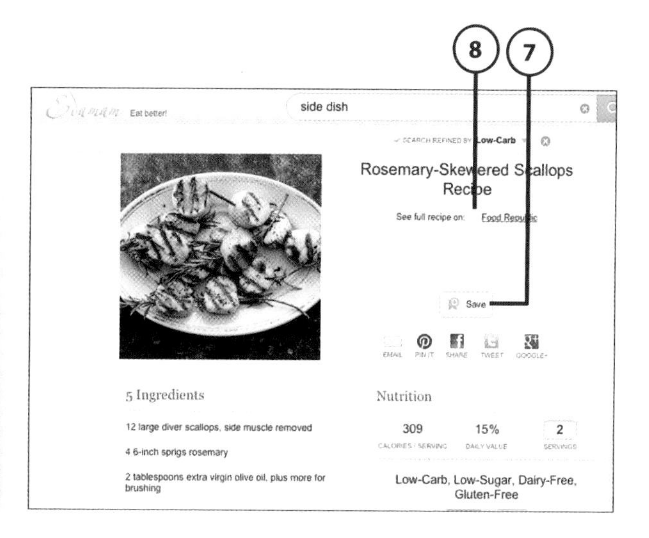

Get Designer Recipes and Delicious Groceries at PlateJoy

PlateJoy is a subscription-based service that offers meal plans designed for your specific time constraints and customized ingredients. First, you take a lifestyle quiz and tell PlateJoy about yourself. PlateJoy designs custom meal plans and organizes your ingredients into a shopping list that you can print or access on your phone. You follow the recipes and cook the food. It's that easy. PlateJoy accommodates a variety of specific diets including vegetarian, low carb, paleo, and gluten free. To learn more, visit platejoy.com.

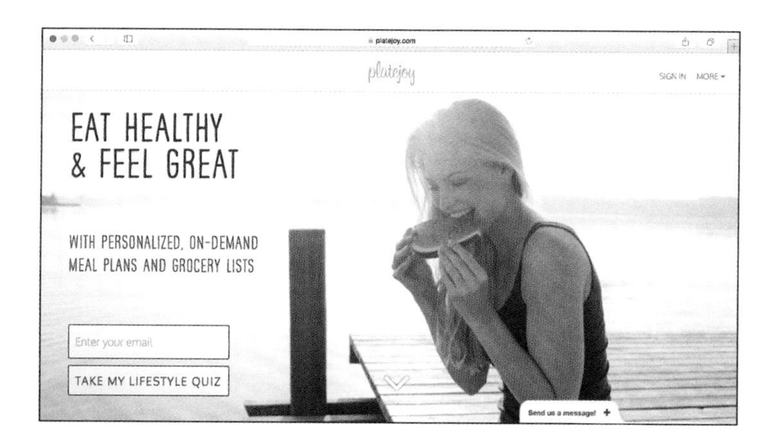
platejoy.com
platejoy
SIGN IN
MORE
EAT HEALTHY
& FEEL GREAT
WITH PERSONALIZED, ON-DEMAND
MEAL PLANS AND GROCERY LISTS
Enter your email
TAKE MY LIFESTYLE QUIZ
Send us a message!

Let PlateJoy design custom meals and create personalized shopping lists for you.

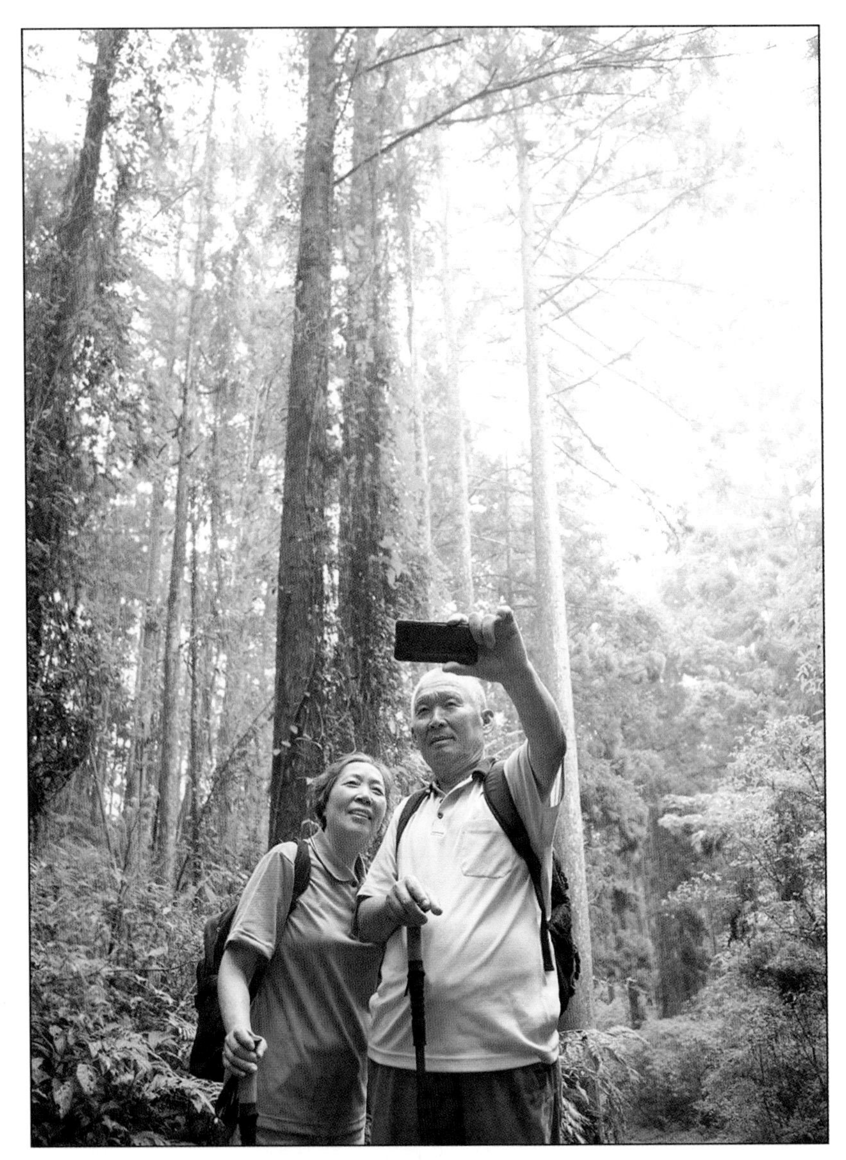

Credit: © Tom Wang/Fotolia.com

Track your daily exercise activities, and achieve your health and fitness goals by using apps and creating a fitness plan. Get to know some innovative walking canes.

In this chapter, you learn how some of the most popular health and fitness apps made by Apple, Fitbit, Google, Samsung, Withings, and more, motivate you to get in shape and stay fit. You also learn about some unique walking canes that offer special features and add a layer of safety while you continue to live an active lifestyle.

3

→ Tracking Your Daily Activity
→ Tracking Steps
→ Tracking Flights of Stairs Climbed
→ Monitoring Walking and Running Distance
→ Tracking Biking Activity
→ Creating a Fitness Plan
→ Achieving Health and Fitness Goals with More Apps
→ Getting to Know High-Tech Canes

Keeping Active and Fit

Many apps are on the market that empower you to set daily goals for the number of steps taken, flights climbed, distance run or biked, and more. You may already have a smartphone with one of these apps preinstalled. Many of the health and fitness solutions in this chapter don't require that you purchase a fitness tracker to get started. If working out is already a part of your daily routine, you'll get to know some resources that can help you get more out of your routine by acting as a workout partner or personal trainer. If you're integrating exercise back into your lifestyle or for the first time, apps can help customize a fitness routine. If you use a cane or may need one, some apps have capabilities you may not have considered that help you stay active and safe at the same time. Let's start with some of the basic functions of health and fitness apps, which include tracking steps and flights climbed.

Tracking Your Daily Activity

Tracking your daily fitness activity is a great way to stay motivated and strengthen willpower. Fitness apps and trackers can help you set your own goals and help maintain a pace that will keep you on target to meet those goals. The simple act of keeping a record of your progress can motivate you to do better the next day. If you ran or walked two miles today, a fitness app can motivate you to go farther or faster tomorrow by showing you how many calories you burned. Maybe you just want to best your previous results. Regardless of the metric, this data-driven approach lets you know exactly how much you're doing per activity and can motivate you to run and walk farther, use the stairs instead of the elevator, and bike farther each week. If your smartphone is almost always with you, having a mobile fitness app onboard is practical and at times inspirational.

The examples you are about to read are a mixture of apps that can be used by themselves on your smartphone, in connection with other apps, or with a fitness tracker. If you want to use your phone and app only, consider a sport armband. A sport armband lets you slide your phone into it and fastens around your upper arm while you work out, usually using a Velcro strip. You can easily find these by searching online for "sports armband." Some are made for multiple devices, but tack on the name and model of your smartphone to your search just to be certain you get one for your specific device. Also, take your arm circumference into consideration before you make a purchase.

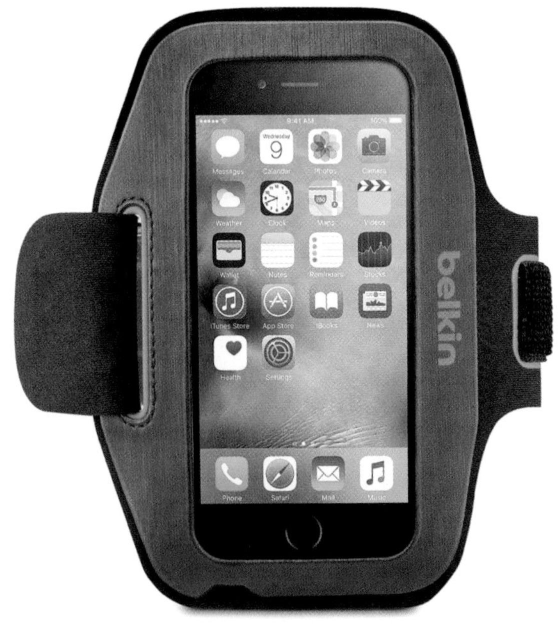

© 2016 Belkin International, Inc.

An example of an iPhone 6S sports armband

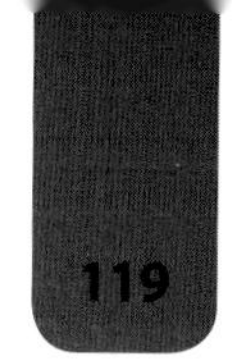

It's Not All Good

Activity Detection Accuracy

Some apps and devices require you to put them into a specific exercise mode such as running, walking, or biking. Others use the sensors in your device, smartphone, and/or tracker to automatically determine which activity you are performing. Neither of these methods gets it right 100 percent of the time. Trackers and apps that automatically detect which activity you are performing can get it wrong sometimes. You may be running or cycling, but your app or tracker may register it as walking. Your smartphone and tracker might differ on how many steps you have taken. Keep these occasional inconsistencies in mind when trying these devices.

Tracking Steps

If you don't use a pedometer, you probably have no idea how many steps you take in a day. For reference, there are roughly 2,000 steps in a mile. Ten thousand steps a day, roughly 5 miles, has been the popular baseline goal for maintaining a healthy weight and is recommended by the American Heart Association. Some fitness trackers use this as a default value. Ask your doctor for a specific baseline for your personal health needs to get you started. A fitness app and/or tracker can help you know approximately how many steps you take in a day.

Apple Health App

If you have an iPhone 5s or later that runs iOS8 or later, you can use the preinstalled Apple Health app to track your steps. The information is neatly presented in graphs. Beginning to track your steps is easy. The following examples are shown on an iPhone.

1. Tap the Health app on your iPhone.

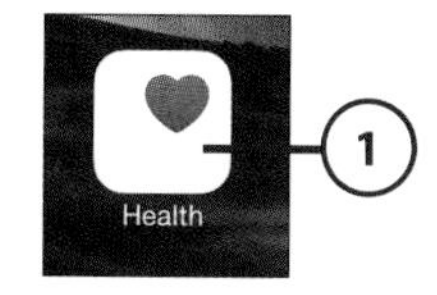

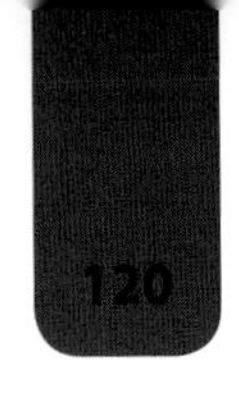

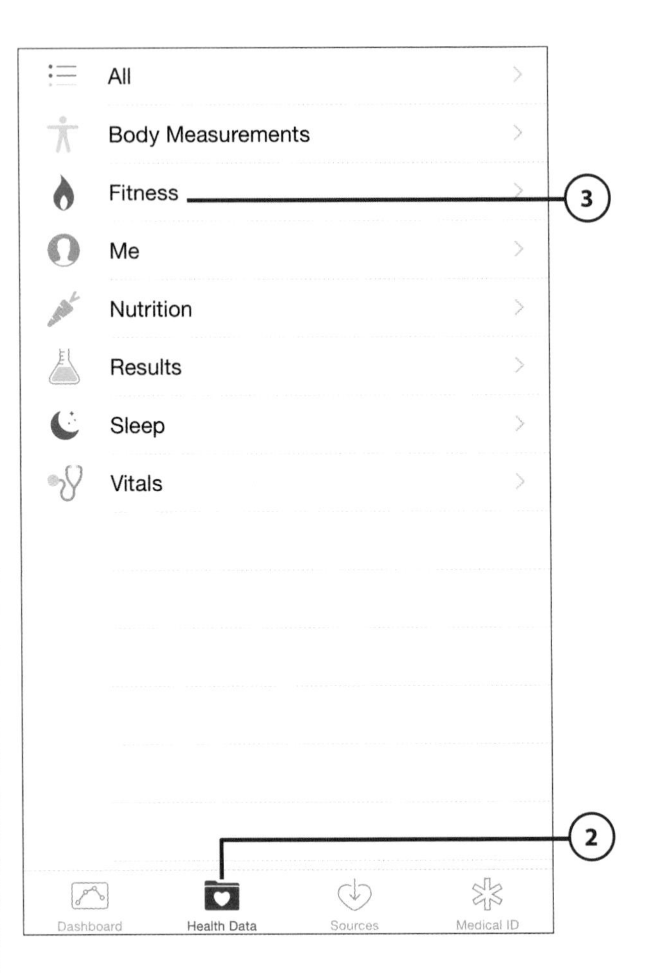

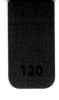

2. Tap Health Data.
3. Tap Fitness.

More Tracking Capabilities

The Health app offers much more than just step counting. The Health Data screen provides options to track health information like body measurements, fitness stats, nutrition, blood glucose, inhaler usage, sleep analysis, and much more. When you download compatible apps and trackers that can connect with the Health app, much of this health data is imported for you.

4. Tap Steps.

Health Data
Fitness
Active Calories
Cycling Distance
Flights Climbed
NikeFuel
Resting Calories
Steps
Walking + Running Distance
Workouts
4

Tracking Other Apps in Health

You can show data from other apps on the Health dashboard. Tap the Sources tab at the bottom of the screen to view the Apple Health–compatible apps you have installed on your iPhone. A list of compatible devices such as the Apple Watch appears here as well. Under Sources you can tap on an app in the list and give it permission to display in the Health app. From the Health data tab, you can enable Show on Dashboard to view that information in the Health app. To find apps that are compatible with Health in the App Store, go to the Health & Fitness categories and search Apps for Health.

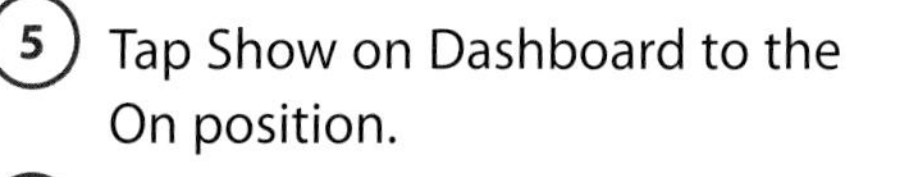

5. Tap Show on Dashboard to the On position.
6. Tap Dashboard to view your step data on the main screen and start stepping. The Health app is able to detect which activity you are performing.

Fitness
Steps
Day Week Month Year
Steps 1,478 steps
Daily Average: 320 Yesterday, 11:29 PM
Show on Dashboard
Show All Data
Add Data Point
Share Data
Unit steps
5

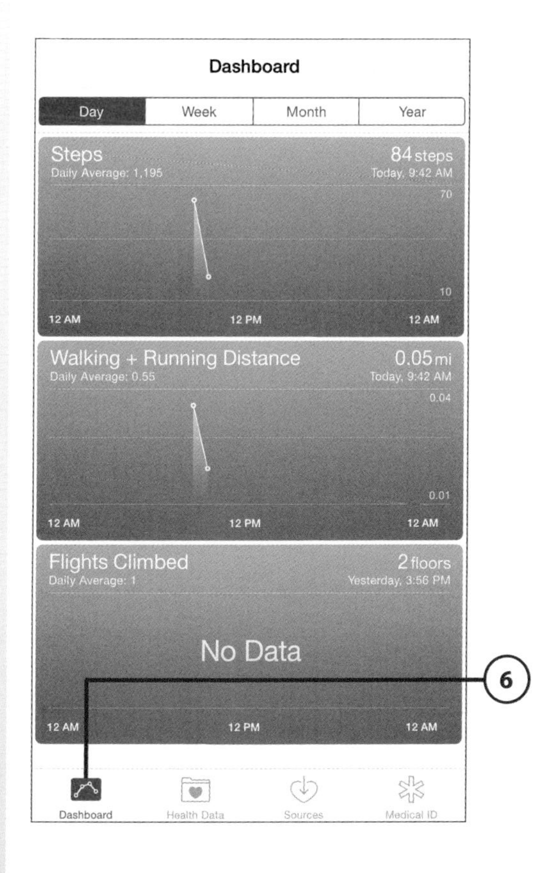

>>>Go Further

THE APPLE ACTIVITY APP AND THE APPLE WATCH

When you sync your Apple Watch to your iPhone, the Activity app appears on your phone desktop. The Activity app lets you set fitness goals and shows your progress. It provides a snapshot of daily activities using three rings: the Stand ring (Blue), the Move ring (Red), and the Exercise ring (Green). This visual design makes it easy for you to monitor your daily activity with a glance at your Watch. The Stand ring shows you how often you have stood up and moved for at least a minute. Your goal is to stand at least 1 minute every hour. The Move ring tracks the calories you've burned and if you have met your daily calorie burn. The Exercise ring shows you how many minutes of brisk activity you have completed in a day. The goal is to accumulate 30 minutes of brisk activity. Your objective is to close each ring each day. Data collected with the Activity app is automatically shared with the Health app. The Activity app on your Apple Watch is also how you can access your step count.

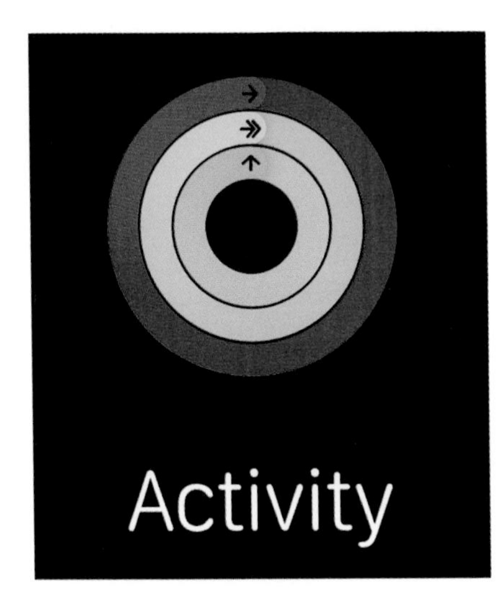

The Apple Activity app

Fitbit

Depending on the device that you have, you don't need a Fitbit tracker to manage some basic activities. You can track steps and distance on your iPhone using only the free app when you carry your phone. MobileTrack uses motion sensors in your iPhone 5s, 6, and 6 Plus to enable you to track steps. As of this writing, Android and Windows Phones require a Fitbit tracker. Pair the Fitbit tracker with the app to unlock all the features Fitbit has to offer. Download the Fitbit app from the Google Play Store, the App Store, and the Windows Phone Store, and then set up an account by answering a few personal questions and verifying your email. Allow the Fitbit app to access your motion activity during the setup process. After the setup, you are taken to the Dashboard where you can access your step information.

Setting Up MobileTrack Account

Use the following steps to set up a new MobileTrack account so you can use the Fitbit app on your iPhone for tracking steps.

1. Tap the Fitbit app on your iPhone.
2. Tap Join Fitbit. A list of Fitbit trackers appears.

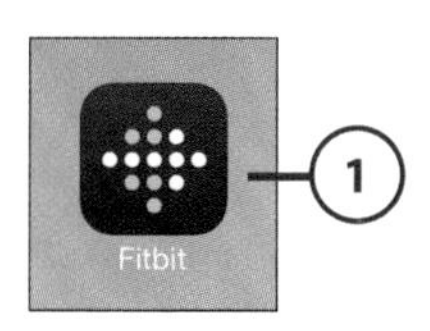

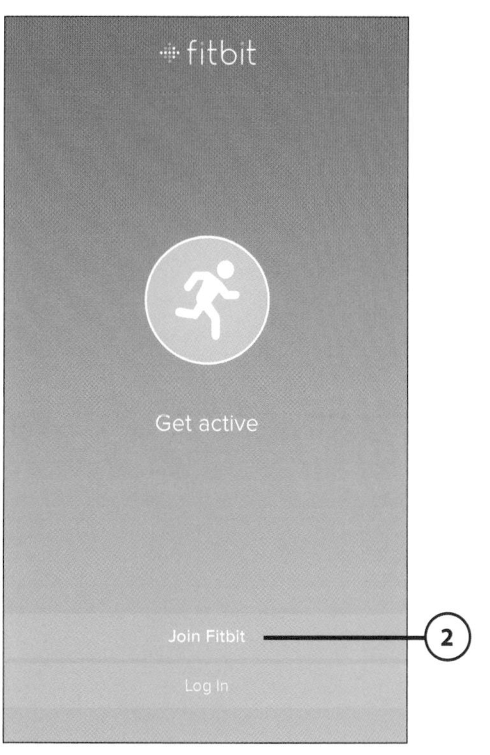

3. Tap No Fitbit Yet?
4. Tap Set Up Your Phone.

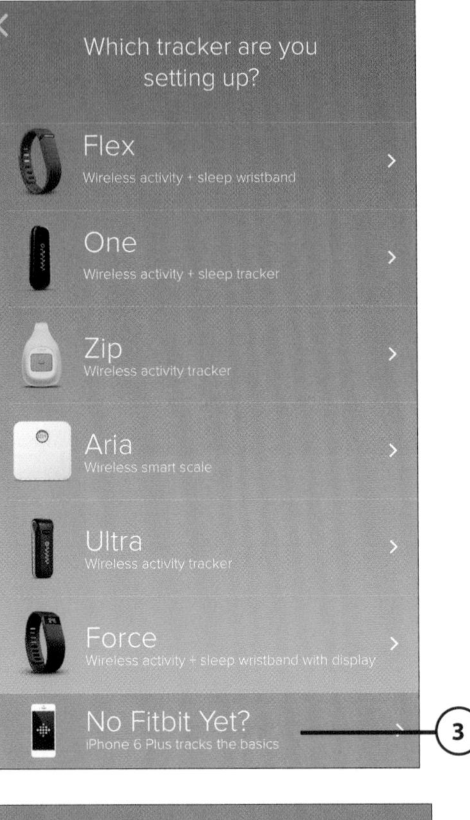

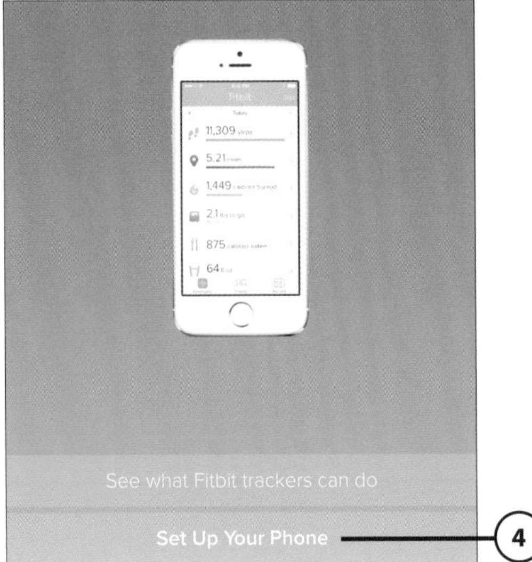

5. Tap Let's Go to fill out some information about yourself. Follow the prompts on the proceeding screens, and then tap Next Step at the bottom of each page. The Main screen appears when you are finished.

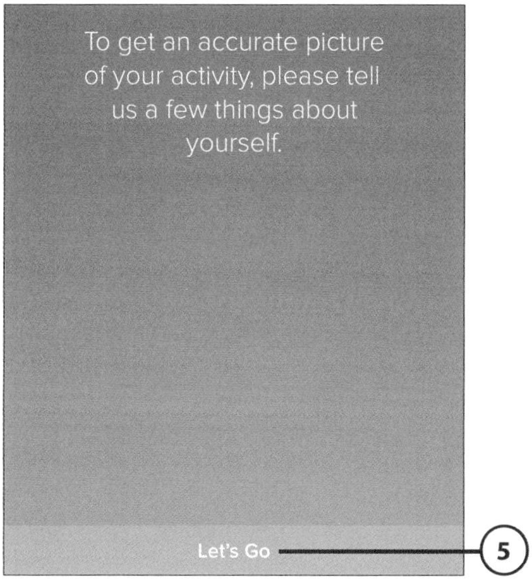

Tracking Activities

After you have set up a MobileTrack account, tracking basic activities such as steps on your iPhone is easy.

1. In the Fitbit dashboard, tap the plus icon in the top-right corner of the screen.

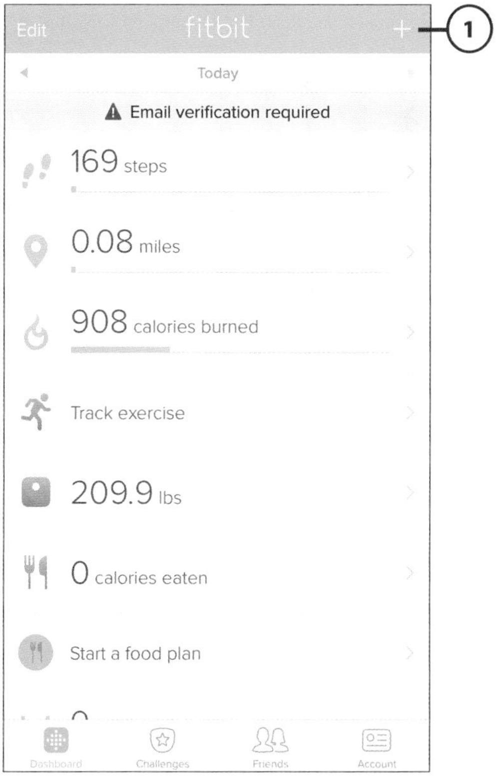

2. Tap Track Exercise.
3. Tap Allow to allow Fitbit to access your location while using the app.
4. Tap in the top field to switch to the activity you want. Walking was chosen for this example.
5. Tap Start to begin the activity.

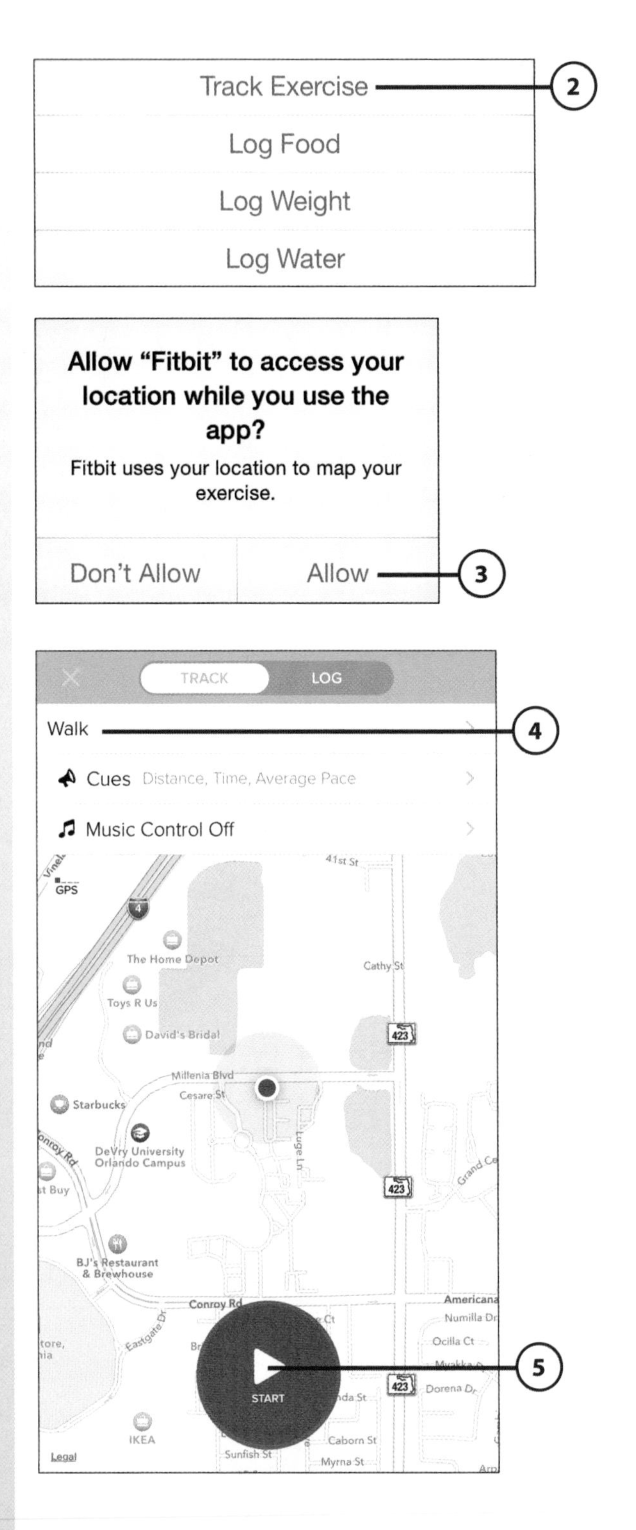

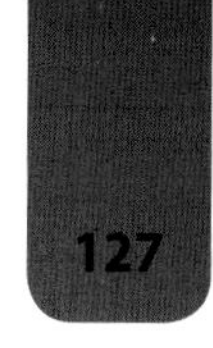

6. Tap the Pause button.
7. Tap and hold the Finish button to view an activity summary that shows your steps along with other data from the activity.
8. Tap Steps. Your steps are broken down into days and weeks. You can view your steps for the day on the graph. The default daily goal is 10,000 steps.

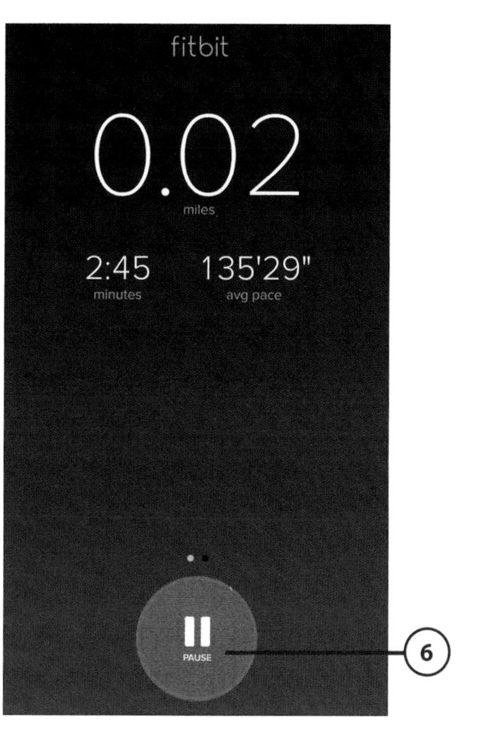

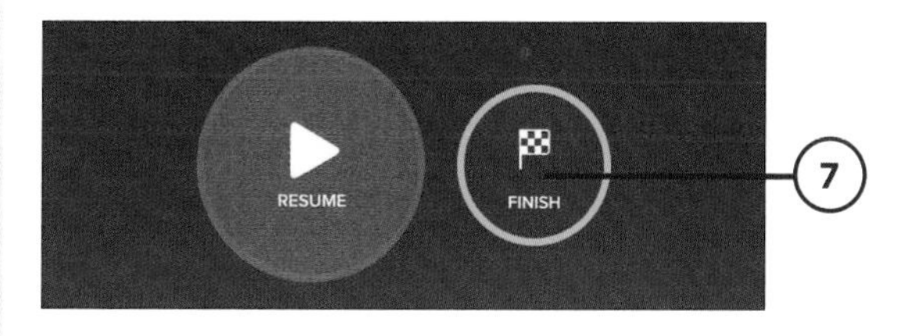

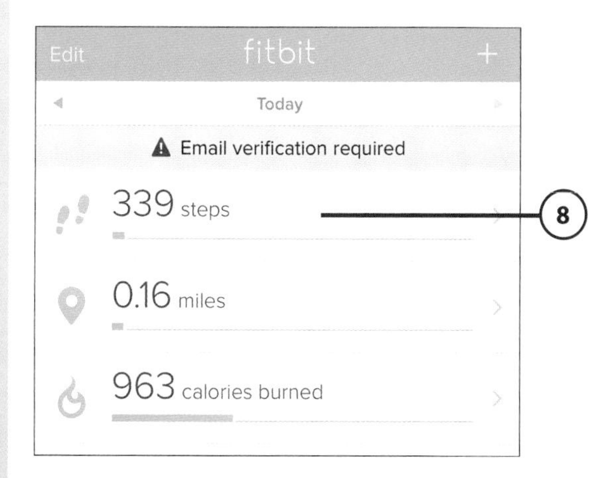

Step Challenges

After you tap Step in the summary, you can tap Challenges at the bottom of the screen to see a page full of step challenges where you can compete with up to 10 people. Challenges range from reaching your own step goal for the day to seeing who takes the most steps in a given amount of time.

It's Not All Good

Smartphone vs. Fitness Tracker Accuracy

As of this writing it is arguable whether the motion sensors in your phone that track your activity, including steps, are as accurate as a dedicated fitness tracker. Keep this in mind when looking for the best resources for your lifestyle. Read about the topic online and perform tests of your own when you go for walks.

>>>Go Further

COUNTING STEPS WITH A TRACKER

Each of the GPS-enabled Fitbit trackers track steps and can share that information with the Fitbit website as well as the app. The Fitbit Charge HR is used in this example. Your "steps taken" are automatically tracked as part of your "all-day stats," so there are no steps to begin tracking. When you sync your Charge HR, your stats are uploaded to your fitbit.com Dashboard. You can also monitor your progress using the Fitbit app. To access your steps on your Fitbit tracker, simply scroll through your stats by pressing the button on the side of the Charge HR. The time is followed by a series of icons. Select the icons that look like two footprints to see how many steps you've taken. The default goal for a day is 10,000 steps. Log in to your Fitbit account online or in the Fitbit app to customize your goal.

Google Fit

Google Fit is a free Android app that is optimized for smartphones, tablets, and web portals. Although it can connect with a wide range of apps and fitness trackers (including Android Wear devices) to gather higher-level tracking data, Google Fit doesn't need additional apps and devices when it comes to the basics. The app can use the sensors already built in to your device to automatically detect activities including running, cycling, and walking. You can set goals and keep track of how often you meet them. If you have a current Android device, this app may already be installed. If it's not, download it from the Google Play Store. Setting up your Fit profile includes providing some basic information about yourself and allowing activity detection. The set-up process walks you through step by step.

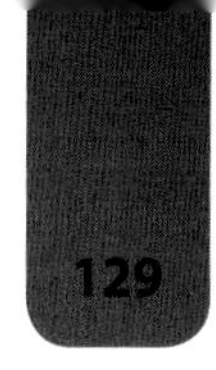

After you set up your profile, follow these steps to track your daily steps with your Android phone.

1. Tap the Fit app on your Android phone. You might need to open the Apps menu to access the app. The main screen opens showing your progress toward your activity goals.
2. Tap inside the circle to cycle through the various activities until you reach "( ) steps today."
3. Tap the Menu button, which looks like three vertical dots in the upper-right corner.
4. Tap Settings.

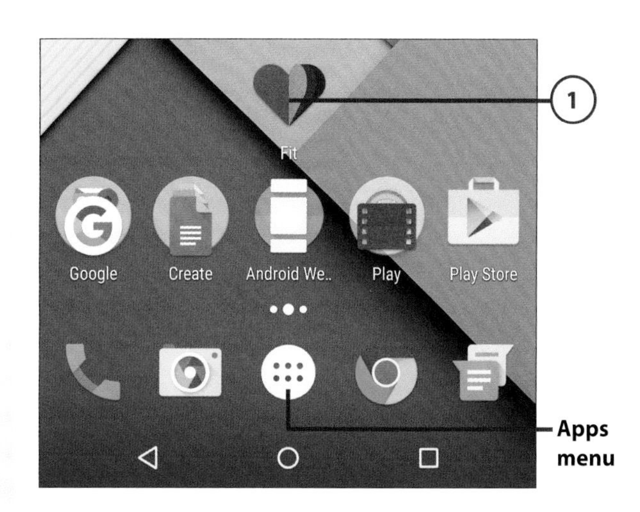

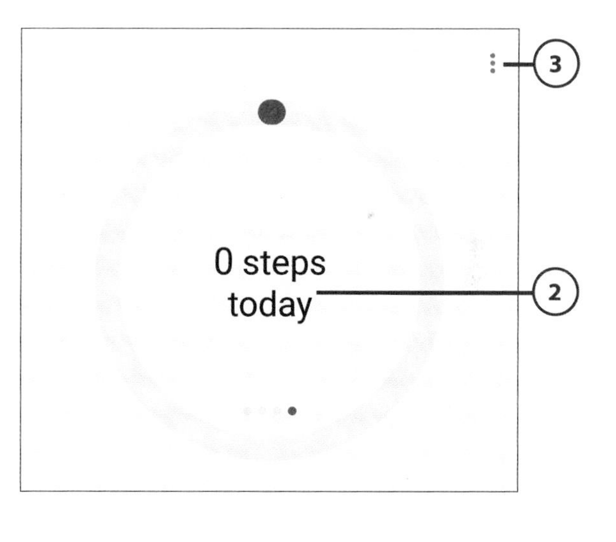

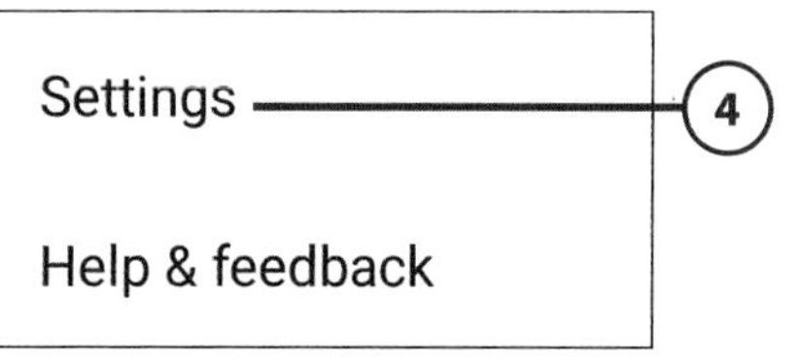

5. Tap the default Active time under Daily goal.
6. Tap Goal Type, and then choose Steps.
7. Enter the number of steps you want as your daily goal, and then tap Save. You are now ready to track your steps and progress to your goal. Go back to the main screen to view your steps.

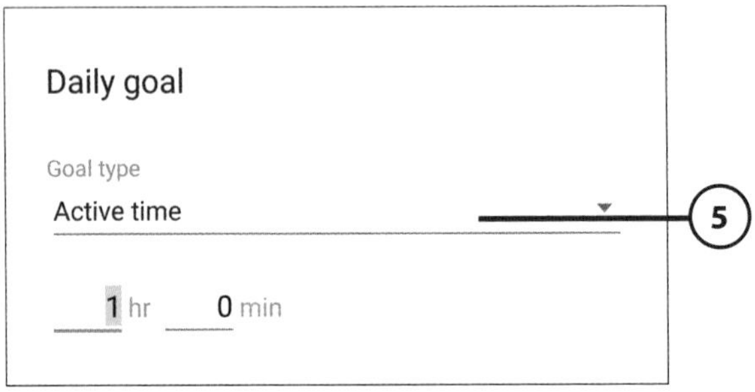

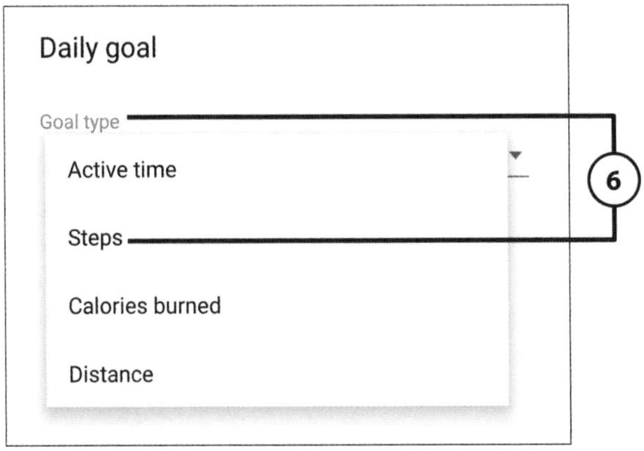

Daily goal

Goal type

Active time

1 hr 0 min

5

Daily goal

Goal type

Active time

Steps

Calories burned

Distance

6

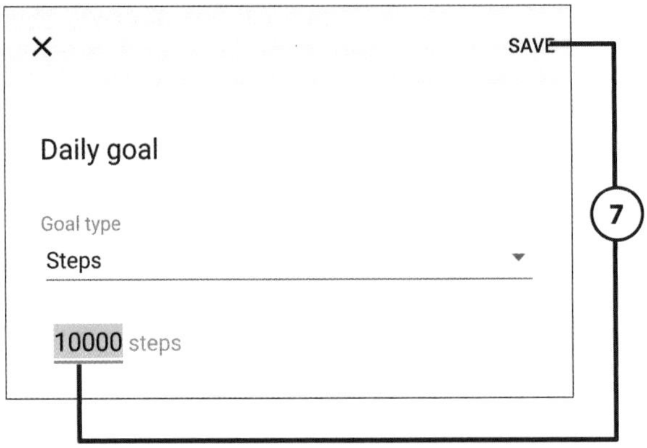

SAVE

Daily goal

Goal type

Steps

10000 steps

7

>>>Go Further

MORE STEP TRACKING CAPABILITIES

Most Android Wear watches come with Google Fit preinstalled. If you have an Android Wear watch, check to see whether you have Google Fit by flicking the screen from right to left and looking for Fit in your apps list. You can use Google Fit solely on your watch without installing it on your mobile device. You will receive Fit cards on your watch with summaries of your activities. You can dismiss a card by dragging it from left to right. Fit cards appear again later in the day or the next day.

Some watch faces display your steps with the time. Tap the steps count to edit your goal from your watch. You can also use your voice to see your steps. If your watch is asleep, tap it to wake it up. Say "OK Google," and then wait for the chimes and say, "Show me my steps." You can access steps taken through the Fit app or on your watch. These numbers can differ.

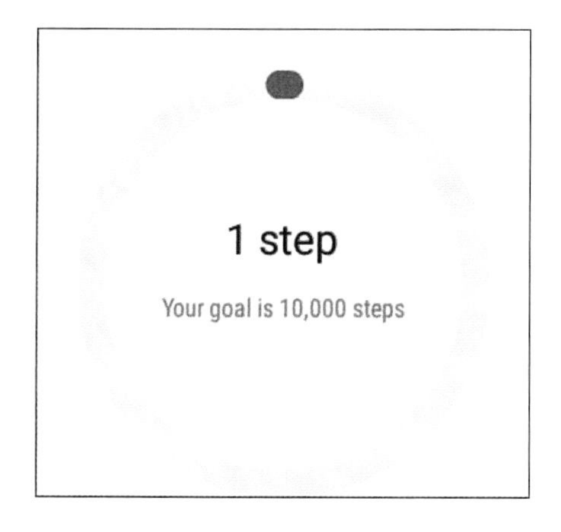

Ask Google to "Show me my steps" to access your step tracker on your watch.

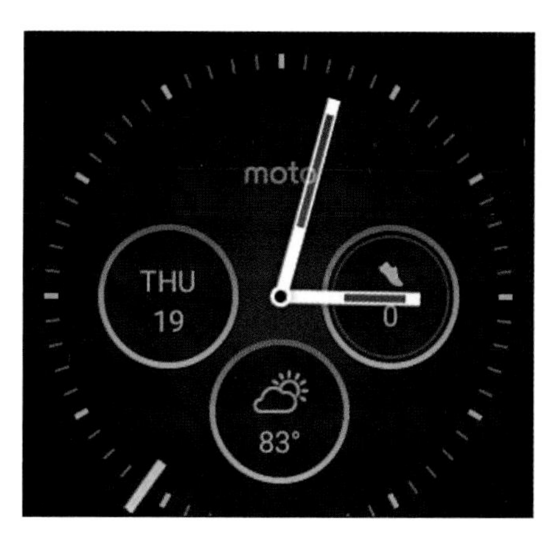

Android Wear watch face with steps counter.

S Health

S (Samsung) Health is a personal trainer and lifestyle companion that enables you to track your fitness endeavors, including your weight, diet, and even sleep. If you have a Samsung phone running Android OS 4.4 or higher, it might be preinstalled on your phone. S Health is free and works with non-Samsung,

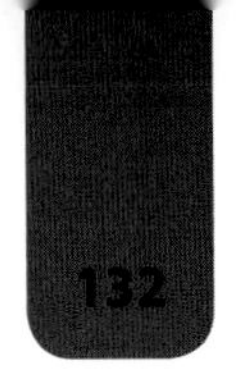

Android phones as well, so you can go to the Google Play Store and download the app. As of this writing, there is no version for Apple (iOS) devices. The app makes it easy for you to track activities including running, hiking, biking, and various exercises by using your phone's built-in trackers. You can track your steps using the Pedometer function that uses your phone's motion sensors.

After you set up your S Health profile, follow these steps to track your daily steps. These steps are shown on an Android phone.

1. Tap the S Health app on your phone. The main screen opens.

2. Tap Steps.

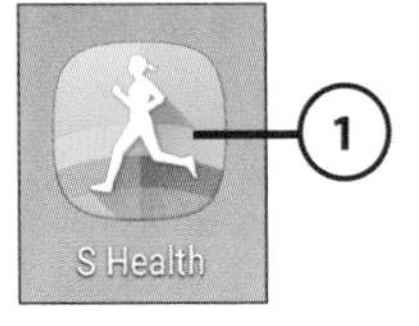

3. Tap More.
4. Tap Set target.
5. Drag the slider to set your daily step goal.
6. Tap the previous screen arrow until you return to the main screen. Now you're ready to start walking.

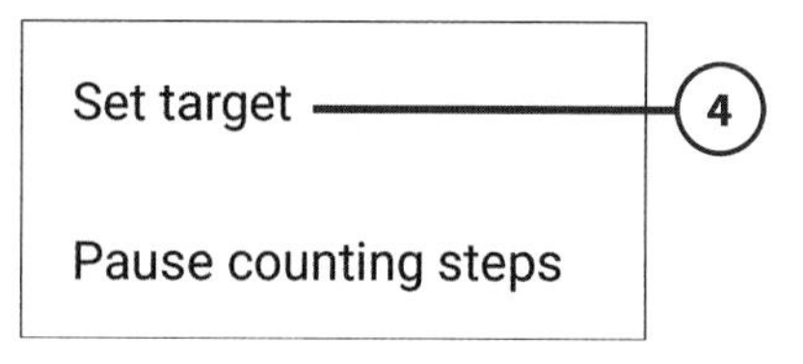

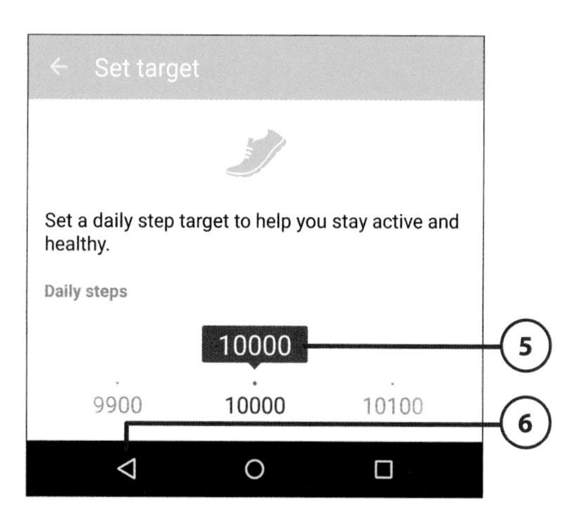

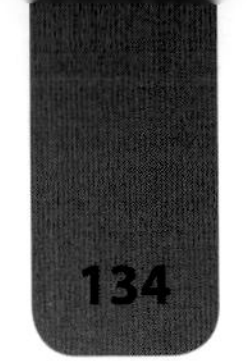

Tracking Flights of Stairs Climbed

Stairs are easily accessible and offer a good cardio workout without a gym membership or expensive workout machines. Some health apps and fitness trackers enable you to count flights of stairs. They are able to do this by using sensors either in your phone or in a fitness tracker. If you want to track flights/floors climbed, look for a fitness tracker that uses altimeter or barometer sensors to sense elevation. Flight climbing capability is nowhere near as common as step tracking, so you'll have to search—mostly mid- to higher-end devices. Fitbit offers many trackers with this ability, as does Garmin. This section offers just a few of the options available for you to start your research. Know that many fitness trackers with these types of sensors will not track flights climbed on stationary workout equipment, such as the Stairmaster, because your body does not change in elevation. While shopping, keep in mind that not all devices with the ability to detect elevation extrapolate that data into flights climbed. Some are made with strictly hiking and biking in mind, so do your due diligence.

Before you get started looking for a fitness tracker for your wrist, you might already possess a device that can track floors climbed: an iPhone.

Apple Health App

The barometer in the iPhone 6, 6 Plus, and 6S allows you to track flights climbed without a fitness tracker. You can show this information on the Dashboard in the Apple Health app, just like tracking steps.

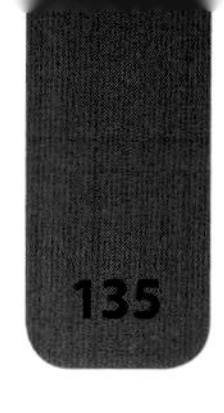

1. Open the Health app, and tap Health Data.
2. Tap Fitness.
3. Tap Flights Climbed.

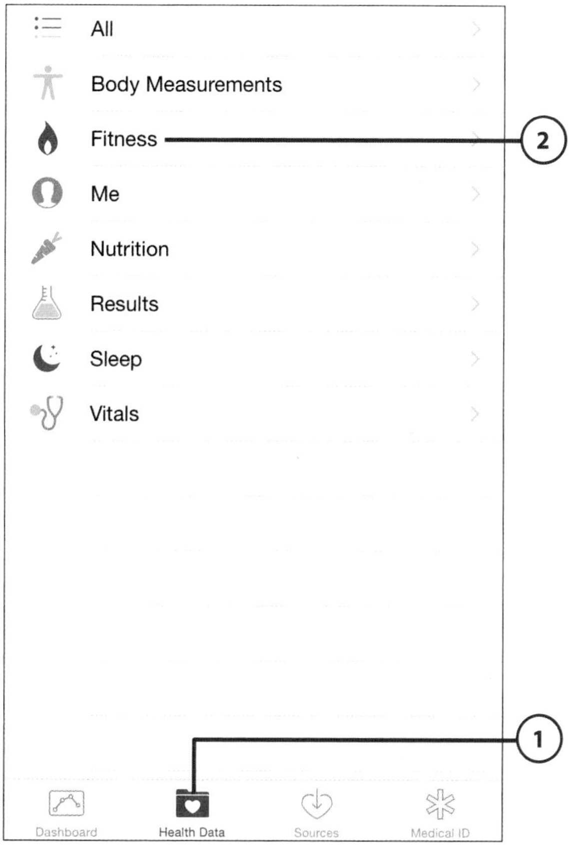

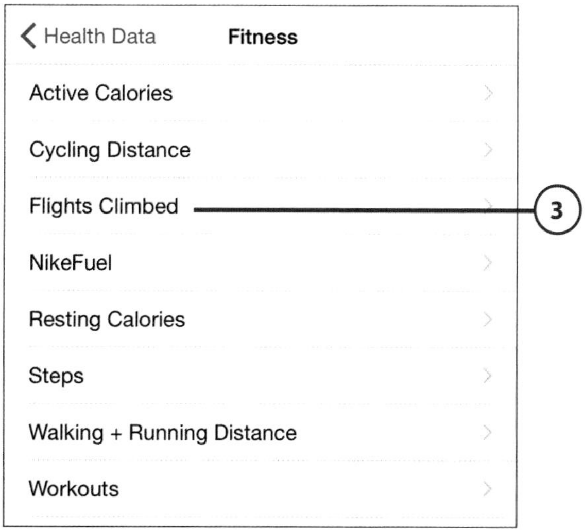

4. Tap Show on Dashboard to the On position. Green should be showing.
5. Tap Dashboard to view your Flights Climbed data on the main screen, and then start climbing flights of stairs. You do not have to be in the app for flight tracking information to be captured. The Health app is able to detect which activity you are performing.

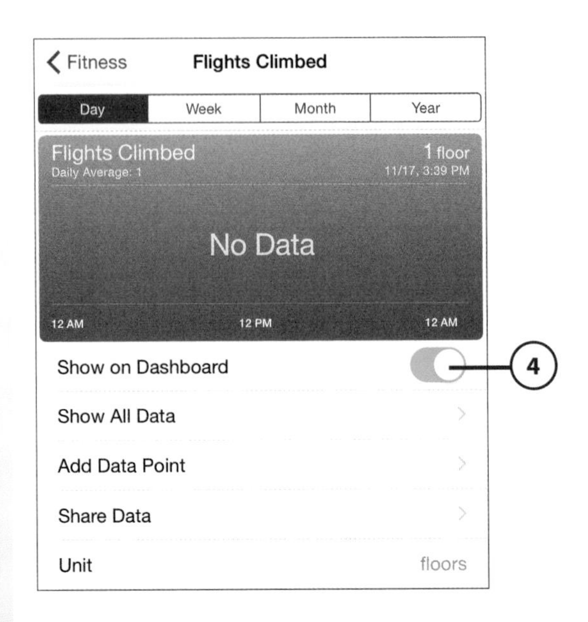

More Tracking Capabilities

As of this writing, the Apple Watch does not track flights climbed.

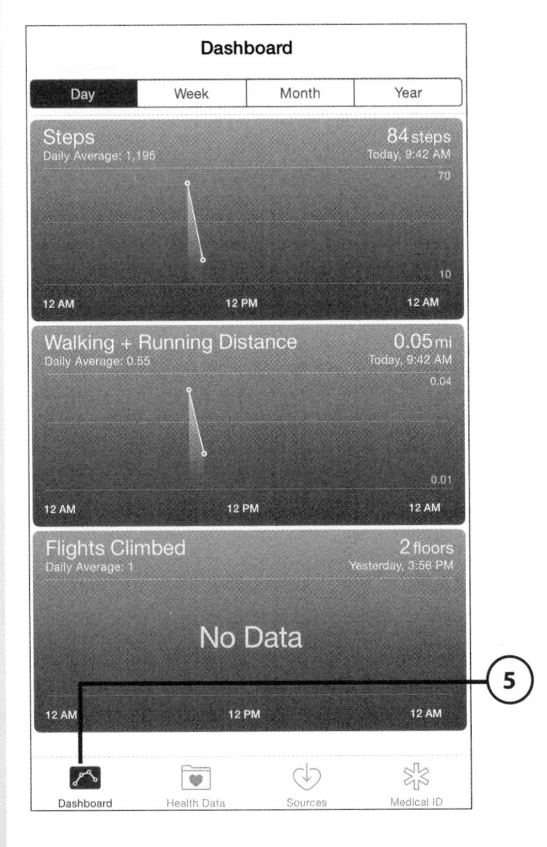

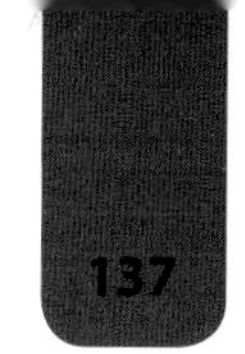

Garmin vívosmart HR

The vívosmart HR is a highly capable fitness tracker. Its tracking capabilities include measuring steps, distance, calories, and floors climbed (using a built-in barometric altimeter). This tracker can also measure activity intensity and let you monitor your progress against activity goals you set. The vívosmart HR syncs with your smartphone using the free Garmin Connect app, and your computer via USB, so you can share your progress and join fitness challenges. This tracker uses a touchscreen so you can use some of the same gestures to navigate as a smartphone.

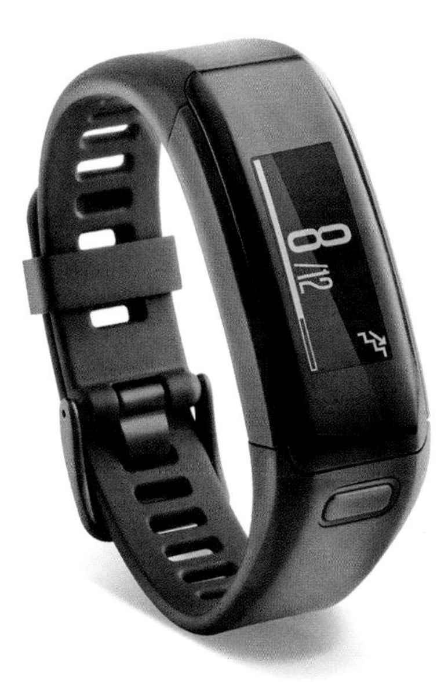

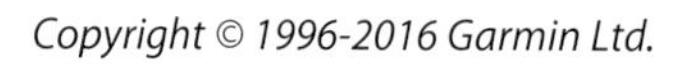

The Garmin vívosmart HR has a touchscreen and a broad range of fitness tracking capabilities.

The icons for the different Garmin vívosmart HR features appear at the top of the screen. You can swipe left or right to scroll through the various features, including floors climbed. The Garmin Connect app is available for Android phones and the iPhone. Garmin Connect allows you to enter a daily goal for floors to climb and view your progress.

>>>Go Further

SMART FEATURES

If you would prefer your activity tracker to have some smartphone features, the Garmin vívosmart HR can receive smart notifications, calls, emails, and calendar and social media alerts. The Garmin vívosmart HR also lets you know when you've been sitting too long, and learns your daily activity level to create a custom step goal.

Monitoring Walking and Running Distance

Tracking distances and duration for walking and running are two of the most common features found on fitness trackers and fitness/health apps. These features are easy to find and inexpensive. Some apps even show you the route you walked on a map. The American Heart Association says "Walking for as few as 30 minutes a day provides heart health benefits." You don't need a gym membership, and walking is a great way to get you started on your quest to become fit. If you're an avid runner, training apps and devices can help incrementally increase your distance so you can be ready for that run.

Most of the resources discussed in this section can be used with or without fitness trackers. Take a look at these options to get you started on your search for the right resource for you.

Apple Health App

The Apple Health app can track your walking and running distances with or without a fitness tracker. Just strap on a sports armband with your iPhone, and then go. The Health app uses your iPhone's built-in motion sensors to track your walk or run.

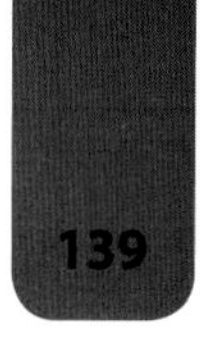

Follow these steps to get started on an iPhone 5s or above.

1. Open the Health app, and tap Health Data.
2. Tap Fitness.
3. Tap Walking + Running Distance.

All
Body Measurements
Fitness
Me
Nutrition
Results
Sleep
Vitals
Dashboard
Health Data
Sources
Medical ID

Health Data
Fitness
Active Calories
Cycling Distance
Flights Climbed
NikeFuel
Resting Calories
Steps
Walking + Running Distance
Workouts

4. Tap Show on Dashboard to the On position. Green should be showing.
5. Tap Dashboard to view your Walking + Running data on the main screen, and then start running or walking. You do not have to be in the app for this information to be captured. The Health app is able to detect which activity you are performing.

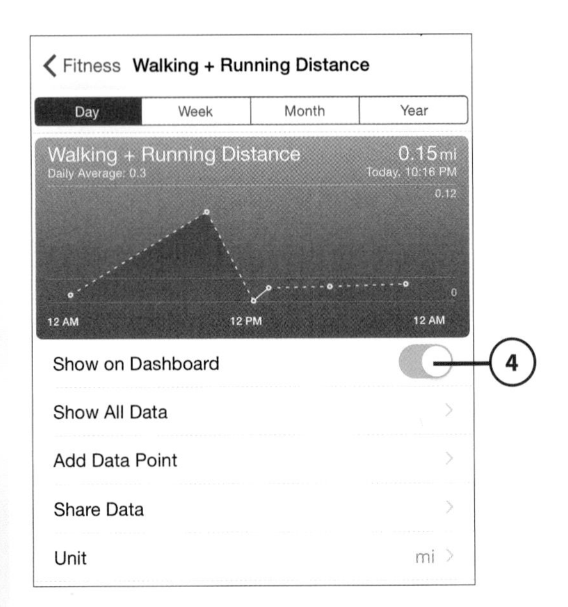

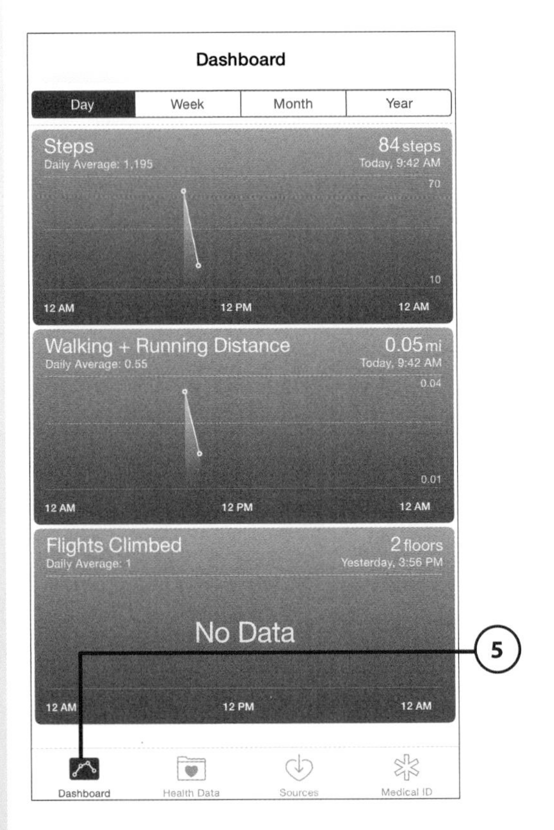

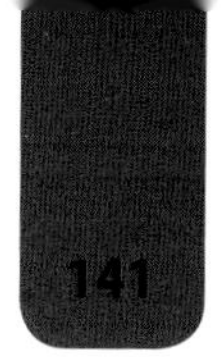

>>>Go Further

USING APPLE WATCH TO TRACK WALKING AND RUNNING ACTIVITIES

The Workout app on the Apple Watch allows you to track your walking and running activities on your watch. Just push in the crown on the side of the watch to access the green app icon with the running man. All data collected is automatically synced to the Health app.

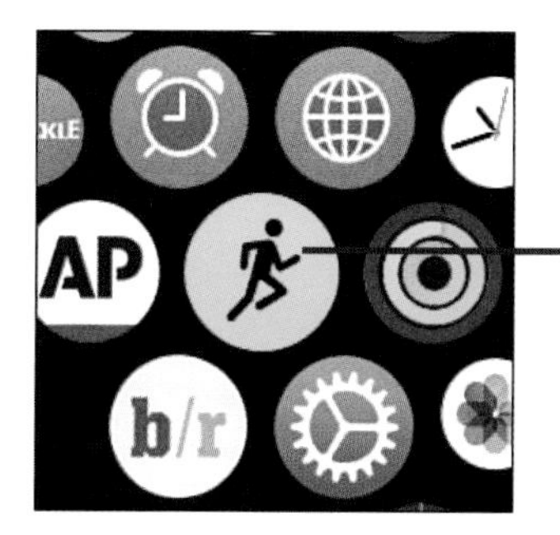

The workout app on your Apple Watch allows you to track walking and running.

Fitbit

The Exercise mode on most Fitbit trackers lets you collect detailed information on your workout, much how like a car's odometer works. Put your tracker in Exercise mode and go for a run. When you complete your run, sync your tracker to your phone or computer and view the new Workout entry that has been added to the Fitbit app Dashboard. The entry provides a summary of your exercise, including distance covered.

Track Your Walk or Run Without a Fitbit Tracker

You can track your walk or run on your iPhone using the Fitbit app. The MobileTrack function enables you to use your iPhone 5s, 6, 6 Plus, and 6s motion sensors to track multiple exercises. Refer to the "Fitbit" section under "Tracking Steps," earlier in this chapter.

>>>Go Further

TRACK YOUR WALK OR RUN USING THE FITBIT CHARGE/CHARGE HR

Press and hold the button on the side of the tracker until a stopwatch icon appears. You'll feel a vibration, and then the timer starts counting. Start walking or running. Press the button to advance through the stats that appear in the following order: Elapsed time, Current heart rate and heart rate zone, Calories burned, Steps taken, Distance covered, Floors climbed, and Time of day. Press and hold the button to end Exercise mode when you are finished. Sync your tracker to your mobile app or computer to view the stats in your activity history.

>>>Go Further

TRACK A RUN AND OTHER EXERCISES ON THE FITBIT SURGE

The Fitbit Surge enables you to track multiple exercises and lets you see your stats on your wrist. You can see more detailed information on your Dashboard when you sync to your smartphone or computer. As of this writing, the Fitbit Surge is the highest end tracker in the Fitbit lineup and is a little pricier than its siblings.

Google Fit

Google Fit makes it easy for you to track your walking and running distance, and more, with or without an Android Wear device. If you have an Android Wear watch with Google Fit preinstalled, you can track your walk or run strictly on your wrist. You get the most from Google Fit when the app is installed on your mobile device, including advanced graphs, maps, and fitness data like calories burned.

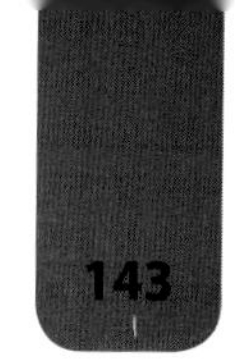

Follow these steps to track your walk or run just using your smartphone with Google Fit.

1. Open the Fit app, and then tap the plus button.
2. Tap Start activity.

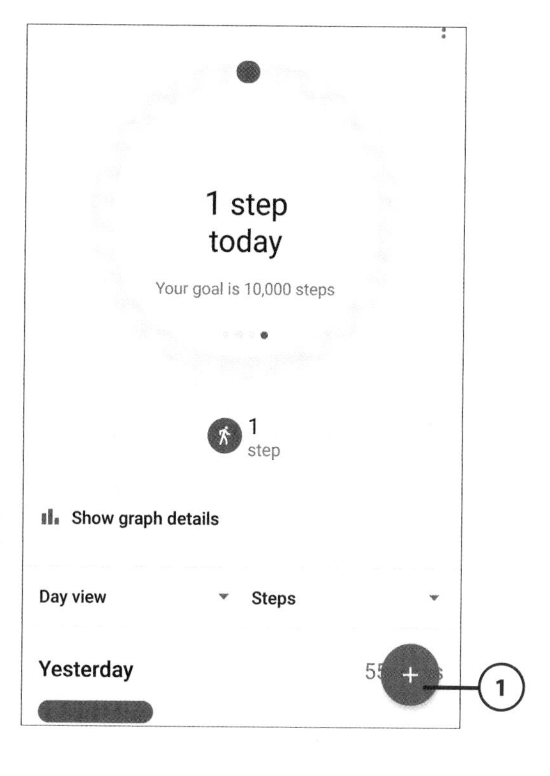

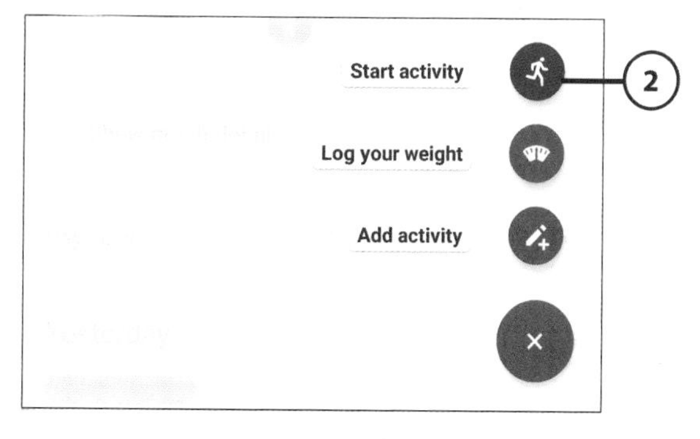

3. Tap Walking or Running. Walking was chosen for this example.
4. Tap Start to begin your walk and view your route on a Google map. You can then tap Pause, and tap Stop to see a summary of your workout.

What activity?

Favorites

Walking — 3

Running

Biking

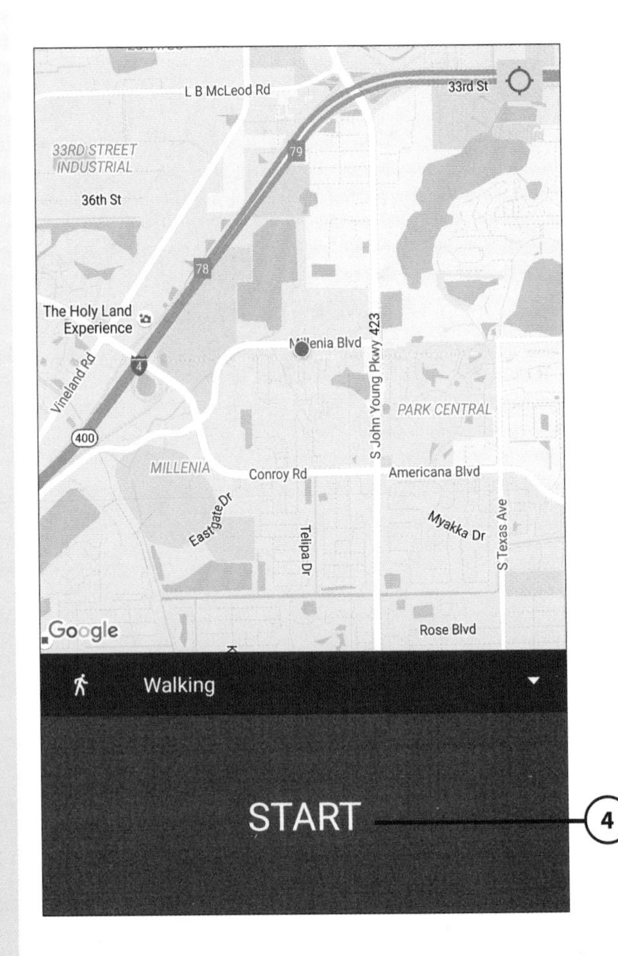

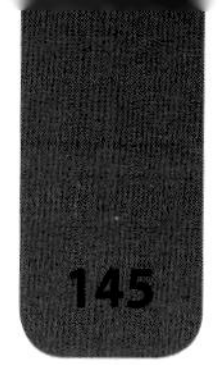

>>>Go Further

USING OTHER RUNNING APPS WITH GOOGLE FIT

Google Fit helps bring all of your health data from compatible health apps into one convenient place. Go to the Google Play Store and perform a search for the term "Google Fit Connected apps" to find apps like MapMyFitness, MyTracks, Nike+ Running, Runtastic, Strava, and much more. You can also shop for compatible apps using the Android Wear app on your phone.

S Health

S Health makes it easy for you to track your daily activities. Whether you are an avid runner, walker, or beginner to both, S Health trackers can help you set milestones and even motivate you using a voice guide. Want to work up to a 5k run? S Health helps you to get there in a regimented, carefully crafted program to help you achieve that goal. S Health is currently available for Android devices, but not for Apple (iOS) devices.

S Health and Android Wear Watches

As of this writing, S Health is not available for Android Wear watches or the Apple Watch, but you can take advantage of its features on Samsung Gear watches.

Download and install the S Health app. The following steps show the app on an Android phone.

1. Open the S Health app, swipe to scroll down to the bottom of the screen, and then tap Manage Items. Note that the tracker for running appears by default onscreen.
2. Tap Walking to the On position. The toggle switch turns blue. Notice the various trackers that are available.
3. Tap the arrow to return to the previous screen. The Walking tracker appears onscreen. The Running tracker appears onscreen by default.

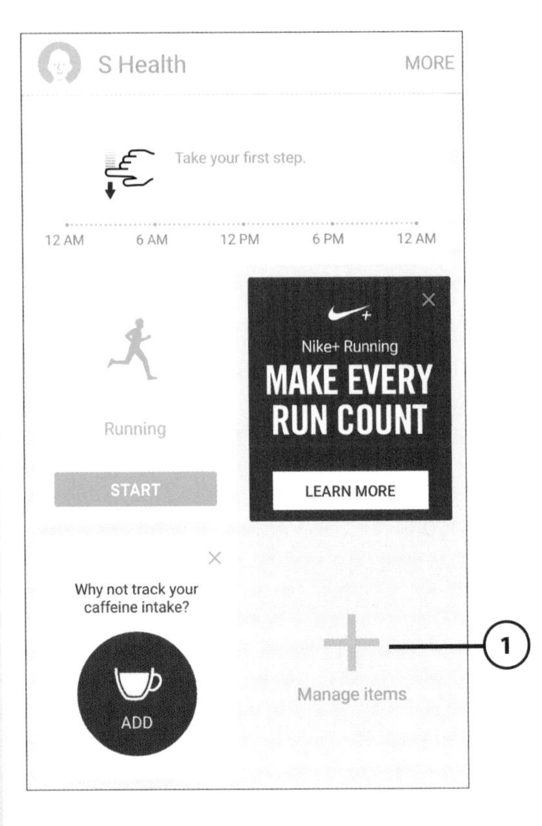

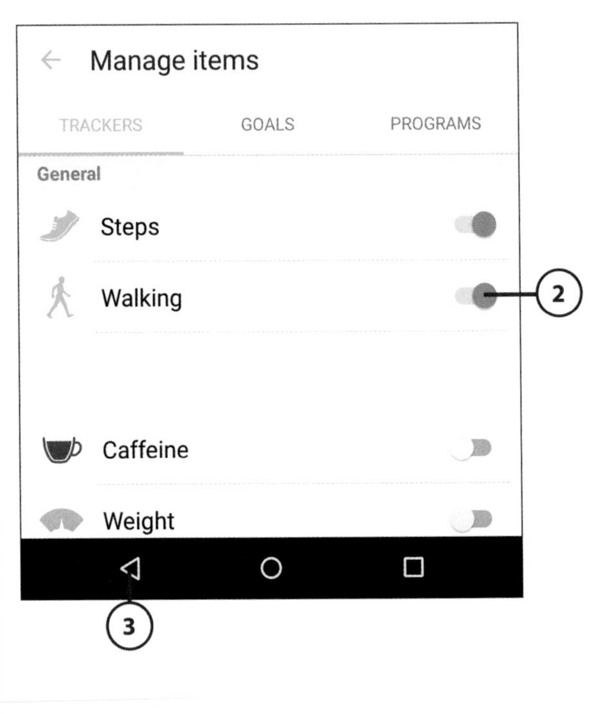

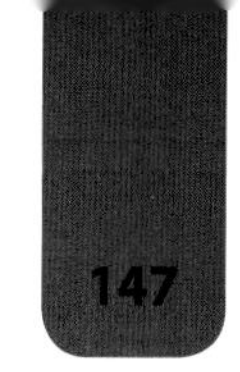

4. Tap Start for the Walking tracker or the Running tracker. The Walking tracker was chosen for this example. S Health pinpoints your location on a Google map.
5. Tap the plus sign to change the distance target.
6. Tap the musical note icon to listen to music while taking your walk.
7. Tap More to hear audio notifications at selected times during your workout, including duration, distance, and other information.
8. Tap Start and begin tracking your walking activity. A countdown starts, and then your activity begins. A Pause button appears, allowing you to pause the exercise. When you are done, you can tap Stop to end the activity and view a summary of your workout.

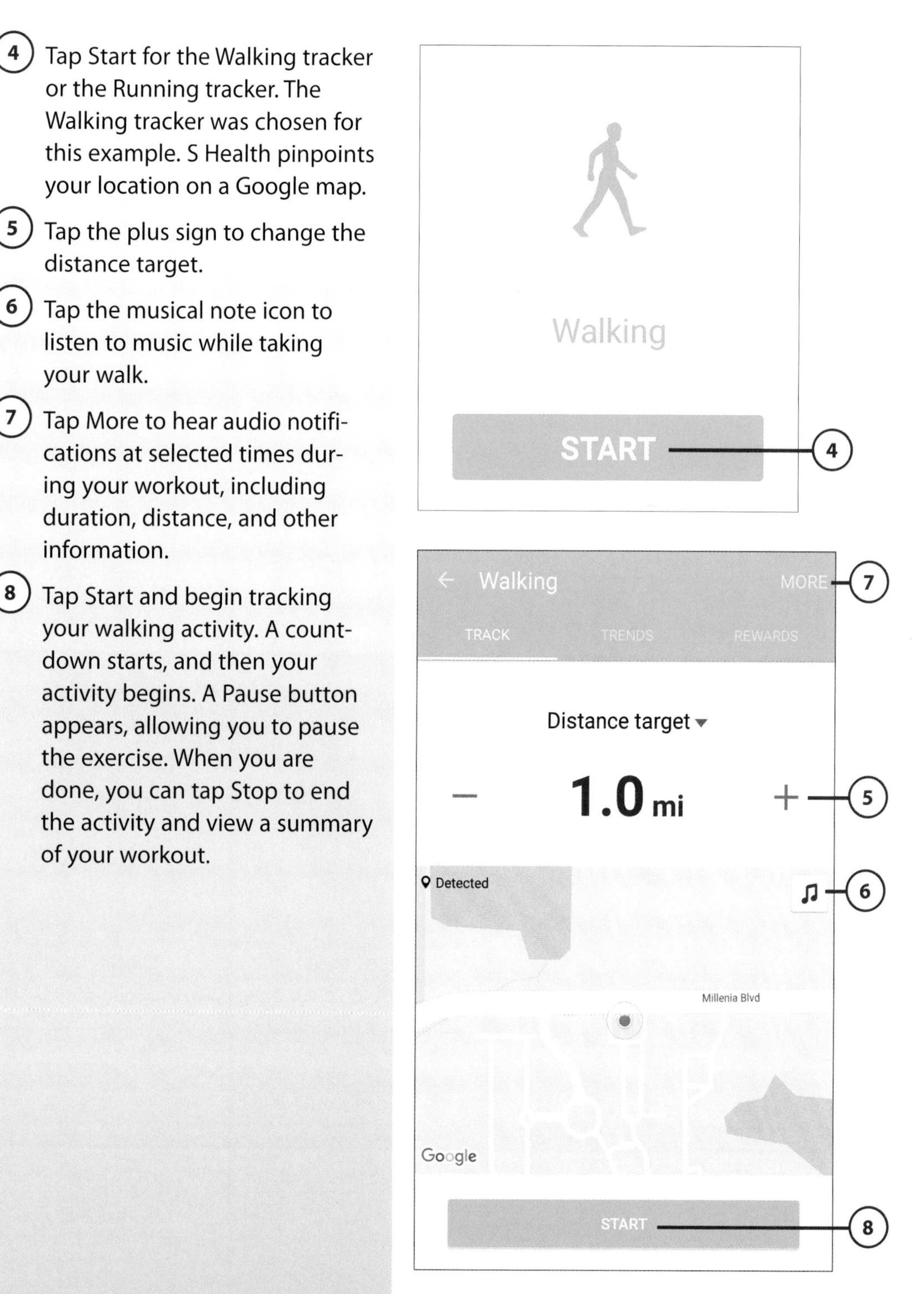

>>>Go Further

TRACK FROM YOUR WRIST

If you don't want to take your phone with you on a walk or run, you can wear the many capabilities of S Health on your wrist. The Gear S2 uses its own cellular plan that can keep you connected while you set activity goals and track your progress. Tap S Health on the Apps screen and rotate the bezel clockwise to access the exercise tracker screen, and then choose options to select the type of exercise you want to monitor. Also, syncing your Samsung Gear watch with an app that is compatible with S Health adds additional features.

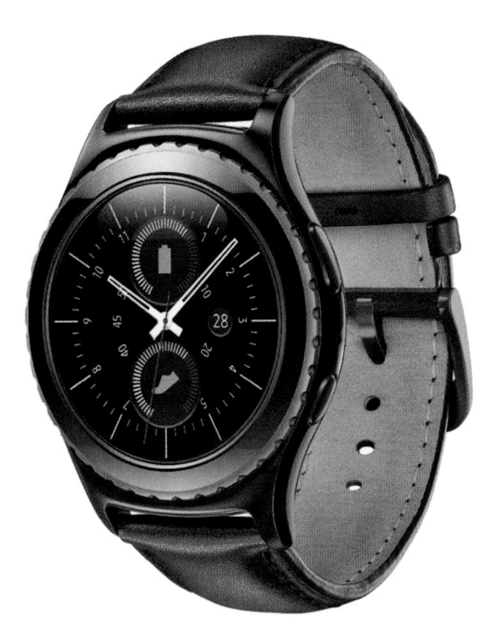

Track your walking activity using the Samsung Gear S2.

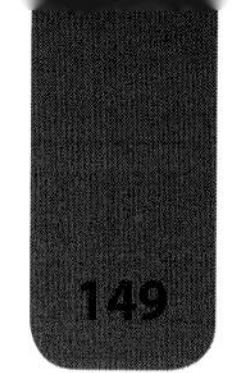

Withings Activité Pop

The Withings Activité Pop is a fitness tracker with the timeless look and style of a refined analog display. If you are looking for a highly capable fitness tracker with the feel of a classic watch, the Withings Activité Pop may be just what you're looking for. It tracks sleeping stages, swimming, and also walking and running distance, speed, and calories burned. The watch uses an analog activity hand that goes from 0% to 100% to monitor progress toward your goal(s). It has an accompanying app named Health Mate that suggests easy changes to encourage you to walk more. If you are walking, swimming, or running, there isn't anything you have to do to start the tracking process. Activité automatically detects surges in activity levels and logs it as running. Set the goals you want to reach in Health Mate and just begin. The Health Mate app is available for Android and Apple (iOS) devices and can also use the sensors in your smartphone to track activities without the tracker. Visit withings.com to learn about Withings products and features.

Download the Health Mate app, join Withings, set up your device, and then follow these steps, which show you how to monitor walking and running activities using the Withings Activité Pop watch and the Health Mate app on an iPhone.

1. Tap the Health Mate app to open it. The default Timeline screen opens.
2. Put on your Withings Activité Pop watch.
3. Go walking. The Withings Activité Pop uses sensors to automatically determine that the activity you are engaged in is walking.

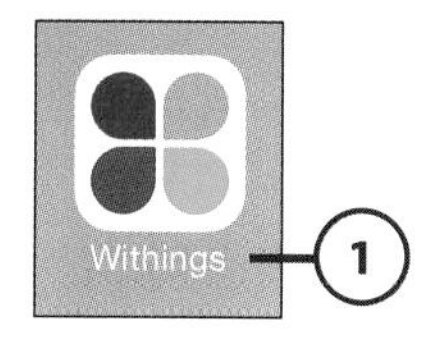

Setting Target Weight and Alarms

Swipe the widget, the top (orange) part of the screen, from right to left to set your target weight. Swipe the widget from left to right two times to set an alarm. The Withings Activité Pop has an embedded gentle alarm vibration to gently wake you.

4. Tap Goal and make sure your Activité Pop is close to your smartphone so that it syncs. Your walking data appears and the activity hand on the watch moves toward completing 100 percent of the default 10,000 steps goal.

Setting a New Step Goal

Tap Goal on the activity screen to set a new step goal.

5. View your walking data in the app.

Storing Your Data

The Withings Activité Pop watch stores your data for 38 hours. Open the Health Mate app regularly to let your data sync so you don't lose any of your data.

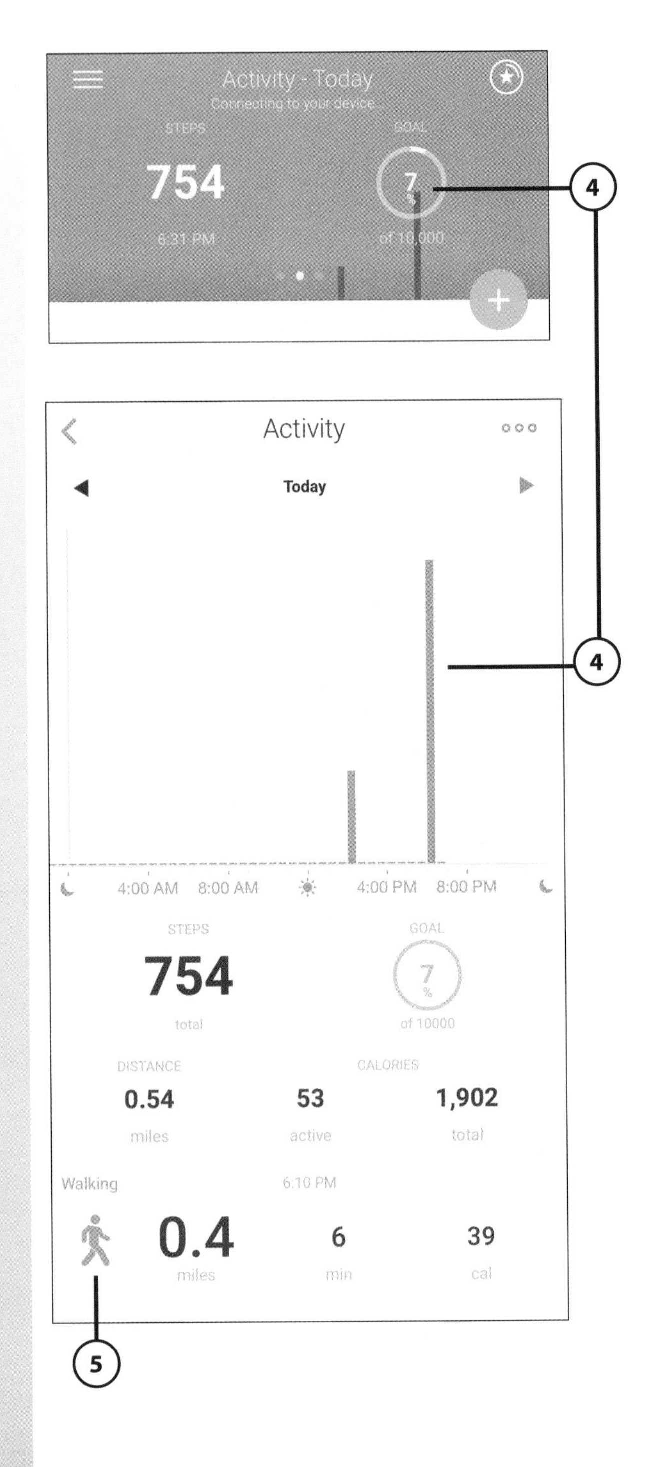

Tracking Biking Activity

It seems like everywhere you go, bike lanes are being created and bike docks are being built. Biking is inexpensive and doesn't require a gym membership; it's a great way to blast calories and drop a pants size. Biking apps, sometimes referred to as cycling apps, and some fitness trackers provide helpful knowledge about your rides. To get the most from your app, you'll need a mobile device with GPS so you can track distance. Apps provide a wealth of information regarding your progress using charts, graphs, and mapped routes. Higher end devices with barometers even allow for information on elevation. Track calories burned, speed traveled, and duration, and even compete with others using an app. What is covered here is just a sampling of some popular apps that are available. Each app offers a variety of bells and whistles. Explore other apps on the Google Play Store and the App Store and search online for the best biking/cycling apps.

Apple Health App

If you have an iPhone, you might already have what you need to track basic cycling data. The Apple Health app can track your cycling distance and calculate your cycling average for the day, week, month, and year.

1. Open the Health app, and then tap Health Data.

2. Tap Fitness.

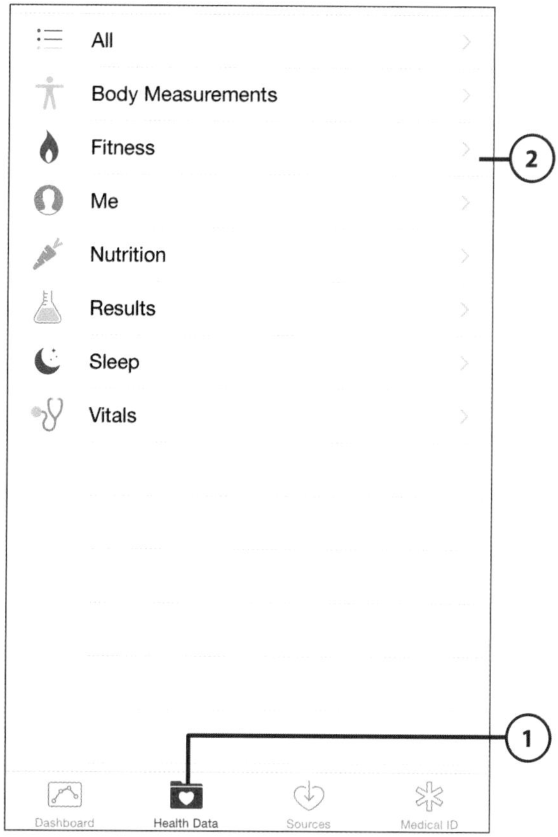

3. Tap Cycling Distance.
4. Tap Show on Dashboard to the On position. The toggle switch should show green.
5. Tap Dashboard to view your Cycling data, and then start cycling. You do not have to be in the app for the data to be captured. The Health app is able to detect which activity you are performing.

Health Data
Fitness
Active Calories
Cycling Distance
3

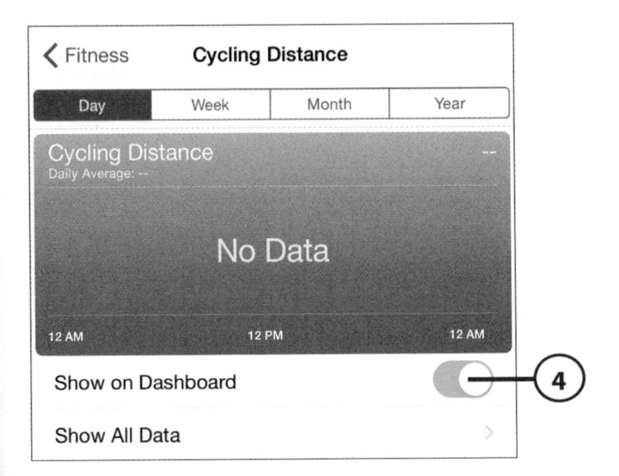

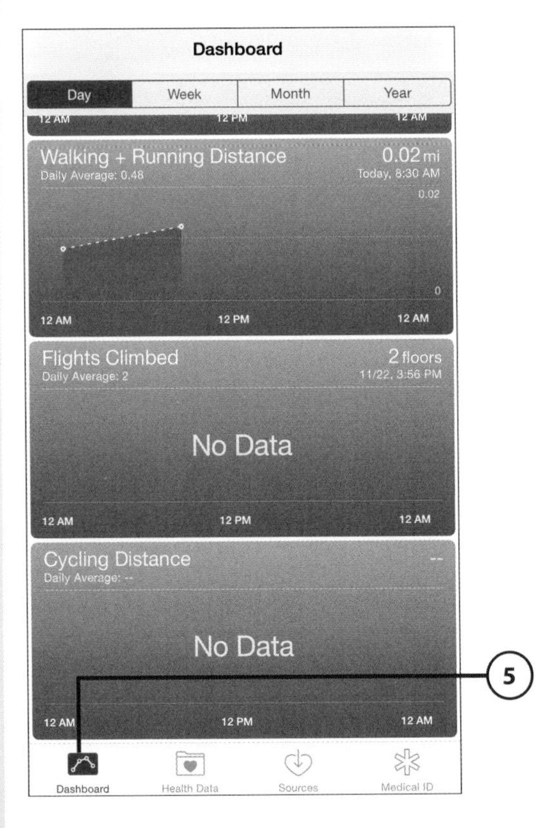

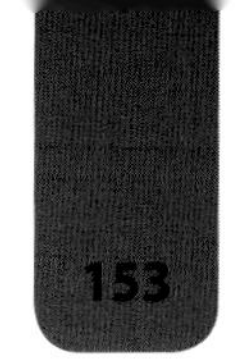

Fitbit

Many of the Fitbit trackers are designed for walking, running, steps, and general household activities. The Fitbit Surge offers GPS bike tracking, which enables you to view summaries including distance, elapsed time, average speed, average heart rate, and calories burned. If you use the Fitbit app, you can see all the stats except elevation. You have to view that stat using your Fitbit account on your computer.

The SmartTrack feature enables the Fitbit Surge to automatically recognize and record your activities such as running or walking, but it does not record GPS data, which is important in biking to calculate distance and other precise stats such as pace. You need to put your Surge into specific exercise modes to get the most precise information. The GPS data will then appear on a map in your Fitbit Dashboard.

>>>Go Further

TRACK YOUR BIKING ACTIVITY USING THE FITBIT SURGE

Press the Home button to access the menu. Swipe to the Exercise screen, and then press the Select button. Swipe to choose the Biking activity, or simply tap the screen. The GPS searching screen appears. Wait for the signal before you begin your ride. Press the Select button to start your ride. Swipe the screen to see the various stats, such as Pace, Heart Rate, Calories, and more. To be safe, you shouldn't check stats while riding. Press the Select button to pause or resume your ride. Press the Action button while paused to exit the exercise and see a summary of your workout.

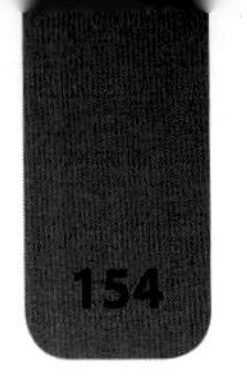

Google Fit

The Google Fit app uses your phone's motion sensors and GPS to track biking distance, duration, and calories burned. You can also view your biking route on a Google map and view elevation data in real time. For the most accurate data collection, put your phone in a sport armband or in a pocket rather than in a backpack or mounted on your bike.

1. Open the Fit app; on the main screen, tap the plus button.
2. Tap Start activity. A list of activities appears.

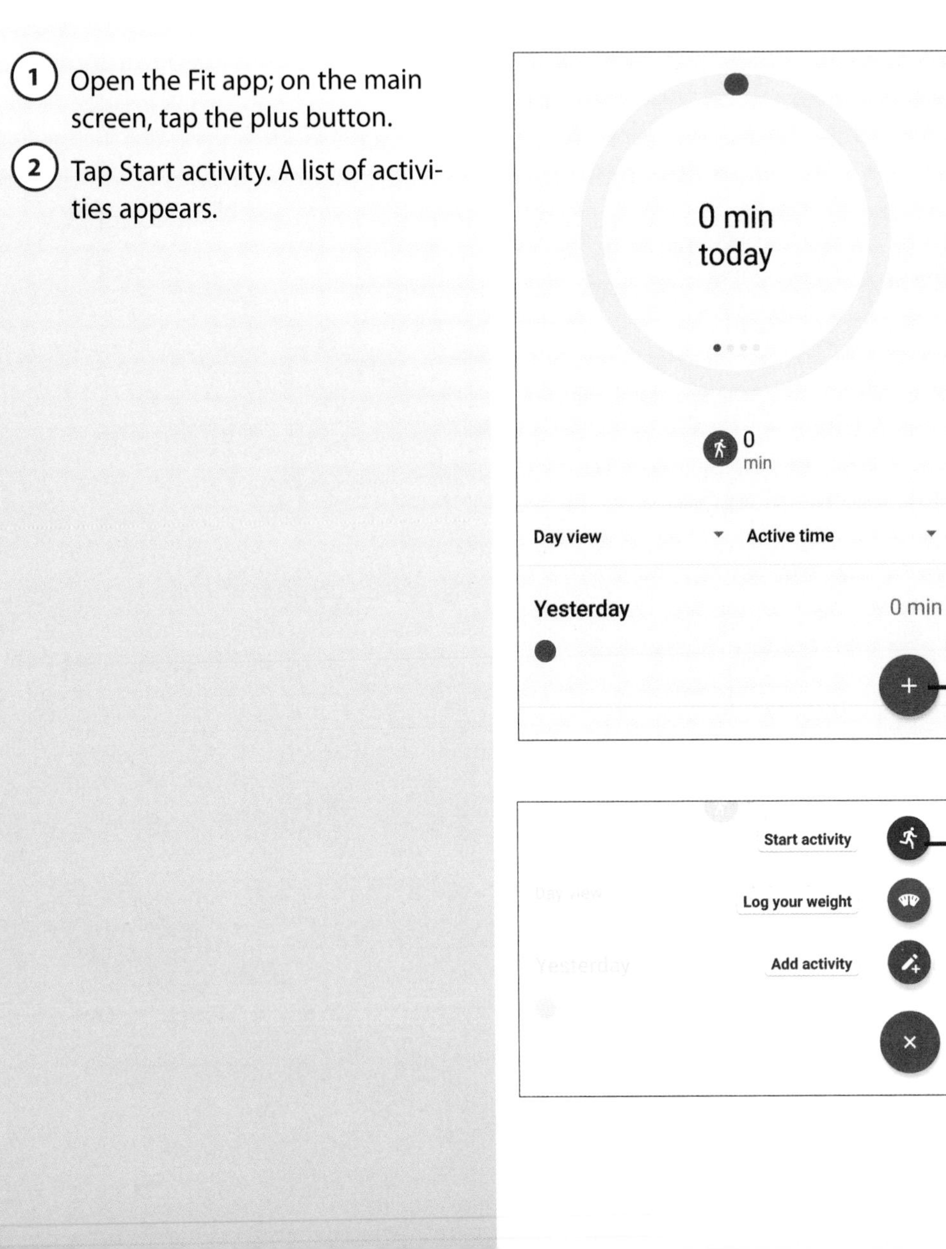

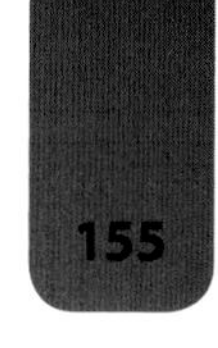

3. Tap Biking.
4. Tap Start to begin biking and view your route on a Google map. A countdown begins and a voice says "Session started."
5. Tap Pause to pause the session.

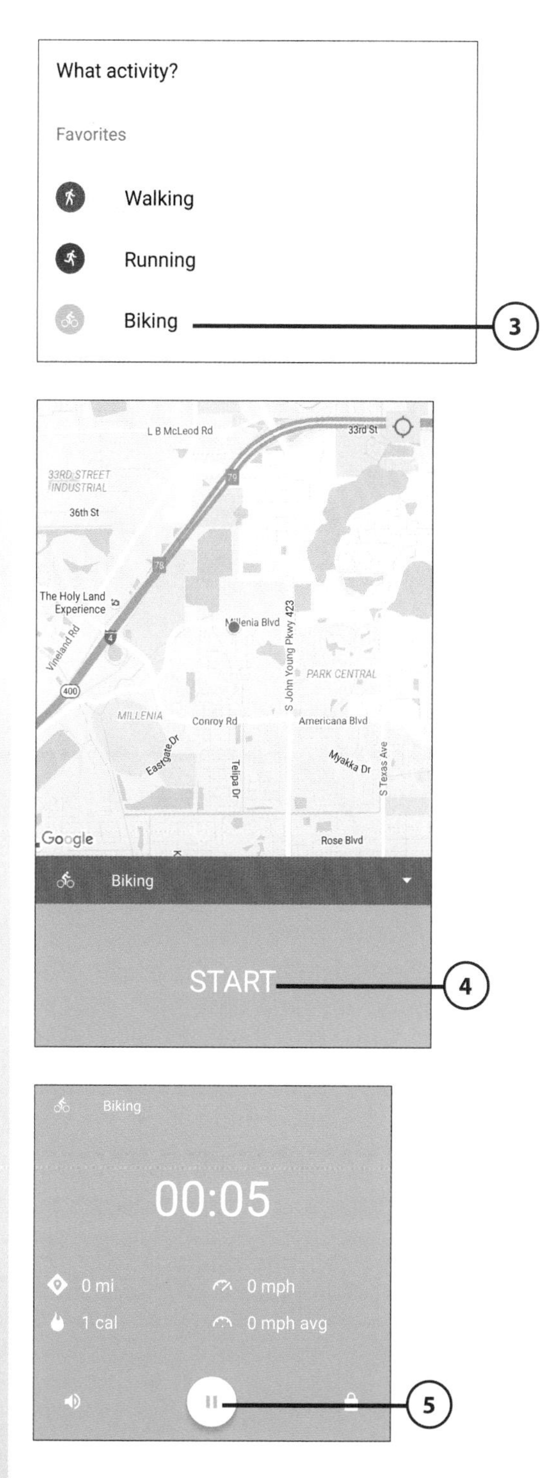

6. Tap the Stop button to stop the activity and view a summary of your workout data.

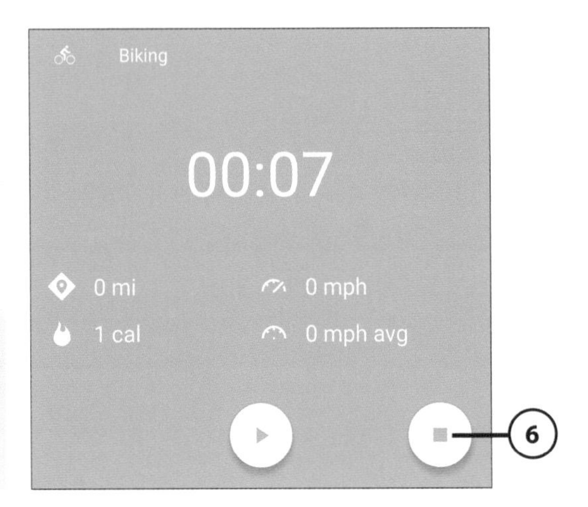

S Health

The S Health app lets you set distance targets for cycling, enables you to monitor trends with graphs, and lets you record and select previous routes. To keep you motivated, S Health also offers audio coaching messages when you select routes and other targets. You can receive audio notifications at intervals during your ride about the duration, distance, and other information. You can even specify the intervals for notifications. For example, the default notification interval is 1 mile, but you can change it to half a mile, 5 miles, 5 minutes, or other options.

1. Open the S Health app, and on the main screen scroll down and tap Manage Items. A list of trackers appears.

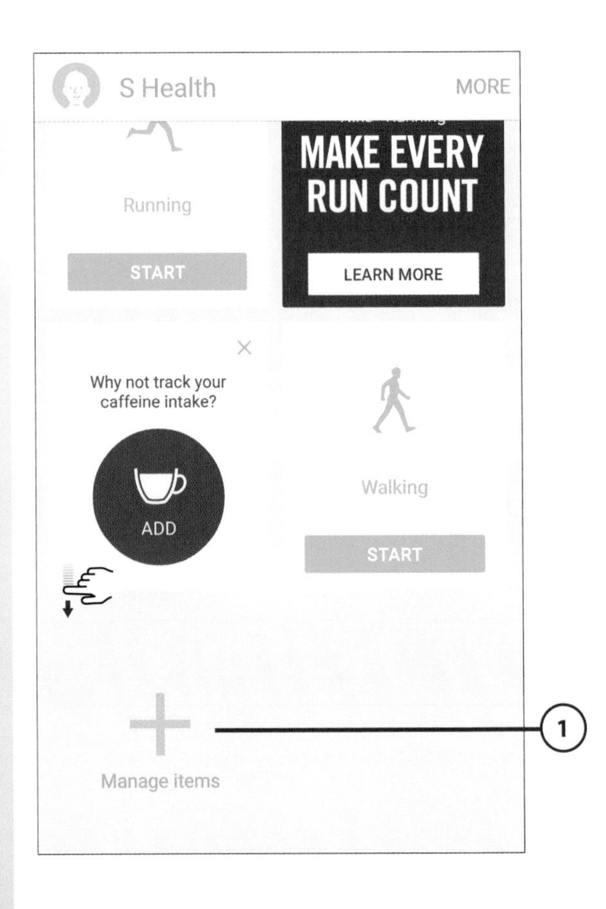

2. Tap Cycling to the On position. The toggle switch turns from gray to blue.
3. Tap the arrow to return to the previous screen. The Cycling Tracker appears.
4. Tap Start for the Cycling tracker. S Health pinpoints your location on a Google map.

Manage items

TRACKERS GOALS PROGRAMS

General

Steps

Walking

Running

Cycling

Hiking

Sports

Food

Water

Caffeine

Weight

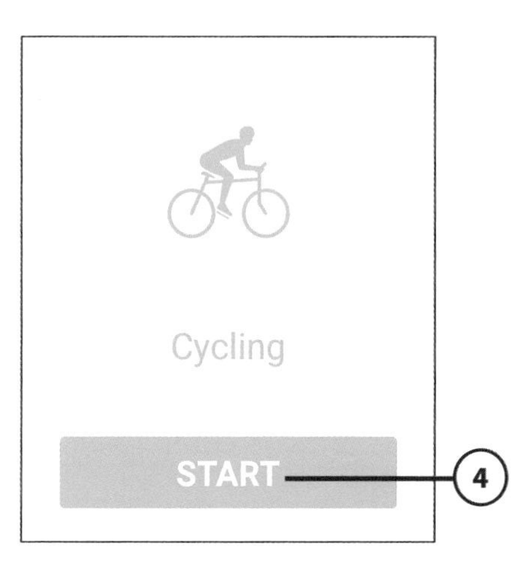

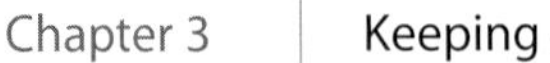

5. Tap the plus sign to change the distance target.
6. Tap the musical note to listen to music while cycling.
7. Tap More to hear audio notifications at selected times during your workout including duration, distance, and other information.
8. Tap Start and begin tracking your cycling activity. A countdown starts, and then your activity begins. A Pause button appears, allowing you to pause the exercise, and then you can tap Stop to end the activity and view a summary of your workout.

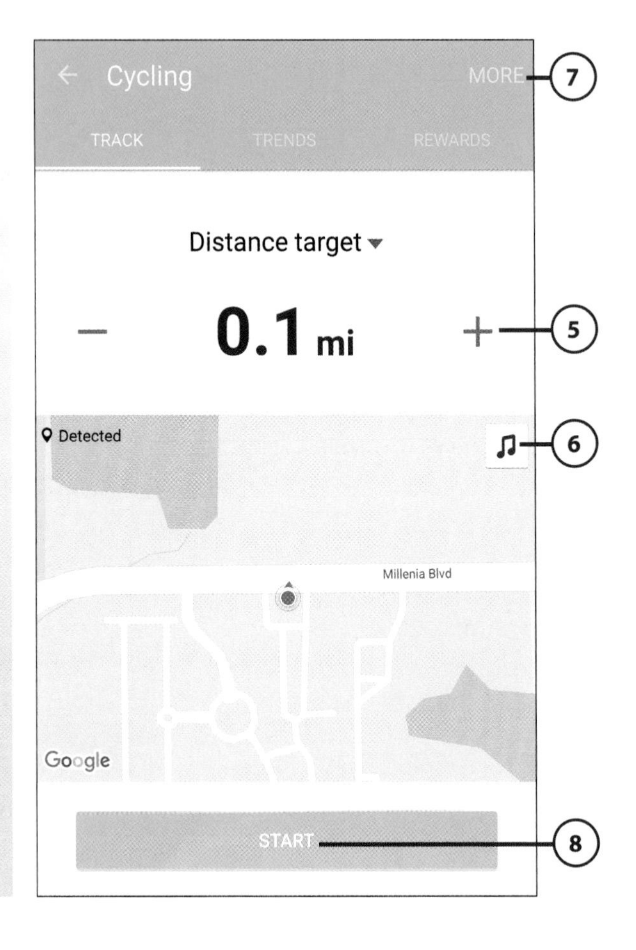

Creating a Fitness Plan

With all the fitness programs to choose from, ranging from Pilates, strength training, aerobics, and more, finding what's right for you can be overwhelming. Apps like FitStar, Fitnet, and many more create personalized workout plans, and all you need to do is provide some personal information, including your goals. We'll talk about some of those apps in a moment, but you need to consider some things as you are creating your fitness plan:

- **Do you have any health conditions?** Consult your doctor before beginning any fitness program, especially if you have a chronic disease including diabetes or a heart condition. Even if you don't have any conditions that you know of, consider having a physical. If you haven't exercised in a long time, sometimes an increase in physical activity can reveal an underlying condition that you didn't know about.

- **Be as honest as possible when assessing your current fitness level.** This helps in creating realistic goals that you can actually accomplish.
- **Have goals and make them realistic.** There's nothing like setting the bar too high to chip away at your motivation and cause you to quit because of discouragement. This is true regardless of your fitness level. If you're an avid runner and want to prepare for a 5K race, there are apps that can help you achieve that incrementally. If you want to lose weight, calorie-tracking apps like MyFitnessPal can help set milestones for how much weight you can lose safely each week, and when you can expect to meet your goal. Setting dates and milestones toward completing your goals provides accountability and the motivation you need to reach your goals.
- **Consider adding variety to your workout.** Variety can keep you from getting bored, but you know yourself better than anyone. Perhaps just a brisk walk or an intense run along your usual route is all you need. Do whatever works for you. We discuss resources that are virtual libraries of workouts for you to try, including Sworkit and Fitnet.
- **What is your budget?** A gym membership and a personal trainer are not required for you to get a good workout, but they can help. Walking, running, biking, and a kettle bell can make for a highly effective workout with the proper guidance.

Now with the previous points under consideration, let's take a look at some apps that can help you create a more refined fitness plan and help you reach your fitness goals.

Achieving Health and Fitness Goals with More Apps

If you have a smartphone, you have the means to obtain more fitness plans and exercises than you can possibly handle. Simply enter some information about yourself—including your height, weight, gender, what activities you like to do, and your current fitness level—to create a custom fitness plan. If you have little time, workouts can be flexible, as well as motivational. Imagine having a personal trainer on hand 24/7 showing you exactly what to do, who can analyze your movements using your device, and make sure you're performing the movements correctly. How about a yoga or personal trainer app that can challenge you to help break through those plateaus? All you need is the will and space. The basement, attic, living room, or lawn will do. Read on to see some apps that can help you create a healthy lifestyle that can last a lifetime.

Get Fit with FitStar Personal Trainer

FitStar empowers you to take your fitness into your own hands and make a lasting change. If you're already in great shape or want to take off a few pounds, this subscription service can tailor a workout especially for you that you'll actually like following. The FitStar app makes it easy for you to access customized HD video workouts when you can't make it to the gym and offers you the guidance you need if you don't have a personal trainer. This program doesn't require you to have a lot of space or an abundance of free time, and no equipment is needed. Visit fitstar.com to watch videos and learn what the program has to offer. The FitStar app is available for both Android and Apple (iOS) devices for free, but you need to pay for the subscription-based FitStar Premium to unlock the apps full potential, which includes unlimited sessions, premium programs, HD Video, and more. The following screenshots are taken on an iPhone.

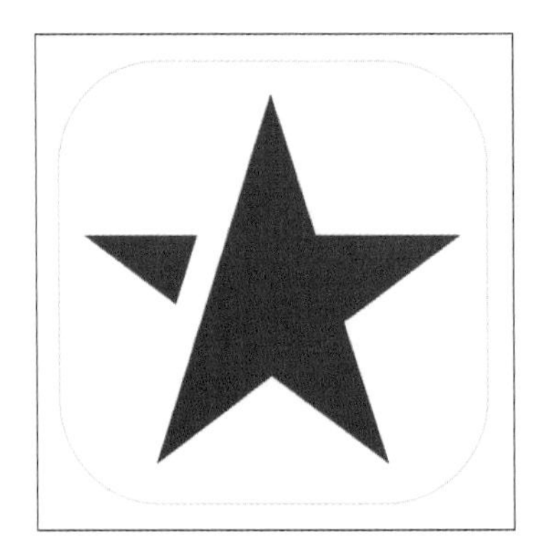

The FitStar Personal Trainer app

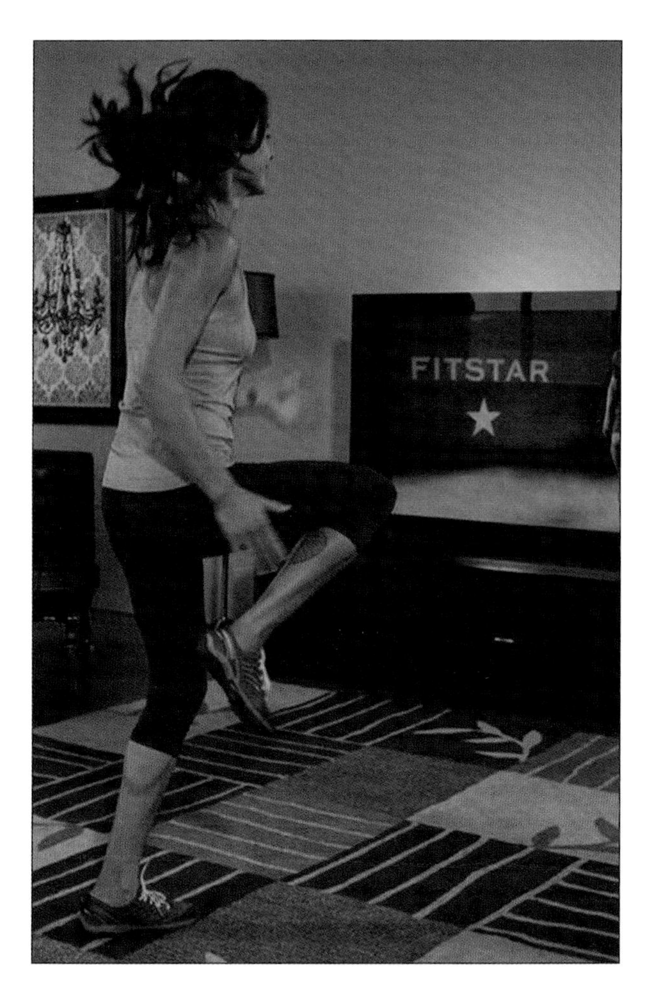

Try FitStar for customized HD video workouts.

If you're coming in at a moderate to high level of fitness, you might find that this program provides just the boost you've been looking for. If you haven't worked out for quite some time, don't get intimidated too quickly. FitStar has the ability to adjust and evolve to a level that can help you along the path to being the fittest version of you.

The FitStar program is dynamic and continually adjusts to your personal needs based on how you're progressing through feedback. After each video session the app asks you questions such as, "How long did you keep up?" and "How hard was that?" so that it can assess your strengths and weaknesses. For example, the app can evolve to understand if you are stronger in your upper body or lower body. FitStar continues to gather information so that each move and repetition is adjusted to fit your level of fitness. You can also find programs for losing weight or gaining strength, and new workouts are added monthly.

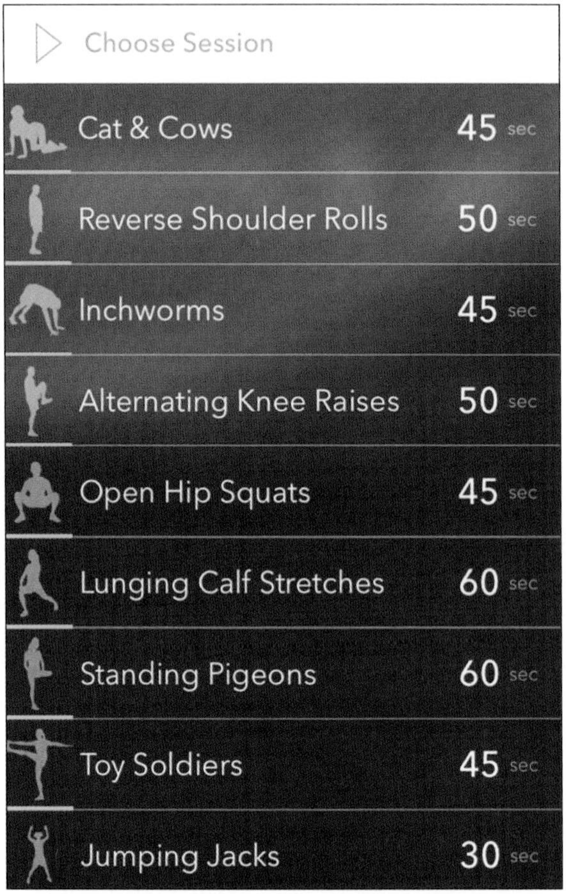

Choose Session

Cat & Cows	45 sec
Reverse Shoulder Rolls	50 sec
Inchworms	45 sec
Alternating Knee Raises	50 sec
Open Hip Squats	45 sec
Lunging Calf Stretches	60 sec
Standing Pigeons	60 sec
Toy Soldiers	45 sec
Jumping Jacks	30 sec

FitStar adapts to your personal level of fitness.

Access More Than 200 Free Fitness Workouts with Fitnet

If you have five minutes, then you have time for a Fitnet workout. The Fitnet app brings video fitness training to your Android phone and iPhone led by real, certified personal trainers, with sessions broken down into 5-minute and 7-minute workouts. Enter your fitness goals, and then receive custom workout plans and personalized guidance, which keep you accountable. Fitnet features

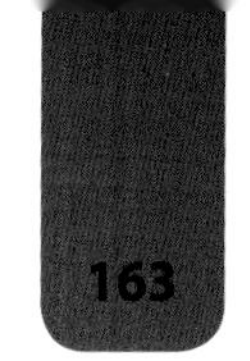

a 7-day plan and weekly goals that keep you on track. Exercises including Yoga, Taiji, and strength and cardio workouts at various levels help to keep you motivated. Choose from a massive collection of workouts to find the perfect one for you and meet your fitness goals. New workouts are posted regularly, and the style and intensity of workout are adapted to you. The following screenshots are taken on an Android phone.

The Fitnet Personal Exercise app.

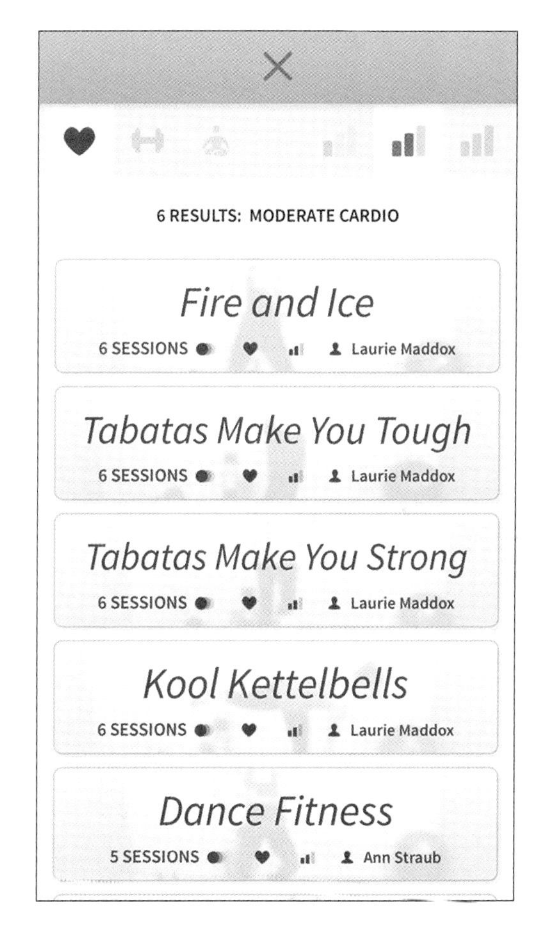

Fitnet offers video fitness training in 5- or 7- minute sessions.

The Fitnet app turns your mobile device's camera into a biometric sensor that provides real-time feedback while you exercise. You can see the trainer and yourself as you work out. The app uses the webcam to analyze your synchronicity with the trainer onscreen and provides webcam scoring based on your performance.

You can find the Fitnet app in the Google Play Store and the App Store. The app is free to download and use, and there are in-app purchases, such as fitness challenges. Visit fit.net to read testimonials and learn more about the app.

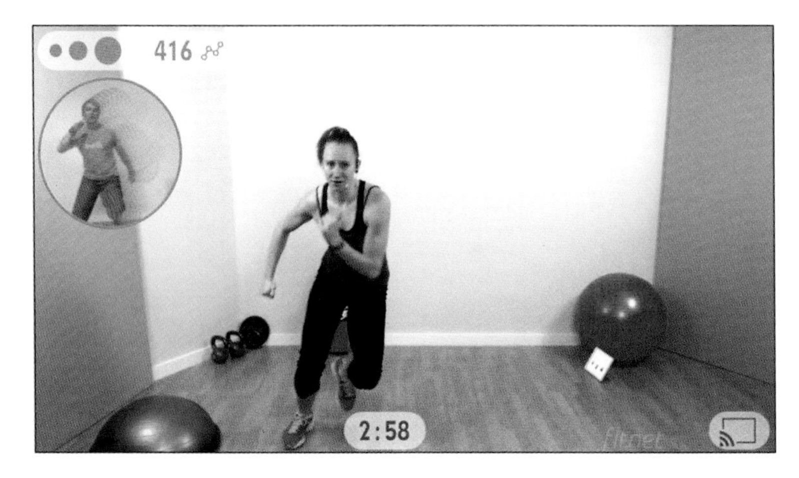

Fitnet uses your device's camera to provide real-time biometric feedback on your performance.

Get the Most from Your Workout with Nike+ Training Club

The Nike+ Training Club app is a collection of more than 100 video workouts and is available to download and use for free for Android and Apple (iOS) devices. You can download only the workouts you want, customize your sessions, and choose drills that are right for your body. All workouts are led by Nike Pro athletes and designed by Nike Training Masters. Just press pause if you need to catch your breath. Audio cues, video guides, and step-by-step images help you keep in good form as you perform workouts. You can take each session on its own, but you can also participate in month-long programs to reach your fitness goals. Stream videos from your phone or tablet to your TV using Apple's Airplay or Google's Chromecast, or with an HDMI cable. The app is also full of drill tips, nutritional advice, and challenges. Stay motivated by sharing photos of your workout on your social networks. The following example is shown on an iPhone.

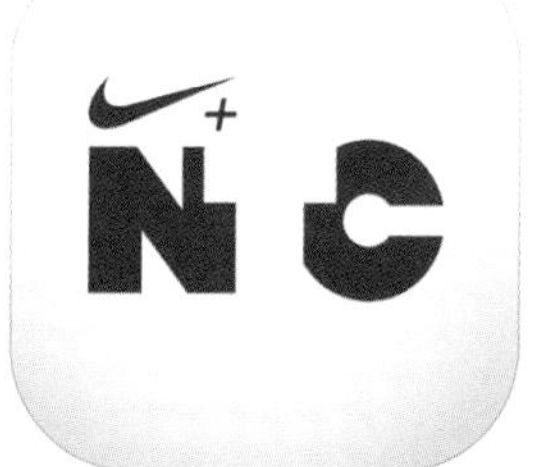

The Nike+ Training Club app.

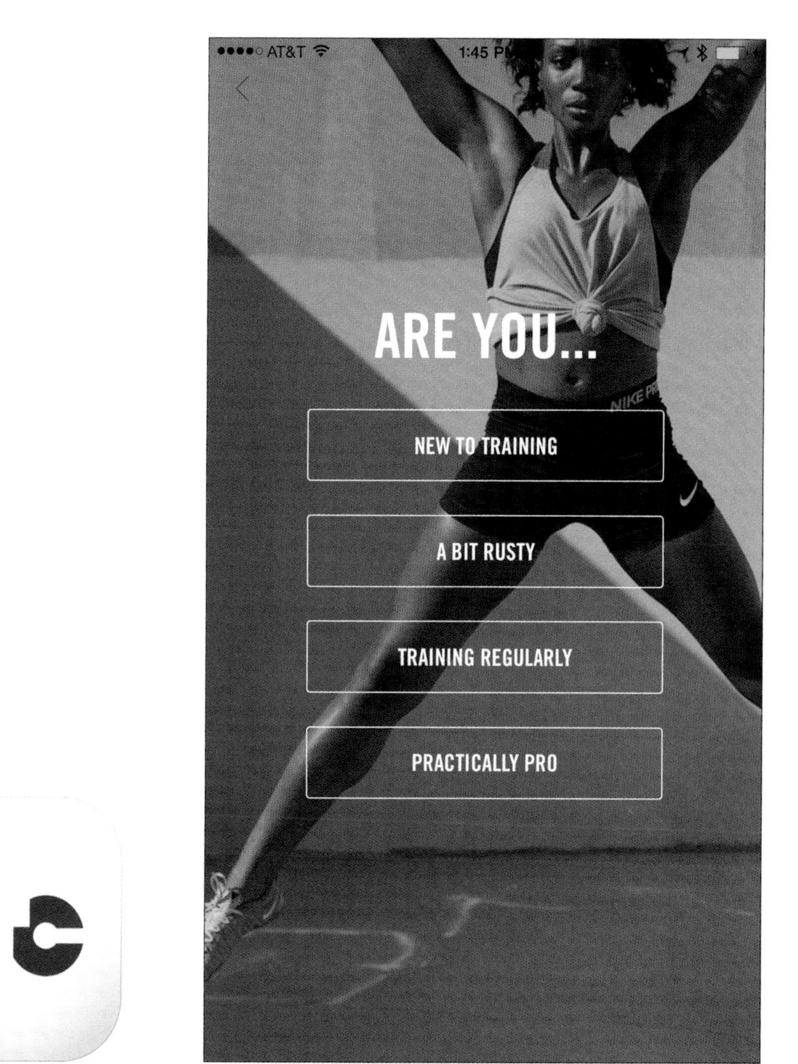

The Nike+ workouts are led by Nike Pro athletes and designed by Nike Training Masters.

Nike+ Training Club helps you design workouts to fit your own personal goals. No matter your fitness level, you can create a four-week program to get lean, get toned, and get strong. The Get Lean Program helps you burn fat and lose inches with high-intensity body-weight programs. The Get Toned program creates muscle definition with longer workouts and light weights. Choose the Get Strong program and use heavier weights to develop full body power without getting bulky. Simply pick a program, select a program level (Beginner, Intermediate,

Advanced), add activities such as running, and then edit the various exercises included in that program.

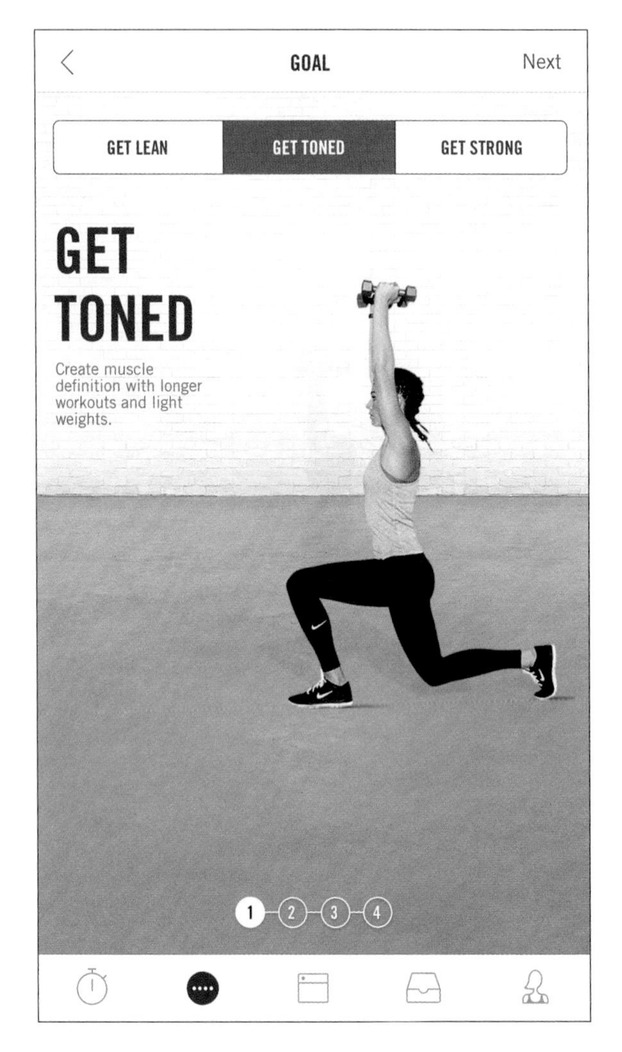
GOAL
Next
GET LEAN
GET TONED
GET STRONG
GET
TONED
Create muscle definition with longer workouts and light weights.
1
2
3
4

Choose to Get Lean, Get Toned, or Get Strong with Nike+ Training Club.

Personalize Your Workout with Sworkit

The Sworkit workout app guides you through video routines that are demonstrated by professional personal trainers. This app comes in a free Lite (scaled back) version and a paid Pro version (full featured). Try the Lite version to see how you like it. This app is great for daily circuit training, cardio and strength workouts, yoga/Pilates, and stretching. Dynamic video routines range from 5 to 60 minutes. Sworkit combines interval training with randomized exercises to maximize each video session. These circuit-training exercises do not require weights or extra equipment, help to ensure that your body doesn't get used to a certain routine, and keep you motivated. Each exercise in the circuit training is 30 seconds long with built-in rest periods. The Sworkit app is available for both Android and Apple (iOS) devices. The following examples are shown on an Android phone.

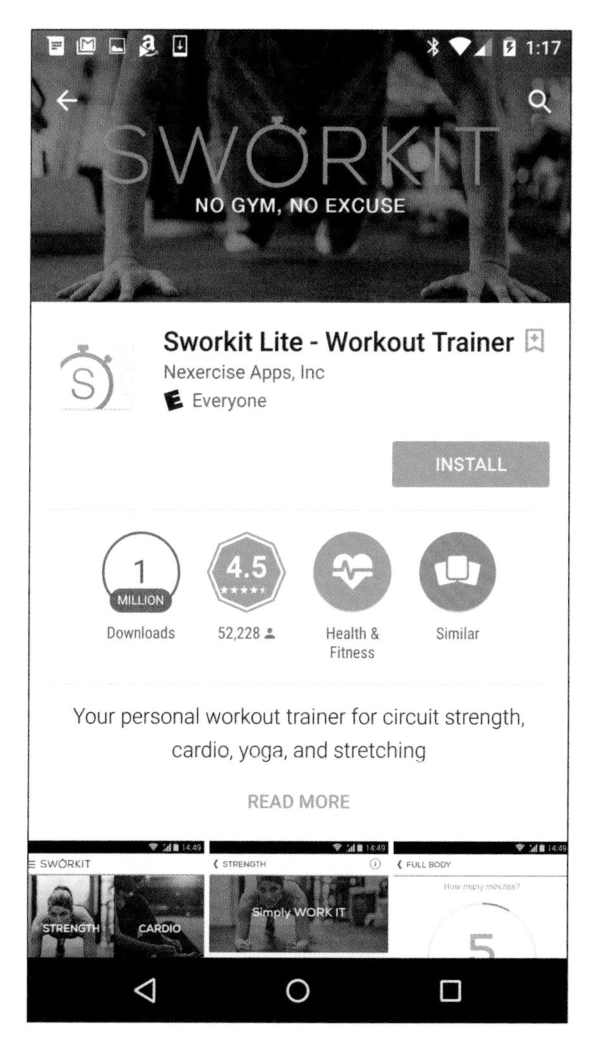

The Sworkit Workout Trainer app

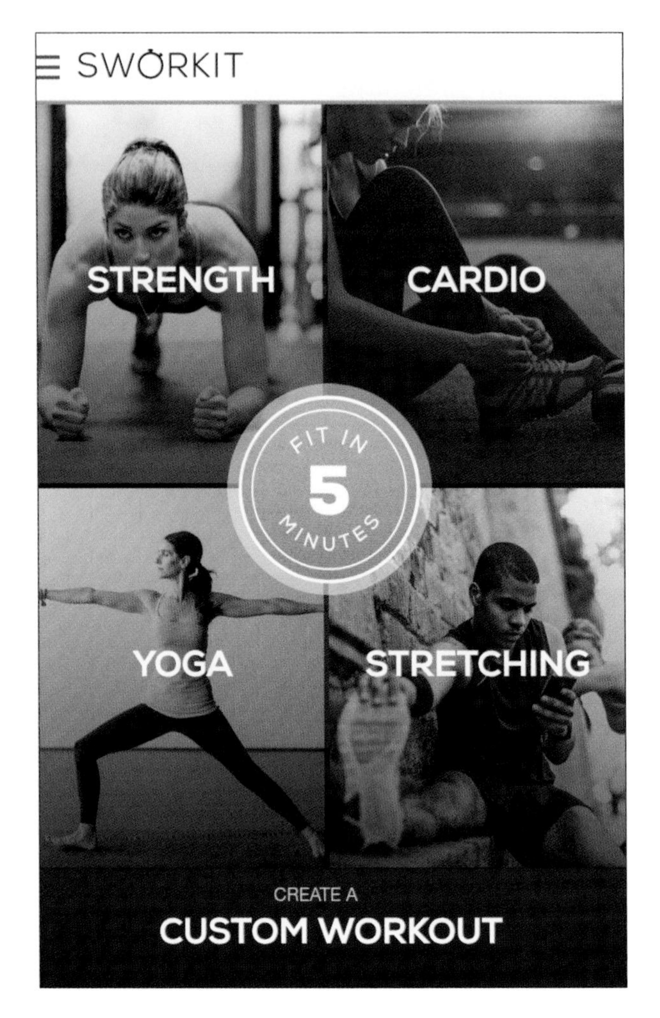

Dynamic videos by professional trainers, ranging from 5 to 60 minutes, keep you motivated.

Think of the Sworkit workout library like the music on an iPod or smartphone music app. Pick any of the videos and create your own exercise playlist. Modify any existing workout for a completely personalized experience. Create new challenges and insert running-in-place and push-ups between every other exercise. Download custom Sworkit workouts including low impact (no jumping),

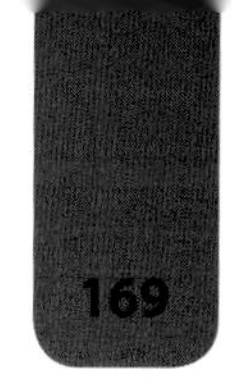

full body, beginner, intermediate, advanced full body, runner's warm-up, office chair stretch, golfer Sworkit, and more. Select a part of the body that you want to work out by choosing from more than 20 workouts, or customize your workout. Use Sworkit to create a workout routine to fit your schedule, and then get to work.

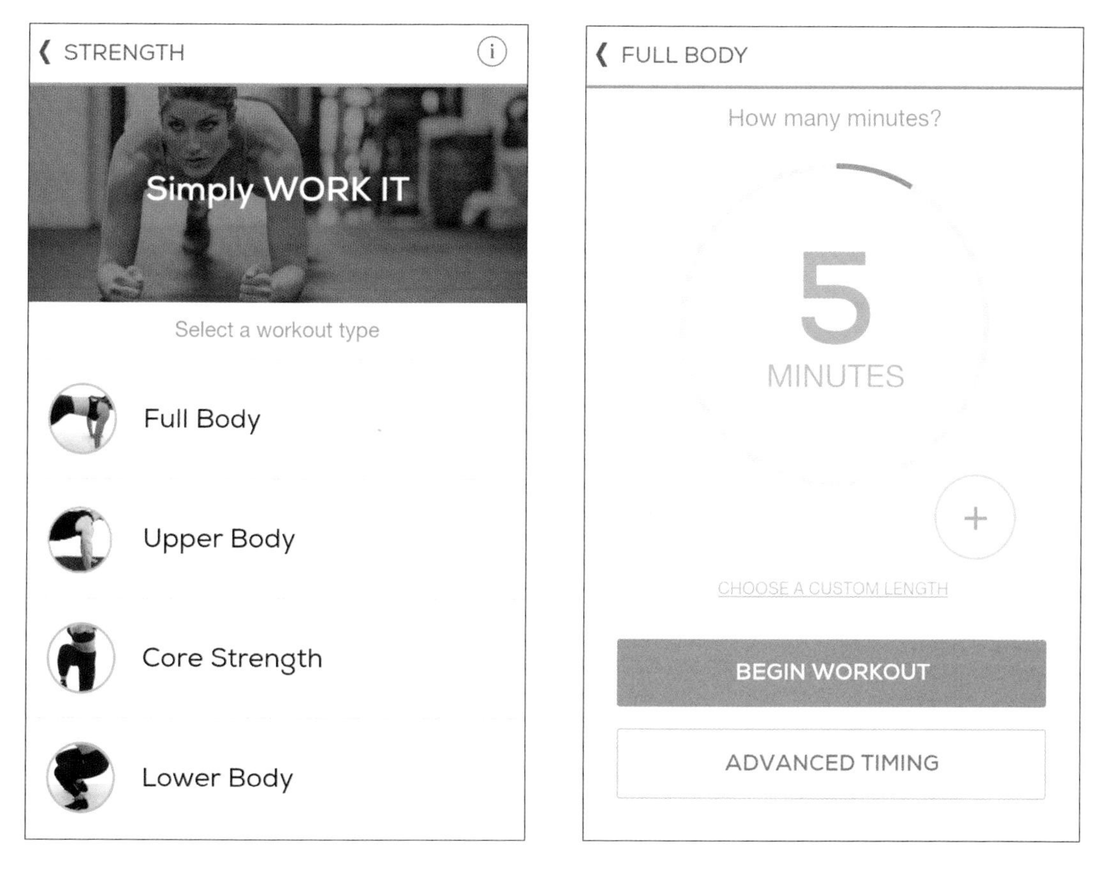

Create personalized workouts from Sworkit's library.

Customize a workout that fits your schedule.

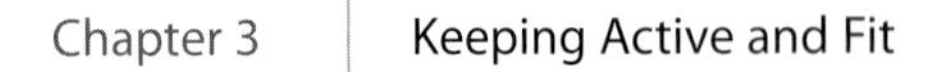

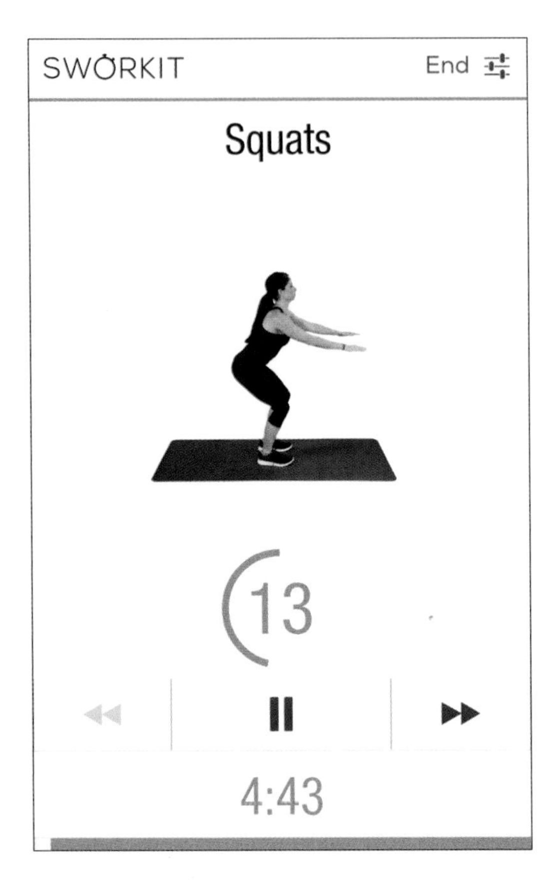

Get to work on your personalized workout.

Maximize Your In-Home Workouts with Wello

Wello is a service uniquely tailored to you, compared to the previous prerecorded video workouts we have discussed. Wello lets you connect with a live personal trainer via two-way webcam from your living room, office, hotel room, or whatever space works best for you. You can also connect with other group members over the Wello video platform. All you need is a laptop or desktop computer with a webcam, a broadband Internet connection, and a little bit of space.

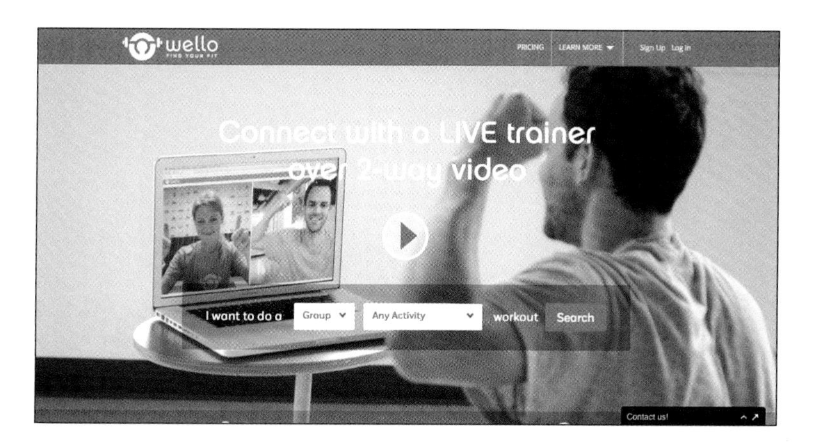

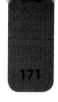

Wello lets you connect with a live personal trainer or other group members via webcam, from your home, or on the road.

Wello offers a wide range of fitness activities including personal training, yoga, Pilates, boot camp, kettlebell workouts, Zumba, martial arts, and much more. Activities are being added every day. You can book 1-on-1 workouts for 30 or 60 minutes, or 60-minute group workouts. As of this writing, Wello offers the choice between 1-on-1 membership plans or small group membership plans, based on how many sessions a month you want to do: 4, 10, or 30. You can also choose to pay as you go for 1-on-1 or group workouts.

To learn more about what Wello has to offer, visit Wello.com. As of this writing, Wello has an iPad app that you can use, but it is still working on its Android app. The following examples are from wello.com. If you visit its site and like what you see, it's easy to get started and connect with a live trainer online.

When you sign up, Wello helps you find the right trainer and get started with your live online workouts. You can search by schedule, price, workout type, trainer style, gender, reviews, plus more criteria to narrow the field and find what fits you. If you don't see a class at the time you want, you can email Wello and the people there will make it happen. Just tell Wello what activity you want to do and when you would like to do it, months or minutes in advance. You can also track your workouts using the Dashboard feature. Before you sign up, visit wello.com to learn more details about operating system, browser, and hardware compatibility. The site also offers a link that you can click to test your video and audio setup so you can prep your physical space to exercise.

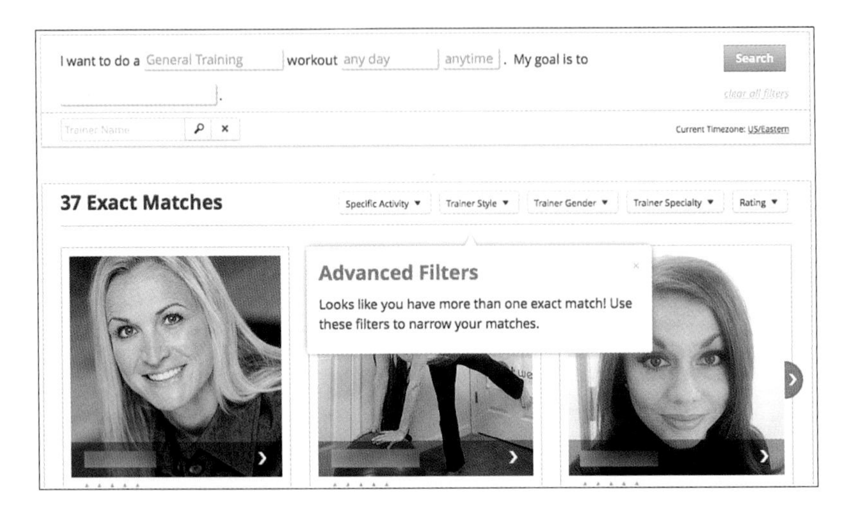

Wello helps you find the right trainer or small group class that fits your needs.

Log Activity with MapMyFitness

With the MapMyFitness app, you can log more than 600 different workouts, record GPS-based activities, and connect with more than 400 devices to import and analyze all of your activities' data. This app has one of the largest selections of activities to track, including running, cycling, walking, gym workouts, cross training, yoga, and much more. Connect your compatible device to view steps, sleep, workouts, and more in a single graph. Record GPS-based workouts and analyze detailed stats such as pace, route, distance, calories burned, and elevation. If you're looking for one app that can handle just about anything you can do and connect to huge list of devices including Jawbone, Misfit, Fitbit, Garmin, and Withings, this may be your go-to one-stop app. Upgrade to Premium and access features like heart-rate-analysis, personal training plans, audio coaching, and Live Tracking. MapMyFitness also lets you share your progress and workouts with family and friends on social media; you can also join group challenges for activities, climb the leader board, and win prizes. MapMyFitness is available for both Android phones and the iPhone and can be downloaded for free. You can use many features for free. You need to upgrade to a paid MVP Membership to access special features, including heart rate analysis, personal training plans, and audio coaching. The following examples are shown on an iPhone.

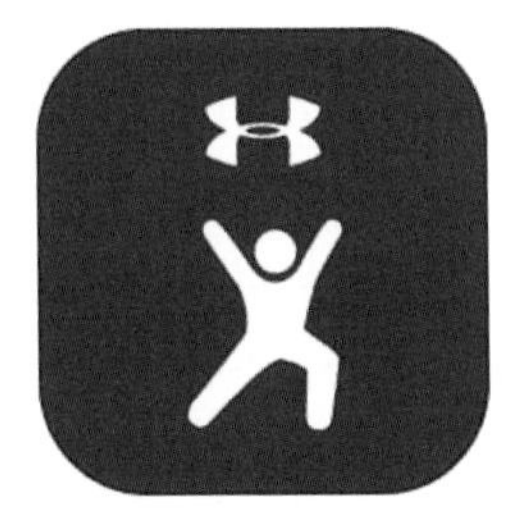

The Map My Fitness app

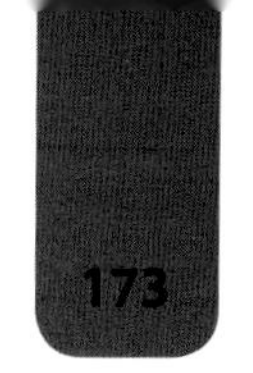

Map Your Route

MapMyFitness can use the sensors in your smartphone and a fitness tracker. Using a GPS-enabled phone, MapMyFitness pinpoints your current location as soon as you select an activity such as Run, Walk, or Road Cycling, and maps your route for that particular activity. After you complete a workout, you can view a summary including distance, duration, and pace, and see your route charted on a map. You can also save a route to use it for future workouts. If you're looking for a new route to run, MapMyFitness can help with that as well. Route Genius scans your current area and presents a list of different routes for you to choose from. Each option is also presented with the distance for each route. To narrow down your search for a new route even further, you can filter options shown in the list by distance.

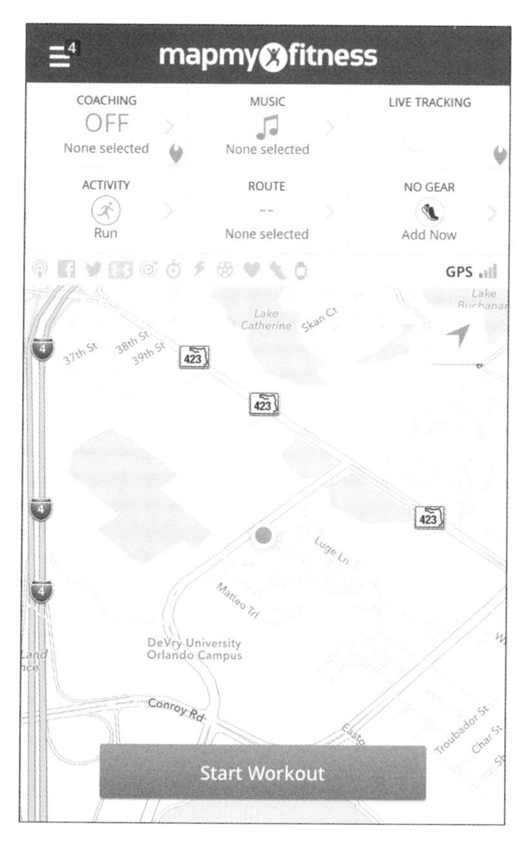

MapMyFitness uses GPS-based data, and you can log more than 600 different exercises.

Try the Route Genius in MapMyFitness to get new ideas on where to walk, run, or cycle in your area.

Track Your Activity

Tracking your activity with MapMyFitness is simple. Just tap Activity on the default main page to choose from more than 600 activities. At first, the Activities list is filtered to only show a few of the activities under the Recent tab. You can tap All to view a comprehensive list of what MapMyFitness has to offer. When you first switch from an activity that utilizes GPS, such as running, to one that doesn't, such as pushups, MapMyFitness alerts you that GPS is not needed for this activity, and then prompts you to turn off GPS. You can do this within the alert message, so there is no need to leave the app. After you have picked a workout, tap Start Workout at the bottom of the screen. The Start Workout button turns into a Pause Workout button. Pause the workout when needed, and the option to finish the workout also appears. You can then view a summary of your activity data, which you can save or discard after each activity.

Record | Activity Type

Recent | All

Sit Ups
Run
Walk
Road Cycling
Mountain Bike
Hike
Run, Treadmill
Stairs
Walk, Treadmill
Dog Walk
Other Gym Workout
Push Ups
Crunches and Leg Lifts
Lap Swim

Choose from a list of recent activities performed or from all available activities.

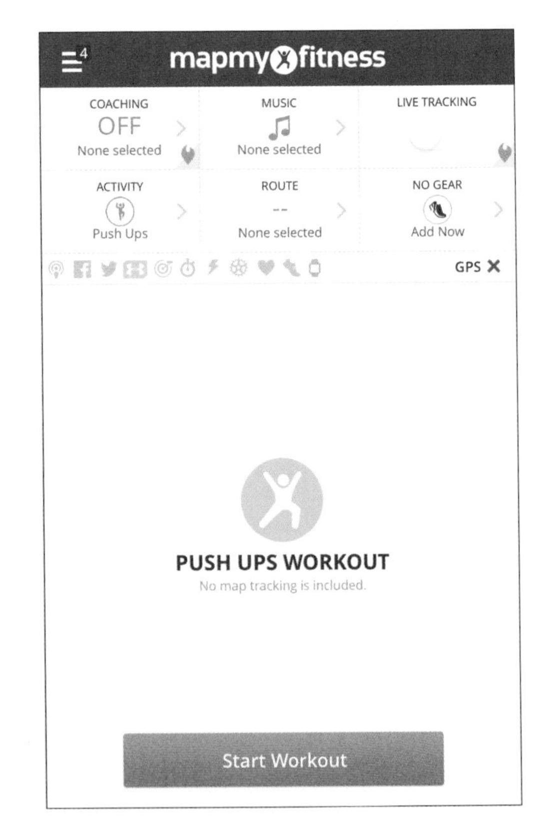

MapMyFitness alerts you when GPS data is used or not.

Improve Your Posture with the Lumo Lift App

The Lumo Lift sensor and app is your digital posture coach and activity tracker. Slouching doesn't only make you look bad, but can actually cause long-term damage. This imbalance in body alignment can strain ligaments and muscles and cause chronic pain in the neck, back, and hips; joint stiffness; and more ailments. The Lumo Lift sensor and app helps you improve your posture long term by reinforcing good posture habits. Here's how it works. Clip the Lumo Lift sensor using the magnetic clasp onto your shirt, right below the collarbone. The sensor can be easily concealed. Lumo Lift tracks your posture and activities, and uses a gentle vibration to remind you to straighten your posture when you begin to slouch. Set goals for good posture hours tracked for the day. Lumo Lift also passively tracks your steps activity, and lets you set a daily step goal, track distance, and view calories burned. Lumo Lift is available for both Android phones and the iPhone. You can download the Lumo Lift app for free on the Google Play Store and the App Store. Visit lumobodytech.com to learn more and purchase the item. You can also purchase the Lumo Lift sensor on amazon.com. The following examples are shown on the iPhone.

Before you begin your goal to better posture, the Lumo Lift needs some information from you.

Connecting Lumo Lift to Other Apps

The Lumo Lift app can be connected with the MyFitnessPal app to transfer your step and calorie info into your MyFitnessPal account. Simply connect the apps via Partners under Menu.

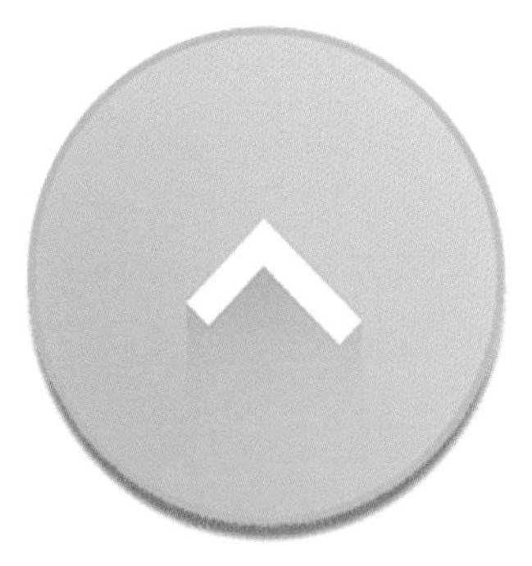

The Lumo Lift app.

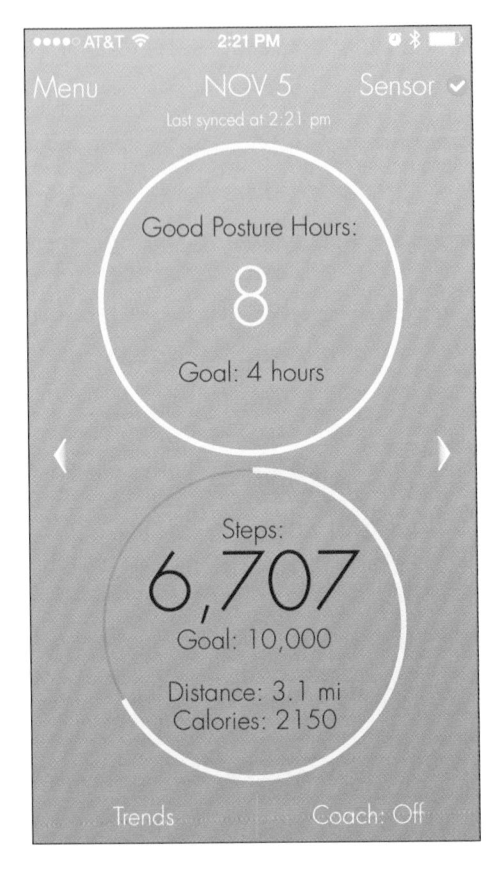

Lumo Lift uses a small magnetic clasp to sense your posture and feeds that data to your smartphone.

Lumo Lift first needs to be calibrated so it knows what constitutes good posture. After calibration, Lumo Lift vibrates to let you know when you have deviated from your standard of good posture. Enable coach vibrations as reminders when you have remained in a slouched position for a specified amount of time. Lumo Lift recommends that this time be two minutes. After two minutes of bad posture, a gentle vibration reminds you to adjust your posture. Track your progress over time using a graph for more insight into your posture habits.

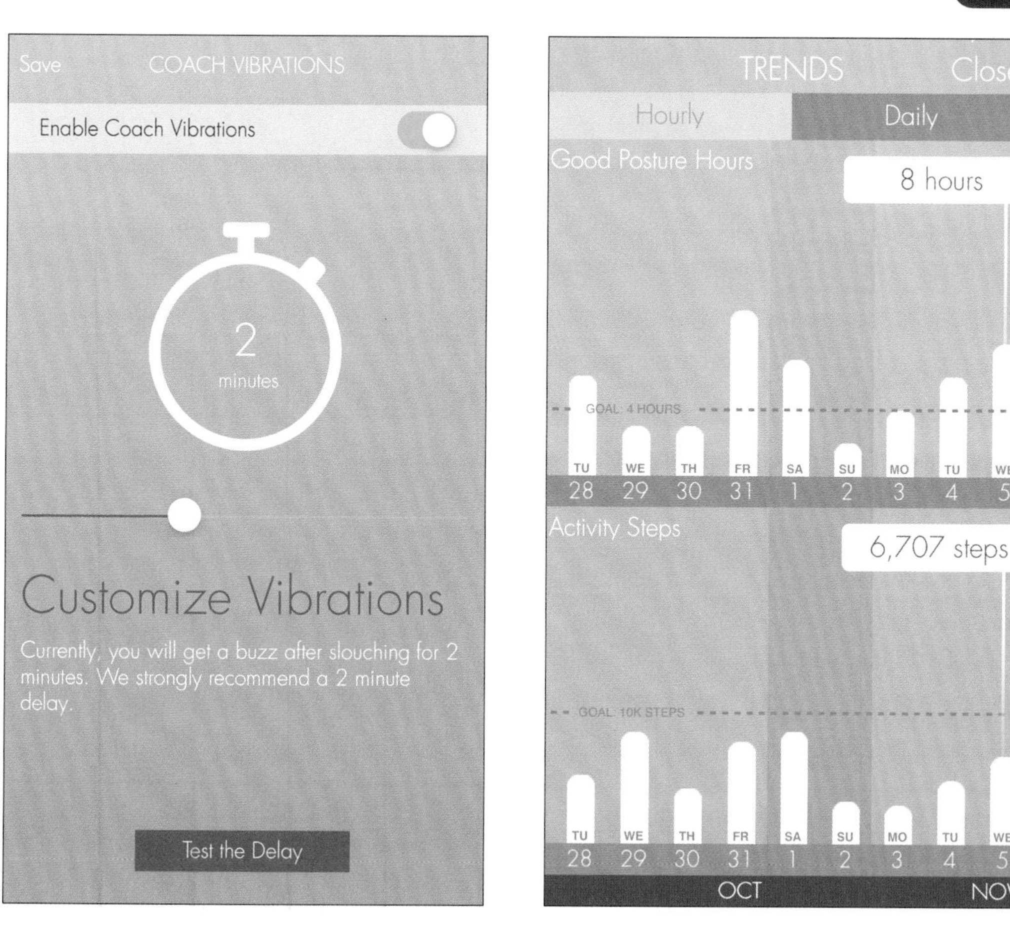

Set reminders to alert you when you have been slouching.

Track both your posture and your steps over time.

Getting to Know High-Tech Canes

If you use a cane on your walks, you should know that technological developments are being made for canes as well. These extra bells and whistles provide an added layer of safety and security when you're out living an active lifestyle. In the world of high-tech canes, there are two types: those that are in development, and those that you can purchase today. There are promises of canes with GPS, and even facial recognition for people who are blind. For now, this section deals with the canes that you can get today.

Secure Folding Walking Cane

The Secure Folding Walking Cane's multifunction features make it a great safety accessory for everyday use. This cane includes an LED flashlight that you can use to light the way in low-light conditions, as well as to make yourself more visible, such as when you're crossing the street. If you're ever in an emergency situation or feel unsafe, the Secure Folding Walking Cane also has a pushbutton panic alarm and a flashing red alert/warning light. When pressed, the pushbutton panic alarm emits a high-decibel alarm sound that draws the attention of others, making it great for situations when immediate help is needed.

The Secure Folding Walking cane requires 2 AAA batteries and has a weight capacity that supports up to 220 lbs. It's made of durable aluminum alloy and is telescopically adjustable from 30"–34" in length. Just like the name indicates, it folds away neatly for storage. Visit padalarm.com or just search online for "Secure Folding Walking Cane" to learn more about and to purchase this cane.

Trusty Cane

The Trusty LED Folding, Walking, Triple Head Pivot Base Cane is a product you might have seen on TV in an infomercial. The three built-in lights (one pointing forward, two pointing down) help light your path in low-light conditions and make you visible to motorists and cyclists. The triple head, extra-wide pivoting base provides more stability on different terrains, enabling you to maintain a more natural stride. The ergonomic grip adjusts to your size, and then locks in to place. It is adjustable from 31"–38" tall and can be adjusted to five different lengths. This cane requires 3 AAA batteries and supports up to 250 lbs. This cane also folds neatly away for easy storage. Point your browser to amazon.com and search for Trusty Cane LED.

© Personal Safety Corporation. Used with permission.

The Secure Folding Walking Cane has an LED flashlight, panic alarm, and flashing alarm light, and it folds for easy storage.

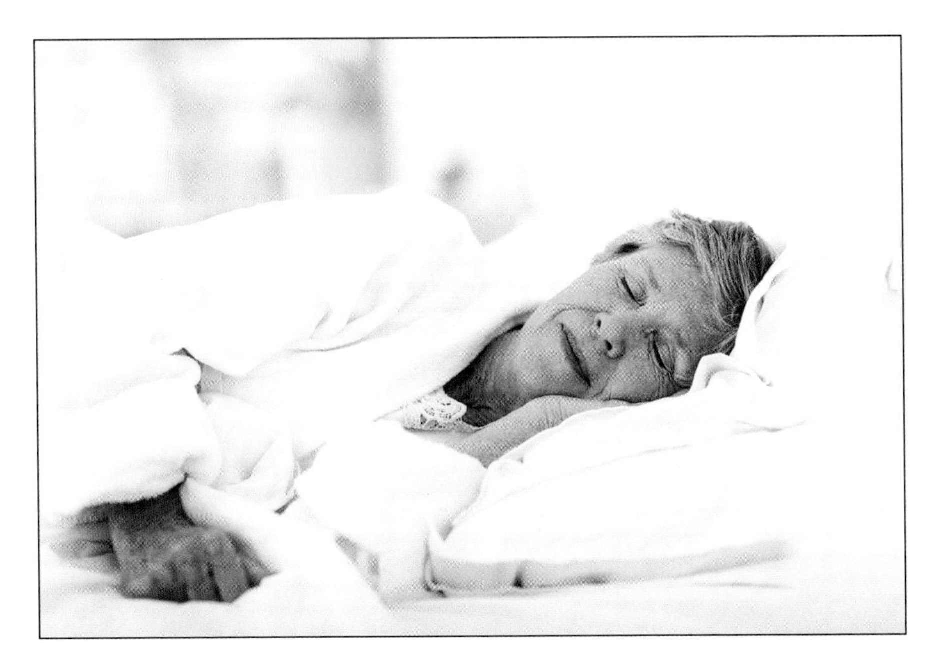

Credit: © michaeljung/fotolia.com

Track your sleep patterns to get a better night's sleep and manage your stress.

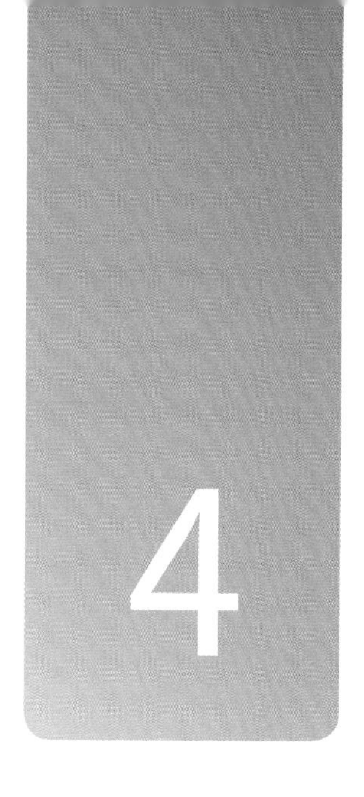

In this chapter, you discover how fitness trackers and apps can help you achieve better quality sleep. You also learn about some resources that help manage your stress level.

→ Exploring Sleep Monitoring
→ Forming Consistent Sleep Habits
→ Tracking Your Sleep with Devices
→ Tracking Your Sleep with Apps
→ Using Apps to Help Relax and Fall Asleep
→ Exploring Meditation Apps

Sleeping Better and Managing Stress

It seems like every other commercial on TV or the radio is promoting another energy drink whose effects take you higher and last longer than the one before. Perhaps the problem is that you're not sleeping enough, or the quality of your sleep is poor. Although a good cup of coffee throughout the day can keep you going, nothing can substitute for getting a good night's sleep and learning to better manage stress. This chapter covers some of the devices and apps that are available to track light and deep sleep stages so that you can see the overall picture in your sleeping patterns and make adjustments when necessary. It also covers some apps to help you incorporate relaxation time throughout a hectic day and help you unwind at night to prepare for a good night's sleep.

Exploring Sleep Monitoring

Scientists have been monitoring sleeping patterns for a long time and agree that a healthy diet, a regular exercise regimen, and good stress management can help you sleep better. The National Sleep Foundation (sleepfoundation.org) estimates that "50 to 70 million Americans are affected by chronic sleep disorder and intermittent sleep problems that can significantly diminish health, alertness and safety." The Foundation also points out that most people don't know when to seek help, unlike with a fever or pain. Connected technology including fitness trackers, apps, smart alarms so you don't wake up feeling groggy, and sleep sensors can provide a data-driven approach toward not only understanding your sleep patterns, but also achieving quality sleep. They can make you aware of a problem so you can get help from your doctor, if needed.

Sleep problems frequently go undetected and can lead to impaired thinking as well as health concerns. Using sleep analysis tools can help you be more aware of your sleeping habits and patterns, so that you can make informed choices about sleep. Improving your sleep habits might help you be more alert, which can translate to avoiding accidents and other safety threats, and can greatly diminish even chronic health issues such as depression, hypertension, diabetes, and stroke, according to the National Sleep Foundation.

It's Not All Good

Non-Clinical Sleep Trackers

The non-clinical sleep trackers shown in this chapter are not as accurate or extensive in their results as formal sleep studies performed by qualified sleep specialists. Sleep studies use a wider array of parameters and equipment with higher levels of precision than sensors found in fitness trackers, smartphones, and smart alarms. Also, sleep trackers that automatically detect whether you are sleeping can sometimes interpret other actions as sleeping, such as sitting on the couch watching television, or even when you set the device on a table instead of having it on you. Vet all products before purchasing by reading consumer reviews online and reading the FAQs provided on the manufacturer's websites.

Forming Consistent Sleep Habits

Before we get into sleep trackers, let's talk about some habits that can help make this connected technology most effective.

- **Try to stick to a set sleep and wake-up schedule, even on the weekends.** This helps to calibrate your internal clock to know when it's time to fall asleep.
- **Put away the smartphones, computers, and tablets hours before you go to sleep.** Bright lights and especially blue light, emitted by electronics and energy-efficient light bulbs, stimulate the brain and make it more difficult to get to sleep.
- **Don't take naps if you know you have a hard time sleeping at night.** Naps can make you stay up later than usual and interrupt your set sleep schedule.
- **Exercise.** The National Sleep Foundation says, "People sleep significantly better and feel more alert during the day if they get at least 150 minutes of exercise a week." This equates to just over 20 minutes a day and can be vigorous or moderate.

These are only a few good habits to incorporate into your lifestyle for a better night's sleep. To learn more go to sleepfoundation.org.

Tracking Your Sleep with Devices

There are a variety of items you can use to track your sleep, including smart watches and fitness bands, as well as technical devices dedicated more specifically to sleep tracking. Consider what goals you have for your sleep and what type of information would be most helpful to you as you review a few of the many options.

Track Sleep Patterns with the Withings Activité Pop

The Withings Activité Pop activity tracking watch automatically detects when you are sleeping and keeps track of light and deep sleep stages, the number of times you wake up during the night, and how long you've slept. This device doesn't require you to do anything but wear it as you sleep. The following examples are shown on an iPhone.

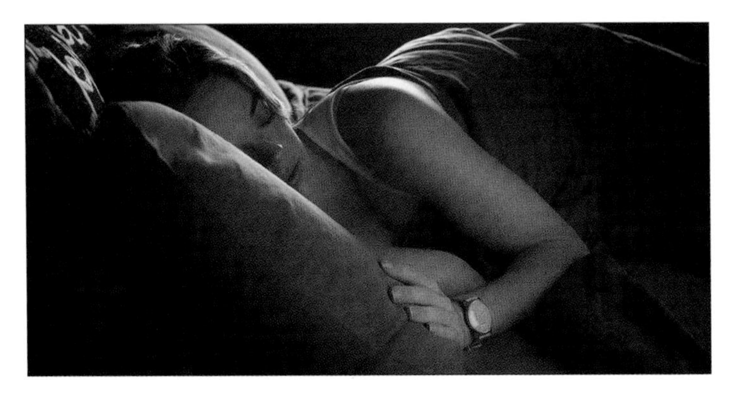

The Withings Activité Pop

Just go to sleep with your watch on, and it will register in the Timeline on your Dashboard in the Health Mate app as an activity when you awake. Use the Health Mate app to view your collected sleep data. The Health Mate app is available for both Android phones and the iPhone. Visit Withings.com to learn more and to purchase the Activité Pop. You can also find it on Amazon.

Follow these steps to access your sleep information using the Health Mate app with your Activité Pop.

1. Open the app on your phone and place it in close proximity to your Activité Pop watch so it can sync. Health Mate opens and reveals the Timeline on your Dashboard. You can see in the orange widget that the app is connecting with the watch.
2. After the device and phone sync, tap the Sleep (Activité) data that appears. A summary of your sleep information appears.

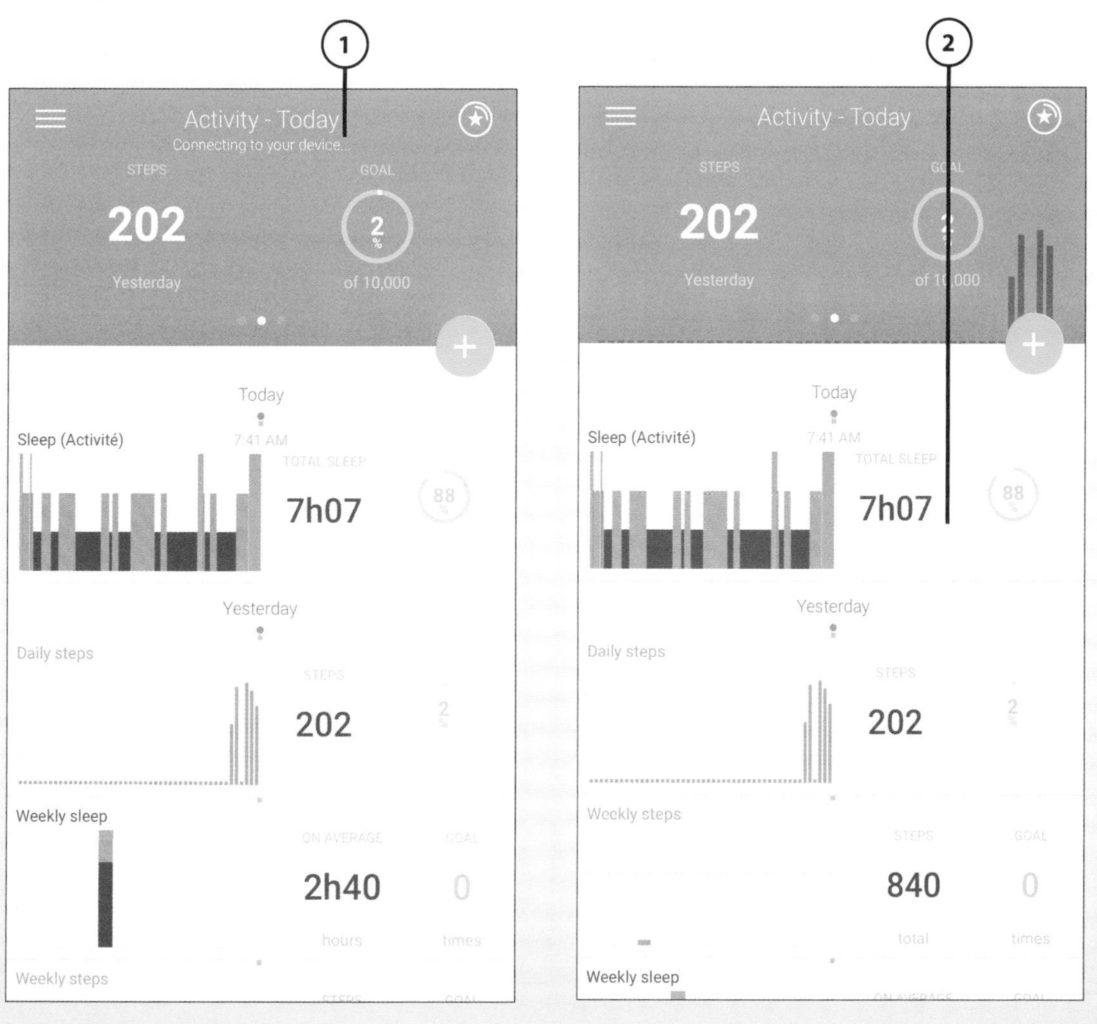

(3) View the summary of your sleep information.

(4) Tap the menu that looks like three horizontal circles in the upper-right corner to view your information by Day or Week. Withings also provides tips for achieving higher quality sleep and answers to questions you might have about the sleep cycle.

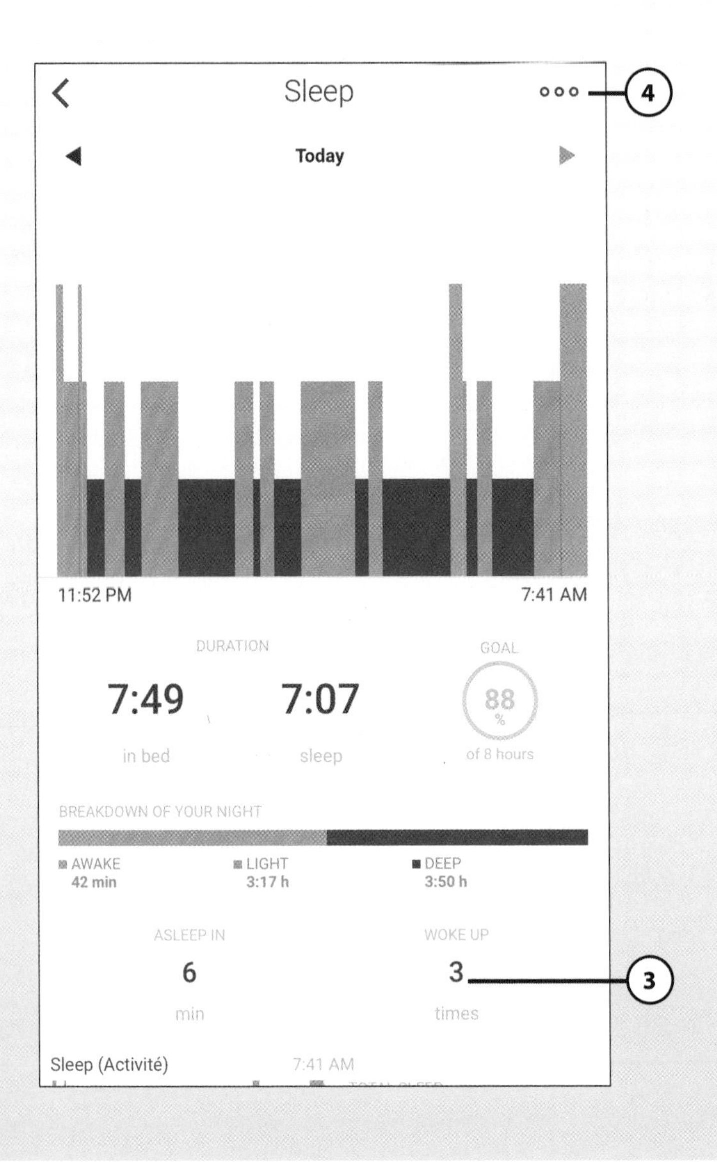

Reading the Graph and Other Data Points Collected

- Time spent awake is represented in orange.
- Duration of light sleep cycle is represented in light blue.
- During of deep sleep cycle is represented in dark blue.
- Other data points collected include time spent lying down, total time spent sleeping, percentage of an 8 hours sleep goal, and number of wake-ups.

Setting an Alarm

When you set an alarm, your Activité Pop can wake you with a gentle vibration. Swipe the orange widget from left to right at the top of the Dashboard to set an alarm.

>>Go Further

CONSIDER THE AURA CONNECTED ALARM + SLEEP SENSOR

Withings also makes a smart alarm that might be your ultimate sleep aid. The Aura is marketed as using optimized colors to promote the release of sleep hormones, plays sounds to induce sleep, and even comes with an optional sleep sensor that fits under your mattress so you can track your night's sleep in the Health Mate app. The sensor and app enable you to visualize your full sleep cycles. The Aura Total Sleep System offers a Smart WakeUp function that can adapt to your internal clock using the sleep sensor. Aura uses its gentle light and sound program to bring you to your optimal state in which to wake. Visit https://www.withings.com/us/en/products/aura to learn more.

Get Insight with the Beddit Sleep Tracker

The Beddit Sleep Tracker uses an ultra-thin force-activated sensor to measure your nighttime activity. Here's how it works. The Beddit sensor recognizes the natural fall in resting heart rate and respiratory rate as sleep. It also recognizes waking events and when you're not in bed, which affects the quality of your sleep. There is nothing to wear. Just place the Beddit Sensor under your bed sheet, and then sleep on it. The Beddit Sleep Tracker consists of a sensor and an app to track your sleep data.

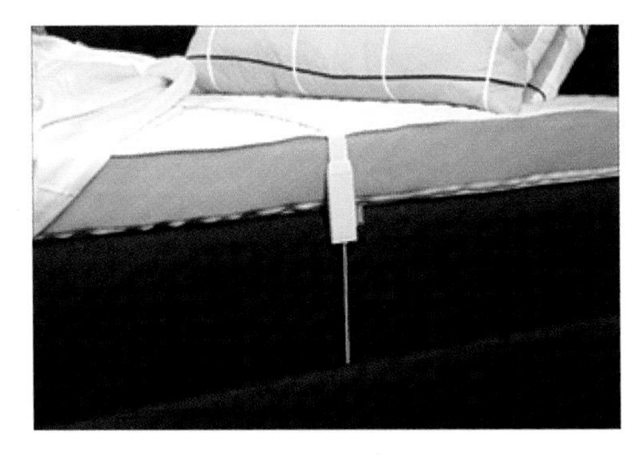

The Beddit Sleep Tracker

Each morning you can view your Beddit SleepScore in the Beddit app. Your score is dependent on how you sleep and uses a scale ranging from 0 to 100. The scientists at Beddit have examined thousands and thousands of nights of sleep of other Beddit users around the world and pinpointed a zone for good sleep. They call it the Green Zone. You can see whether you reached the Green Zone by viewing your Beddit SleepScore.

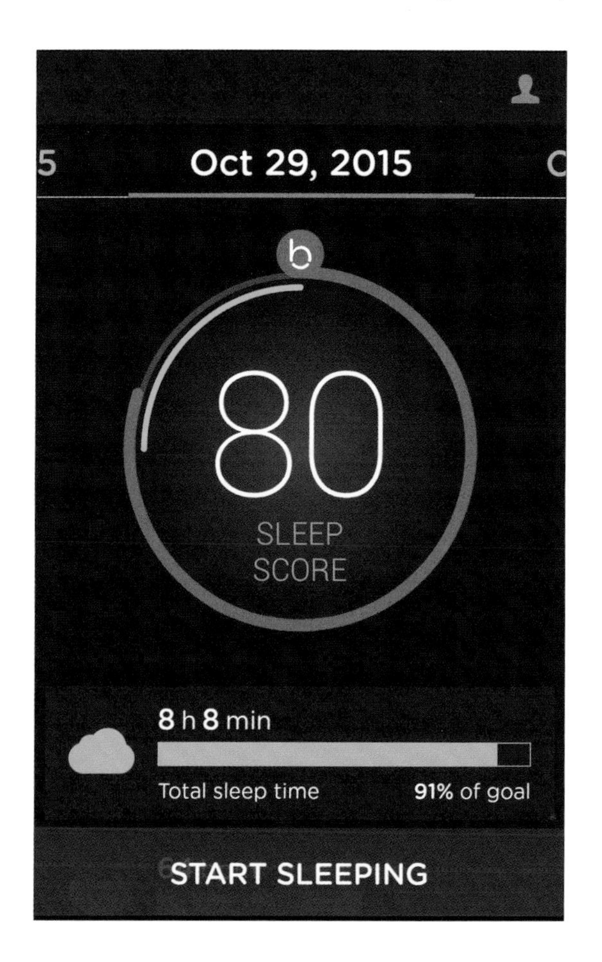

The Beddit app also provides detailed sleep graphs for you to view your sleep data. You can access the most important parameters of your sleep, including average respiration rate, total sleep time, time to fall asleep, and sleep efficiency. Visit beddit.com or Amazon.com to learn more and purchase the Beddit Sleep Tracker. The Beddit app is available for Android phones and the iPhone by downloading from the Google Play Store and the App Store.

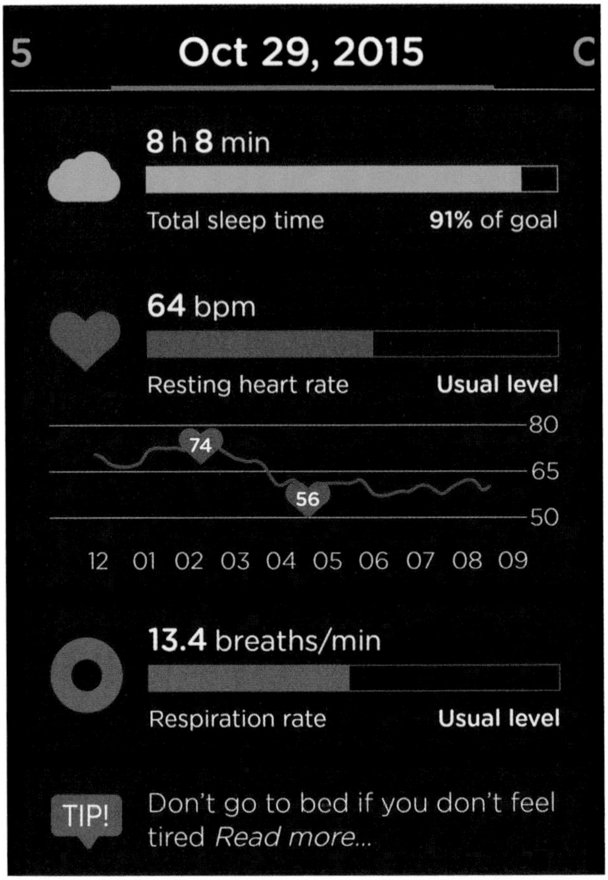

Oct 29, 2015

8 h 8 min
Total sleep time 91% of goal

64 bpm
Resting heart rate Usual level
80
74
65
56
50
12 01 02 03 04 05 06 07 08 09

13.4 breaths/min
Respiration rate Usual level

TIP! Don't go to bed if you don't feel tired *Read more...*

Focus on Sleep with the Fitbit Flex Band

As of this writing, all Fitbit trackers can track sleep with the exception of the Zip. Your tracker can help you see how many hours you sleep, to better understand the quality of your sleep and your sleeping patterns. The default sleeping goal for each tracker is 8 hours. The National Sleep Foundation says that adults and older adults can require anywhere from 5 to 10 hours of sleep, with a recommended range of 7 to 9 hours. You can change this goal to fit your needs using the fitbit.com Dashboard or the Fitbit app, monitor your sleep progress with a focus on meeting your goal. You should have a good notion about how much sleep you need to feel at your best during the day. However, consider consulting with your doctor before setting a new goal to make a more informed decision.

Monitor How Well and How Long You Sleep

Your Fitbit tracker is equipped with two modes for tracking sleep: Normal and Sensitive. The Normal mode registers significant movements as being awake. Normal is appropriate for most users. For more detailed information, choose Sensitive. Sensitive mode records nearly all movement as time awake. If you are a sound sleeper, this mode might work best for you. You can adjust your sleeping mode by going to your Dashboard on Fitbit.com. You must sync your tracker to your computer by using the supplied wireless sync dongle for the change to take place. The dongle is a small device that fits into the USB port in your computer. You can also sync your Fitbit to the Fitbit app on your phone.

Follow these steps to put your Fitbit Flex tracker into sleep mode.

1. When you are ready to go to sleep, tap your Fitbit Flex rapidly for two seconds to enter sleep mode. Two blinking lights alternate to signify that you are in sleep mode.
2. When you wake up, tap your Fitbit Flex rapidly to exit sleep mode. Your tracker will vibrate, and all five lights will flash three times and then display a sweeping light pattern.
3. View a daily and week-by-week summary of your sleep information on your Dashboard on fitbit.com or the phone app.

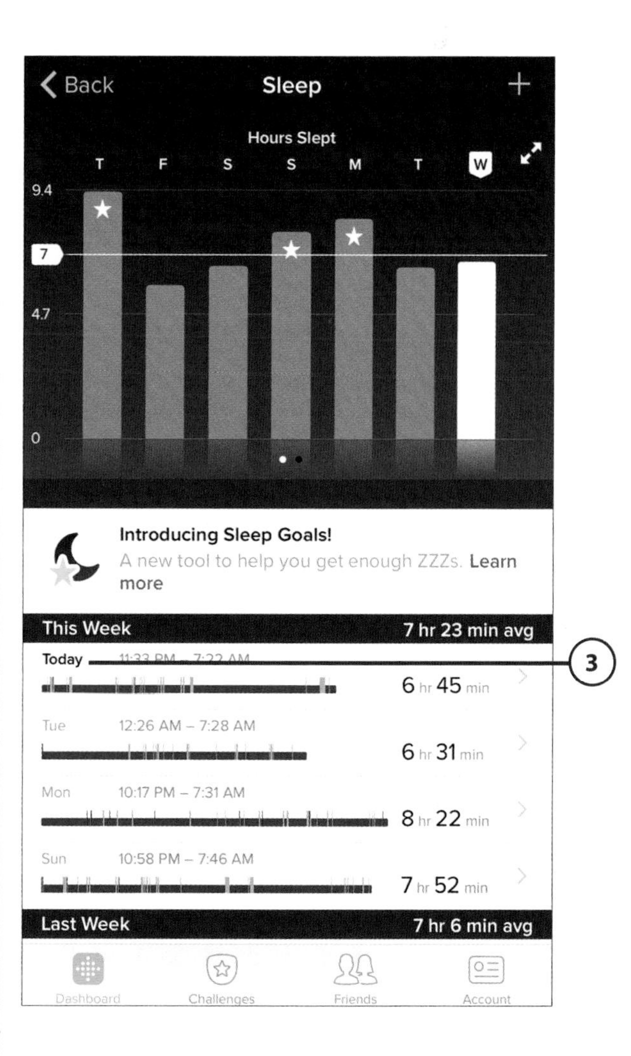

Automatic Sleep Detection

All Fitbit trackers except the Zip and the Fitbit One can automatically track your sleep without putting them into sleep mode. You just sleep and wake up. Note that automatic sleep mode may count time when you are still, like on a couch watching a movie, as sleep time.

Set a Silent Alarm

The Fitbit Flex vibrates and the center light flashes when a silent alarm goes off. You can set eight gently vibrating silent alarms on your Flex. Alarms can be set to recur every day or on specific days of the week. You can set up silent alarms from the Fitbit app and your computer on your Fitbit Dashboard. Simply go to fitbit.com, and then log in to your Fitbit account. Tap the settings icon that looks like a gear at the top right of the screen, and then tap Settings. In the settings you can choose your device, add an alarm, enter a time for the alarm, and then choose how often the alarm is to occur. Fitbit works with Android and Apple (iOS) phones. Visit fitbit.com for more information and to purchase a Fitbit device. You can also purchase Fitbit devices at a sporting goods or electronics retailer, or search the Internet.

Tap the Settings icon to set up alarms from your Fitbit Dashboard.

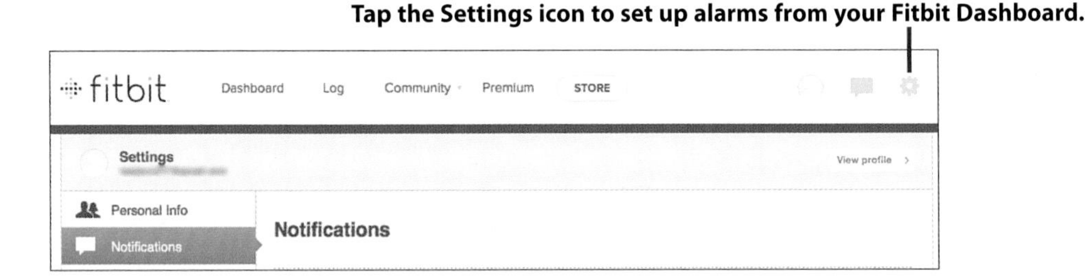

Improve Sleep Patterns with the Jawbone UP3 Tracker

All the Jawbone UP trackers track your sleep by monitoring micro movements to determine whether you are awake, in light sleep, or in deep sleep. The data is stored on the tracker and can be accessed by the UP app, which is available for Android phones and the iPhone. Multiple UP apps are available in the Google

Play Store and the App Store, so make sure you download the one for your device. The model each app accommodates is located next to the title.

The Jawbone app doesn't just provide an overall view of the quality of sleep you get each night—it gives you direction. The Smart Coach feature provides suggestions to maximize your sleep and improve the quality of your days. The UP app gathers information about you, your lifestyle, what you eat, and your activity level, and then uses those factors to provide tailored recommendations. It might suggest some better-known tips, such as keeping your bedroom dark and cool, as well as some lesser-known ones.

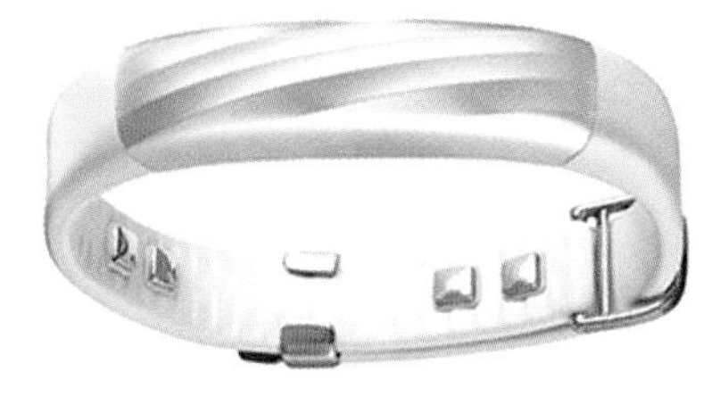

Jawbone UP3

Track Your Sleep Patterns

The Jawbone UP3 (as well as the UP2 and UP4) has Automatic Sleep Detection. It detects when you fall asleep at night and when you wake up in the morning. Your sleep data appears in a graph on the home screen of the UP app when you sync your tracker with the app. The UP3 and UP4 trackers recognize detailed sleep stages including REM (rapid eye movement), along with light- and deep-sleep stages. The UP3 also monitors passive heart rate (PHR) when your body is still for a more comprehensive view of your health. Talk with your doctor about what a healthy passive heart rate should be.

Download and set up your Jawbone UP account, and then use the following steps to access your sleep stats in the UP app. These examples are shown on an Android phone.

1. After your Jawbone has synced to the UP app, open the app, and then tap the purple sleep progress bar. The progress bar shows how long you slept and the percentage of your sleep goal you achieved. The default goal is 8 hours.
2. A summary of last night's sleep appears, including Deep Sleep, Light sleep, Fell asleep, REM Sleep, Awake for, and Wake up data.

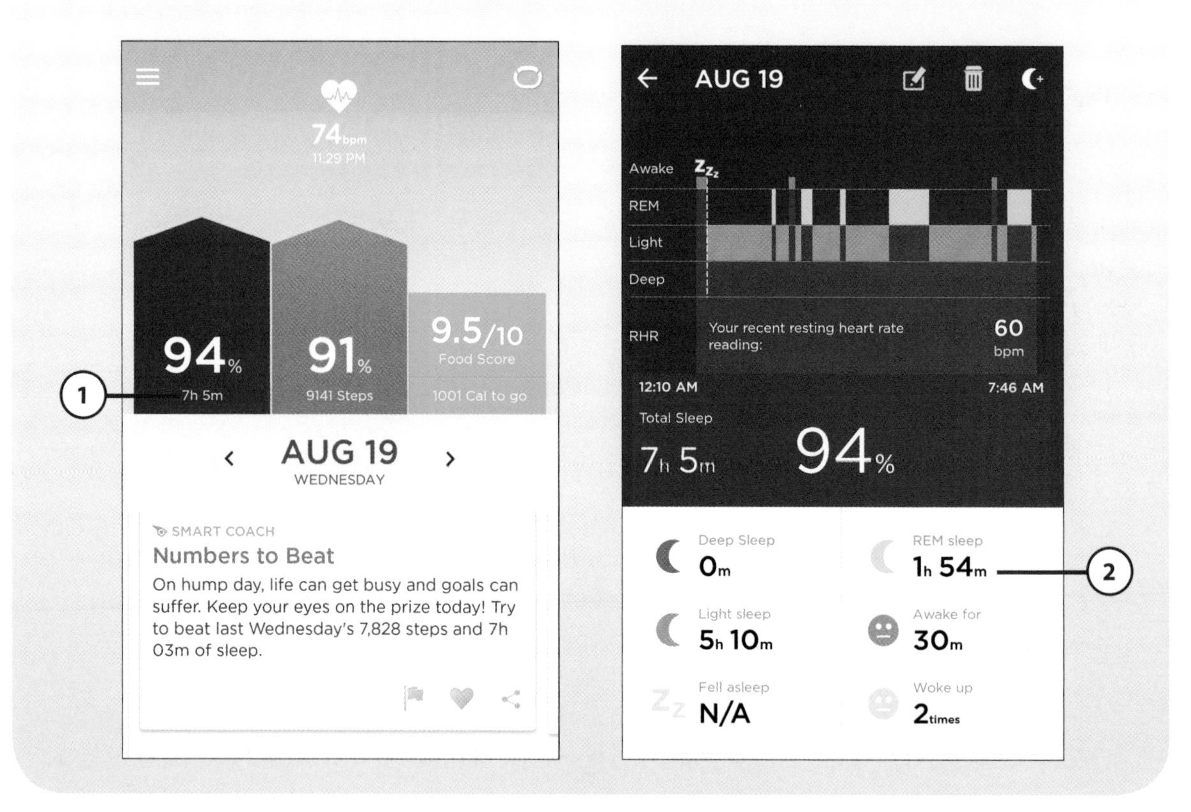

Track Sleep with the Microsoft Band 2

The Microsoft Band 2 can track your sleep, including length and quality of sleep, using motion sensors and your heart rate. You can track sleep with the Microsoft Band 2 in two ways: use the Sleep Tile, or let the band automatically detect when you're sleeping. A tile represents a set of features; for example, use a tile for tracking a run, a workout, or an incoming email message.

You might want to consider using the Sleep Tile instead of automatic detection for three reasons. First, as of this writing, notifications still come through during automatic sleep detection. You probably don't want to be woken up by a vibrating alert. Second, detection is activity-based. If you remain inactive for 2 hours, perhaps while reading a book or watching a movie, it will register as sleep. Lastly, automatic sleep detection does not provide sleep restoration analysis, which lets you know if you had sufficient and high quality sleep. You are the best judge of this, but just know that automatic detection mode does not provide this information.

Use the Sleep Tile Function

The Microsoft Band 2 starts to automatically detect your sleep after two hours of inactivity, even if you don't manually turn on sleep tracking. Follow these steps to use the Sleep Tile function to view summaries of your sleeping patterns.

1. Press the power button on your Band, and then swipe left until you see a tile with a crescent moon.
2. Tap the crescent moon icon.
3. Press the action button to start tracking your sleep, and then go to sleep.

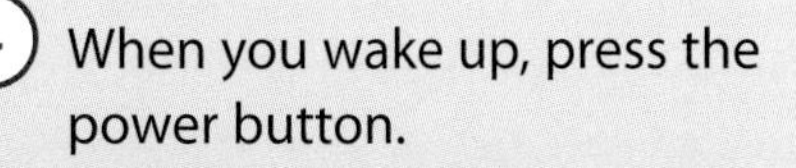

4. When you wake up, press the power button.
5. Press the action button when the Sleep screen appears.
6. Tap Yes to stop tracking your sleep (not shown).

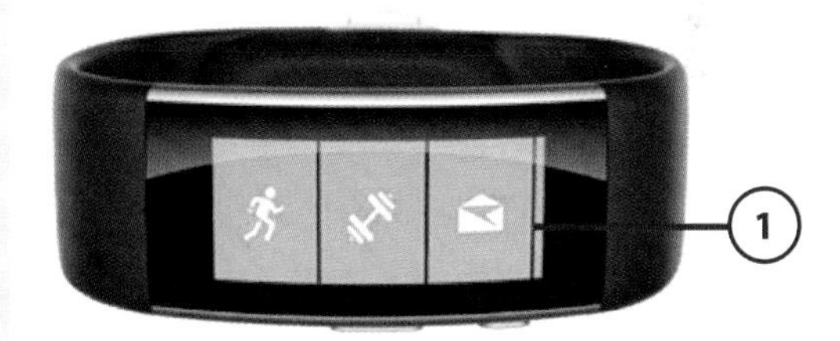

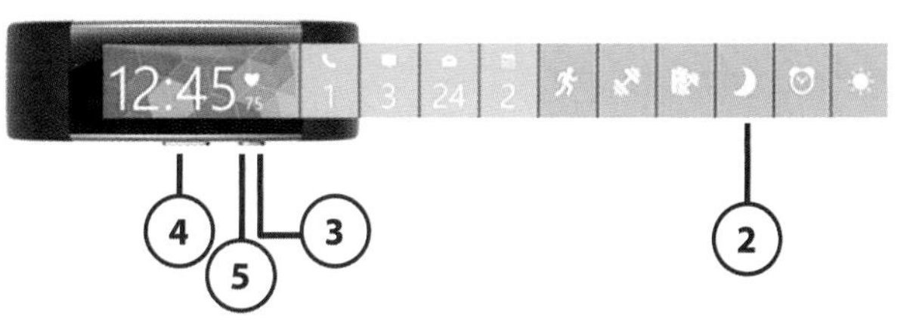

View Sleep Summaries

The Sleep Tile data shown on your Microsoft Band 2 includes the following information: Date, Length of sleep, Time in bed, Sleep efficiency, How many times you woke up, and even calories burned while you sleep. After you track your sleep, swipe the Sleep Tile to the left to view a summary. The free Microsoft Health app provides comprehensive summaries with graphs regarding your sleeping patterns. The graphs display the amount of restful sleep, light sleep, and resting heart rate. You can even view how long it took you to fall asleep and whether the overall quality of your sleep was good, using the Sleep Restoration feature. If you want to go into greater detail with your sleep summaries, use the online dashboard at dashboard.microsofthealth.com in your web browser. There you will find more explanations regarding your data and what it means. It also does sleep comparisons and sleep averages for the month. The Microsoft Health app is available for Windows Phones in the Windows Phone Store, the Google Play Store for Android phones, and the App Store for the iPhone.

Follow these steps to view your Sleep graph and the Heart Rate graph. This example is shown on an iPhone, but as of this writing, the procedure is the same on a Windows Phone.

1. With the Microsoft Health app open showing your sleep summary, tap the crescent moon icon to view your Sleep graph.
2. Tap the Heart Rate icon to view the Heart Rate graph.

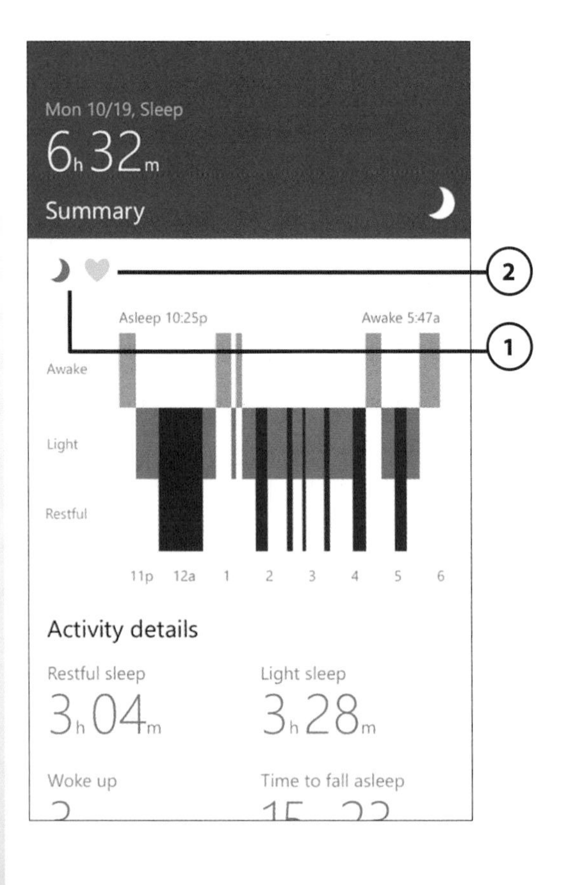

Setting a Smart Alarm

You can set a smart alarm on your Microsoft Band 2 to a daily wakeup time based on your body's natural sleep cycle. Whatever time you choose to wake up, the band monitors your wakefulness a half hour prior. The purpose is to wake you during a light sleep cycle so you can wake feeling your best, not groggy.

Tracking Your Sleep with Apps

There are many apps available that can help track and analyze your sleep. An app may be a good option if don't already have a fitness device that tracks sleep. You should consider, however, if you can safely plug in your phone and place the phone on your bed without causing a tripping hazard in the night, or if you need to receive incoming calls during the night. Consider some of these examples.

Monitor Sleep with the Sleep as Android App

The Sleep as Android app provides sleep-tracking capabilities for your phone, without the necessity of a fitness tracker, although it does work with Pebble, Android Wear, and Samsung Gear smartwatches. We'll be exploring its capabilities using your phone as the tracking device to collect sleep cycle information. The app can send you bedtime notifications, at which time you can use nature sounds to help you fall asleep faster. Then the app can detect and record snoring or talking in your sleep and use a vibration or sound to make you stop. The app also provides sleep deficit stats. The Sleep as Android app has a smart wake-up feature that gets you up in the morning during an optimal sleep phase, so you wake feeling refreshed. Wake up with a gentle alarm, nature sounds playlists, an online radio alarm, or by light. Sleep as Android integrates with Phillips Hue smart bulbs that include features such as a Sunrise-like wake-up, night light, and lucid dreaming cue. The app is chock-full of sleep advice so that you can improve your sleep quality.

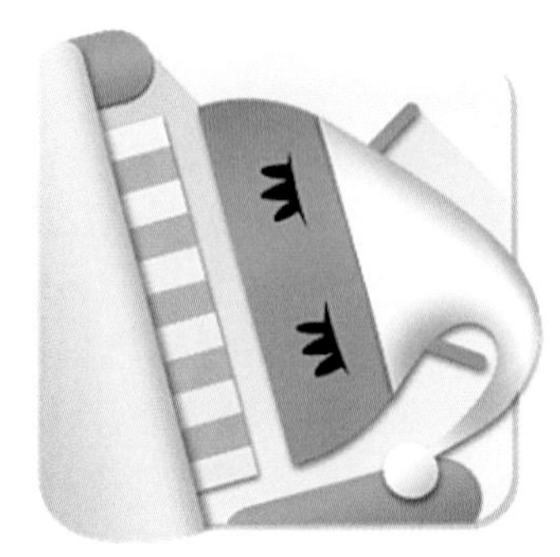

Sleep as Android app

Smart Wake Up

Within a 30-minute window prior to the alarm time you set, the app detects how much you move, and then gently wakes you in a period of light sleep. (More movement is assessed as light sleep.) This period can be set from anywhere between 5 minutes and 50 minutes. For example, if you set the alarm in the app to 7:30 a.m. and choose a smart period of 30 minutes, the alarm goes off between 7 a.m. and 7:30 a.m. during a light sleep, so you don't feel groggy.

Track Your Sleep Cycle and Use the Smart Alarm Clock

When you search for Sleep as Android on the Google Play Store, you will see two versions: a paid Sleep as Android Unlock and a free Sleep as Android version. The Sleep as Android version is a 14-day trial version. Consider downloading the free version to see how you like the app. If you like it, you'll be given the option to upgrade to the paid version. As of this writing Sleep as Android Unlock is not a subscription service, but a license; you just pay the one-time fee.

Download the app from the Google Play Store, and follow these directions to set up the app for tracking your sleep.

1. Open the Sleep as Android app, and tap the plus icon in the upper-right corner of the screen to set up your alarm.
2. Drag the hour and minute hands to set the clock, and then tap to choose AM or PM.
3. Tap Set. A screen opens that lets you further configure the alarm, including setting the occurrence, ringtone, bedtime notification, and more.

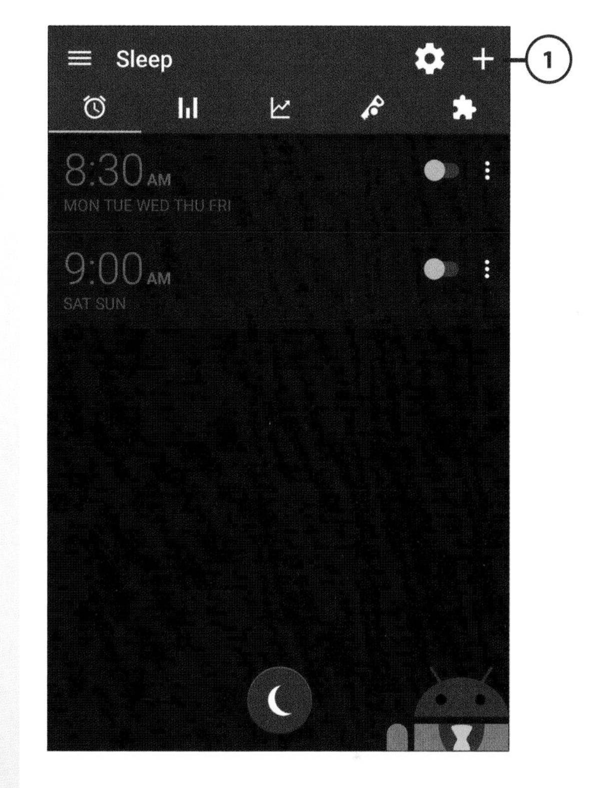

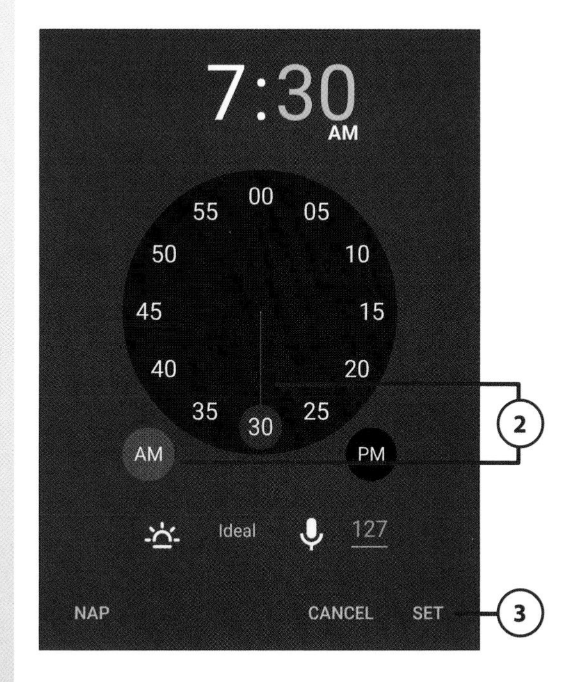

Put Your Phone in Airplane Mode

It is recommended that you turn off your phone's wireless functions by putting it into Airplane mode before you start tracking your sleep. You can do this by dragging down from the very top of the screen to open your phone's settings. Find the icon that looks like an airplane and tap it to deactivate all cellular and Wi-Fi signals. Don't forget to disable Airplane mode when you wake. Keep in mind that you won't be able to receive or make any emergency calls or texts while in Airplane mode. Take this under consideration when deciding whether to use this app.

4. Swipe to scroll down, and then tap Smart Period and tap a window of time, during which the app will wake you at the optimal moment.
5. Tap Done. The Home screen appears.
6. Tap the crescent moon button to start tracking your sleep.

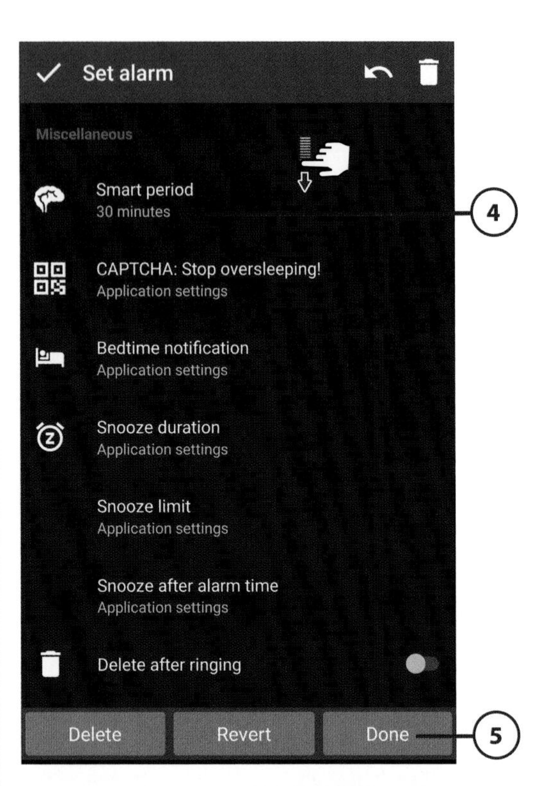

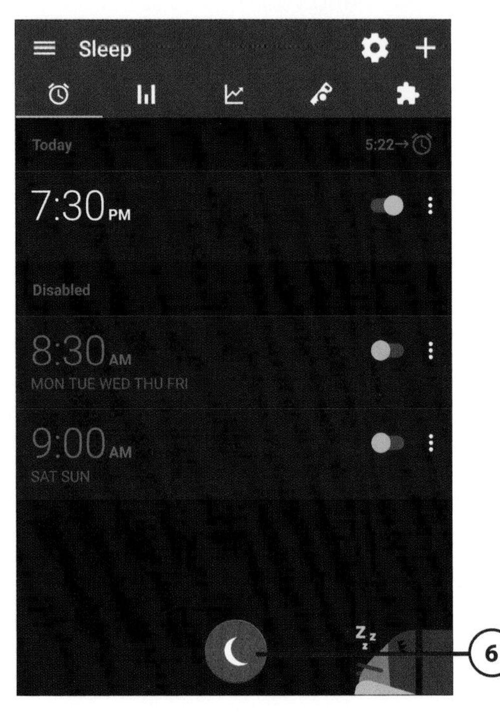

7. Place your phone on the mattress near your body so the app can use sensors in your phone to sense your movement and wake you at the optimal time. After you dismiss the alarm in the morning, you will see your sleep phases, percent of deep sleep, and more.

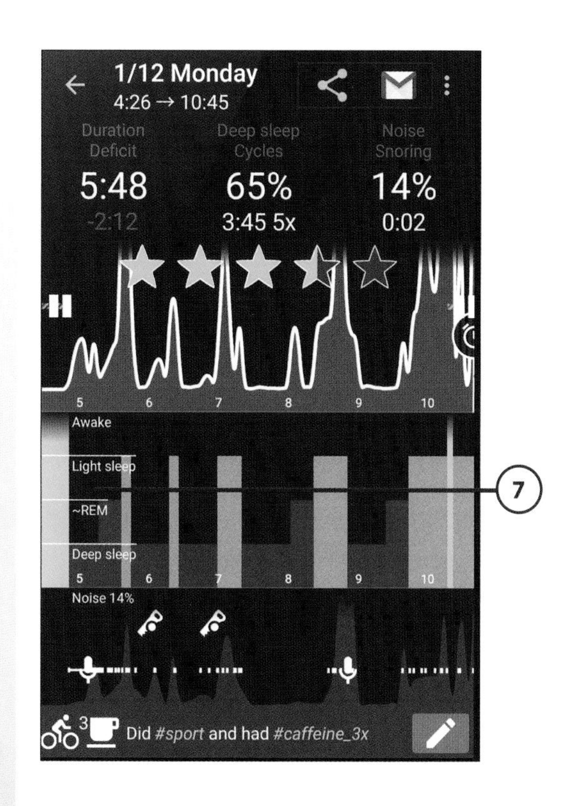

Accuracy with More Than One Person Per Bed

If you share a bed with someone else, the data collected might not be as accurate. The recommendation is to keep your phone very close to your body for the best results, or even use a sport armband in this situation.

Use SleepBot to Get the Sleep You Need

SleepBot is another capable, free app that is a smart motion tracker and sound recorder, available for both Android and Apple (iOS) devices. You can use SleepBot as a simple time log or a comprehensive tracker for sleep. The app supplies you with a detailed sleep history including Wake, Light, and Deep sleep stages. SleepBot also documents variables that might otherwise be overlooked when reviewing sleep quality, such as sounds that might wake you. This app also incorporates a smart alarm that will wake up at the right time, according to your sleep stages, so you feel refreshed instead of groggy. You can also track the amount of hours you slept in comparison to the recommended hours of sleep you need with a feature called Sleep Debt.

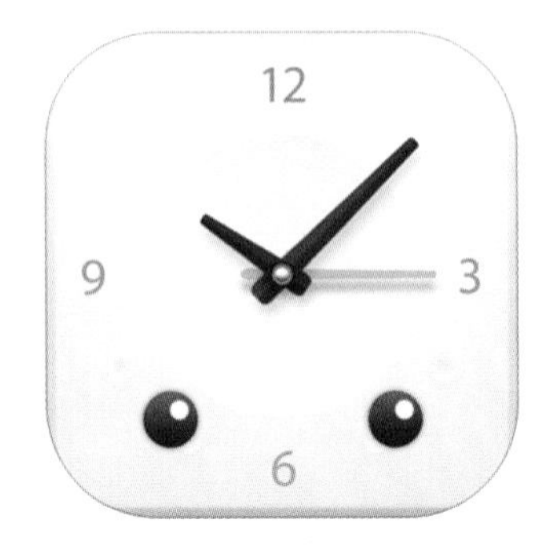

SleepBot app

Improve Your Sleep Quality by Tracking Your Sleep

If you're looking for recommendations and tips on how to improve your sleeping patterns and get a better night's sleep, SleepBot provides actionable items for you to implement right away. The SleepBot interface is intuitive, and it's easy to get started tracking your sleep.

Follow these steps to start tracking your sleep after you download the app. The following examples are shown on an iPhone.

1. Open the SleepBot app, and tap the Home button.
2. Tap the Smart Alarm icon that looks like an alarm clock in the upper-left corner of the screen. The New Alarm screen opens.
3. Swipe up and down to use the scroll wheels to set the time you want to wake up in the morning.

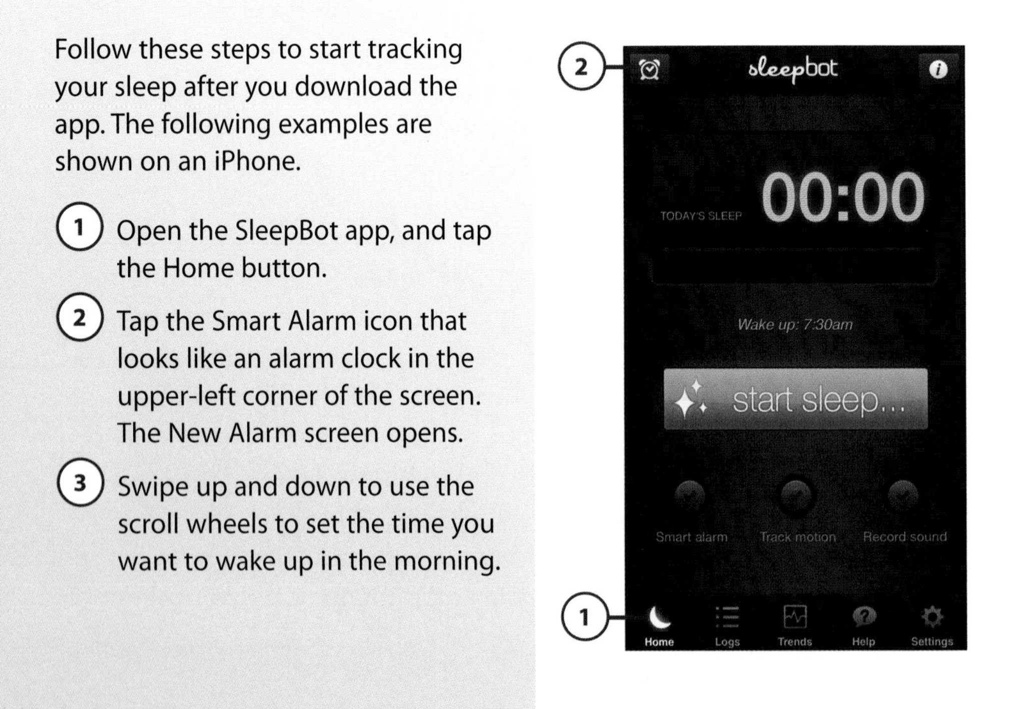

Understanding the Smart Alarm Feature

You can set a smart alarm using the SleepBot app to use a wakeup time based on your body's sleep cycle. Within a 30-minute window prior to the alarm time you set, SleepBot chooses a time to wake you by assessing your wakefulness. For example, if you set the alarm in the app to 7:30 a.m., the alarm will go off between 7:00 and 7:30 a.m. when it assesses you are in a light sleep, so you don't feel groggy.

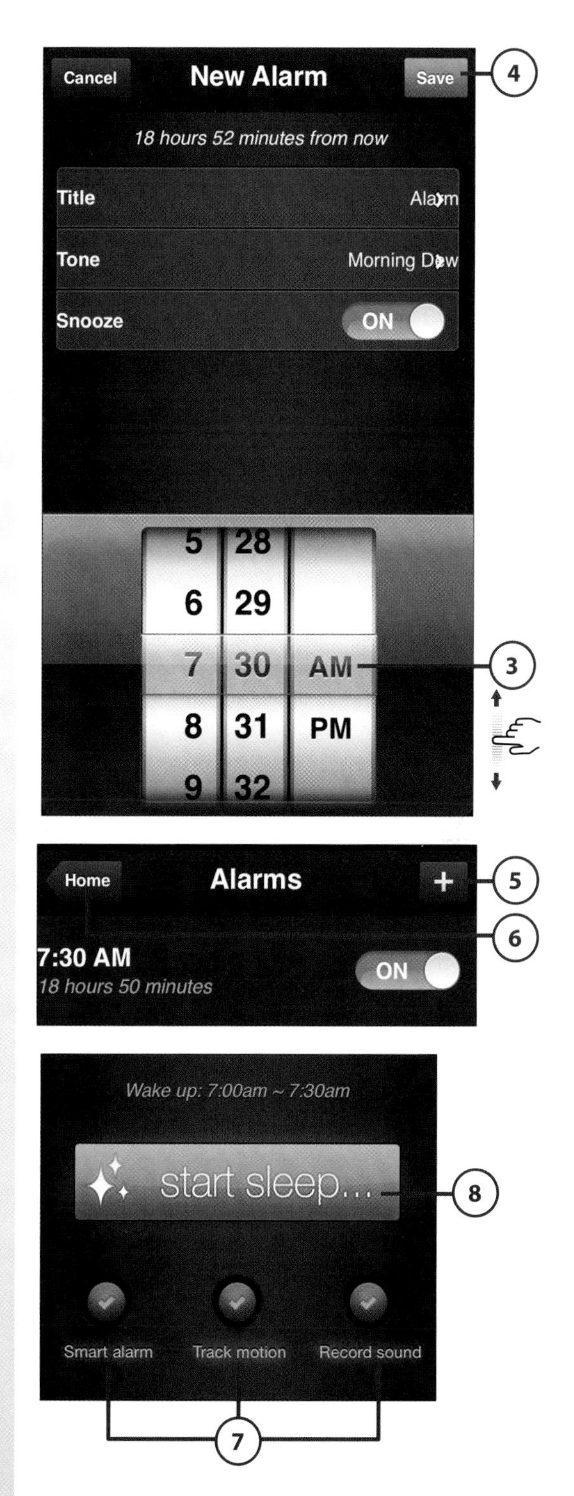

4. Tap Save. A screen listing your alarm displays.
5. If needed, tap the plus sign in the upper-right corner to create additional alarms.
6. Tap Home to return to the Home screen.
7. Choose the options for how you want to track your sleep. You must set a smart alarm first to select the option.
8. Tap Start Sleep to begin tracking your sleep. Your phone will automatically be silenced, turned on Airplane mode, and will turn off music.

Understanding Options for Tracking Motion and Sound

The Track motion option uses the accelerometer in your phone to track your movements throughout the night. Make sure to plug in your phone overnight and don't press the Home or Off/On button on your phone. The accelerometer only works when the display is on. Turn your phone face down next to you on the bed. The Record sound option records snoring, sleepwalking, and other noises, such as a dog barking. You'll be able to play any sounds recorded back when you access your sleep summary.

Airplane Mode and Emergencies

You won't be able to receive or make any emergency calls or texts while in Airplane mode. Take this under consideration when deciding whether to use this app.

9. Place the phone face down, close to your head so that it can record any snoring. If there is more than one person in the bed, SleepBot will still work as long as you have it close to you.
10. When your alarm sounds in the morning, the app exits sleep mode.

Customize SleepBot Settings

SleepBot makes it easy for you to customize settings to match your lifestyle and to tweak your sleep tracking experience. You can change your optimal sleep time from the default 8 hours to more or less time, modify motion and sound sensitivity, change your snooze length, and much more.

1. Tap Settings. The Settings menu opens.
2. Tap in a field to change the General settings. You can tap Ambient noise to the On position and choose different sounds to help you fall to sleep.
3. Tap an option in the Backup Sync field to view the date and time when your sleep data was backed up to mysleepbot.com. You can also choose to sync recorded audio files to mysleepbot.com. Later you'll see how to play back recorded sounds.
4. Tap an option in the Sensors field to tweak motion and sound sensitivity.
5. Swipe to scroll down to view the SleepBot version and rate the app on the App Store.

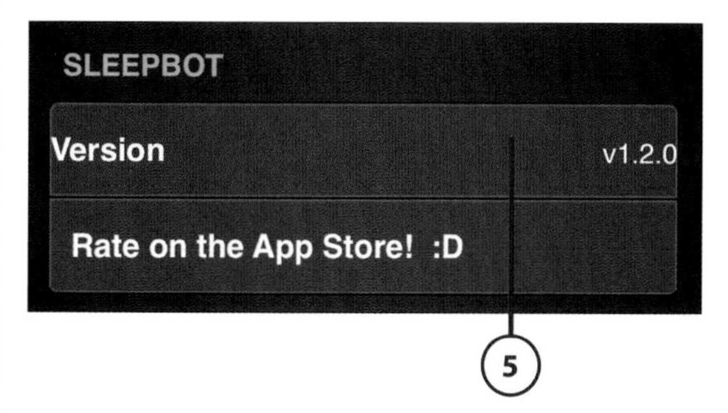

View and Share Your Stats Online and from Your Phone

You can view your sleep stats online as well as on your mobile app. Just visit mysleepbot.com and log in to view your synced data.

Included in your detailed sleep history are sound levels. For example, the neighbor's dog barking in the middle of the night might wake you. Including environmental factors such as this gives you a more detailed history of not just how you sleep, but why you might have fluctuated between Light and Wake stages between 1 and 2 o'clock in the morning. Sounds are graphed as Silent, Quiet, or Loud.

The SleepBot application also includes a sleep Debt Tracker. The National Sleep Foundation recommends that adults and older adults get between seven to nine hours of sleep. When you sleep less than the recommended amount, you accrue sleep debt. For example, if you need seven hours of sleep and you only sleep five, you've accumulated two hours of sleep debt, which starts to add up. SleepBot's Debt Tracker helps track how much sleep you owe yourself over a 10-day period.

Your sleep logs show you how pattern changes affect you in the long term. Your sleep trends enable you to identify positive and negative factors in your long-term sleep analyses. SleepBot also provides actionable information such as tips that help you form good sleeping habits.

Follow these steps to view your sleep data and share it using mail and social networks from the SleepBot app.

1. Tap Logs to view sleeping information including the Date, Sleep, Wake Hours, and Debt.
2. Tap Trends to view graphs of sleep patterns for the past 10 days, Sleep Debt, Shortest Nap, and Longest Sleep.
3. Tap the Share button to share your summaries with family, friends, or a caregiver by email or post to one of your social networks such as a Twitter account.

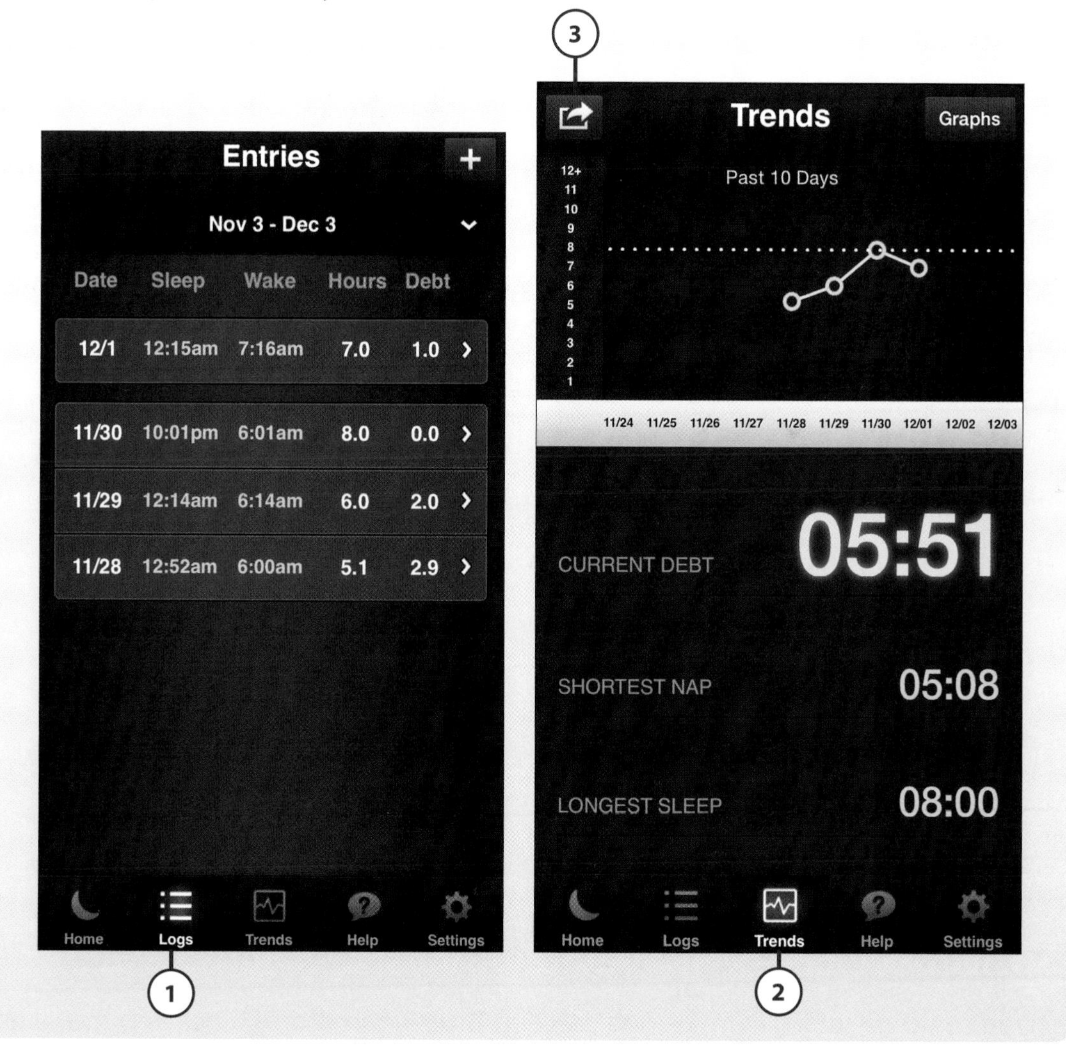
3
Entries
+
Nov 3 - Dec 3
Date Sleep Wake Hours Debt
12/1 12:15am 7:16am 7.0 1.0
11/30 10:01pm 6:01am 8.0 0.0
11/29 12:14am 6:14am 6.0 2.0
11/28 12:52am 6:00am 5.1 2.9
Home Logs Trends Help Settings
1
Trends
Graphs
Past 10 Days
12+ 11 10 9 8 7 6 5 4 3 2 1
11/24 11/25 11/26 11/27 11/28 11/29 11/30 12/01 12/02 12/03
CURRENT DEBT 05:51
SHORTEST NAP 05:08
LONGEST SLEEP 08:00
Home Logs Trends Help Settings
2

Understand Your Sleep with the Sleep Time Smart Alarm Clock App

The Sleep Time Smart Alarm Clock is another app dedicated to waking you up in the morning feeling fully rested. Using the accelerometer in your phone to detect movement during the night, along with some advanced programming behind the scenes, this app can determine which phase of sleep you're in and set off an alarm at just the right moment so you don't wake up groggy. By tracking your level of movement throughout sleep, Sleep Time Smart Alarm Clock generates customized sleep data in easy-to-read charts so you can access your full sleep history and identify sleep trends easily. The Sleep Time Smart Alarm Clock app also includes soundscapes to help you fall asleep faster.

The Sleep Time Smart Alarm Clock app is available for Android phones, the iPhone, and Windows Phones. As of this writing, if you search for this app, the App Store has a paid and a free version, whereas the Google Play Store has just a free version. The free version for Android has to be upgraded to the Pro version for you to access its full feature set. Regardless of which phone you have, try out the free version to see how you like it. The following examples are shown on an Android phone.

Sleep Time Smart Alarm Clock app

Set Alarms and Measure Your Nighttime Sleep Movements

You can set a smart alarm using the Sleep Time Smart Alarm Clock app to wake you up based on your body's natural sleep cycle. Within a ten- to thirty-minute window prior to the alarm time you set, Sleep Time wakes you up during your lightest sleep phase. For example, if you set the alarm in the app to 7:30 a.m., the alarm will go off between 7:00 a.m. and 7:30 a.m. when you are in a state of light sleep, which is assessed by your increased movement, so you don't feel groggy.

Because the Sleep Time Smart Alarm Clock app uses the motion sensors in your phone, like the other smartphone-based sleep trackers, your phone needs to be physically close to you in bed. Lay your phone face down and the display will turn off automatically. Azumio, the developers of this app, say that sleeping in the same bed with a partner or pet might disturb readings. For the most accurate readings in this scenario, Azumio instructs you to keep your phone isolated on your side of the bed.

Download the Sleep Time Smart Alarm Clock app, sign up, and then follow these steps to set smart alarms and begin tracking your sleep through your level of movement.

1. Open the Sleep Time Smart Alarm Clock app, and tap Alarm.
2. Drag the Set button until the clock shows the time you want to set for your alarm in the morning. The alarm can be set no more than 12 hours in advance.
3. Tap the Settings icon that looks like a gear in the upper-left corner to customize settings.

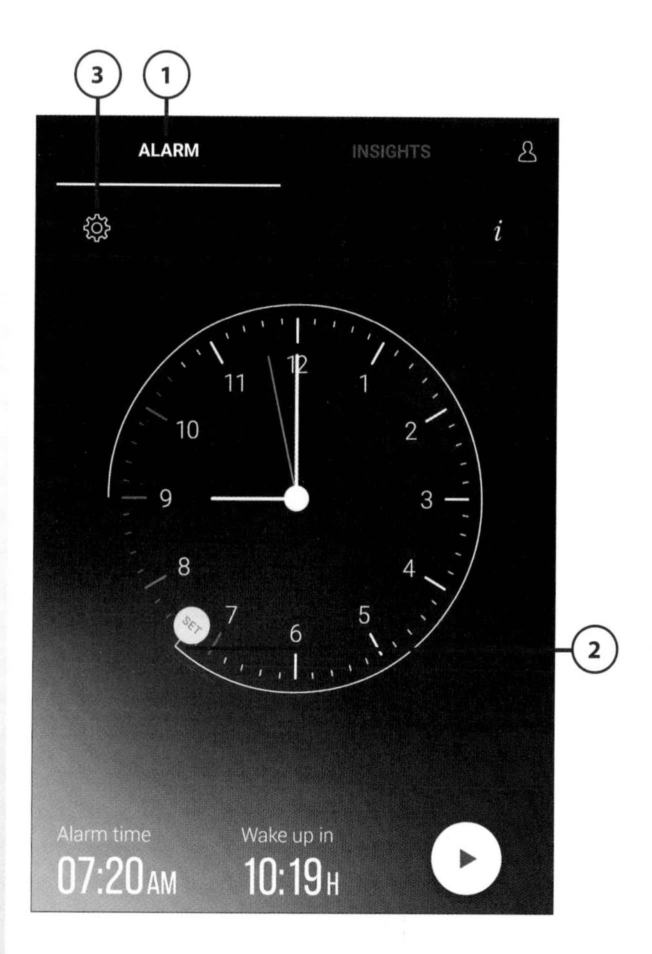

4. In the Settings, you can adjust your wake-up phase from 10 to 30 minutes, turn on a silent vibrating alarm, adjust snooze settings, and more.
5. Tap the arrow to return to the previous screen.
6. Tap Insights after a night of sleep to view your sleep summary.
7. Tap to start recording your sleep. A tip appears.

Sleep Time Settings
GENERAL
Wake up phase 30 min
Ringtone Morning Dew
Vibrate
RINGER
SNOOZE
Snooze
Auto

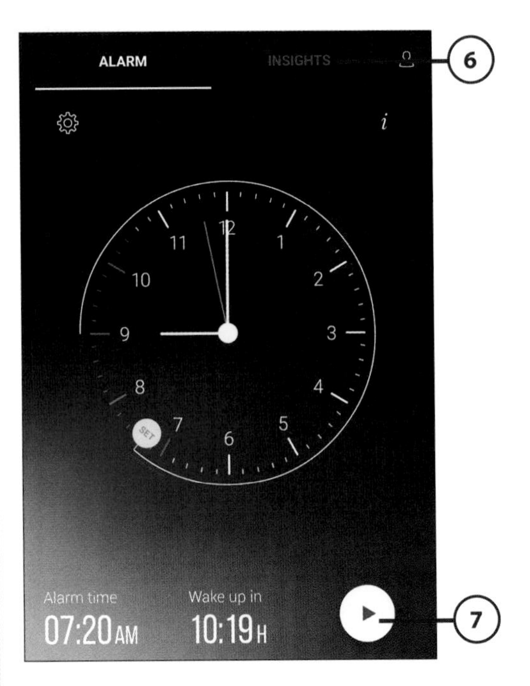

8. Tap OK, Got It, and then place the phone on your bed face down. The display will turn off automatically.

9. When the alarm goes off, press the Hold to Stop button at the bottom of the screen. A countdown appears and then the app exits sleep mode. A summary of your sleep appears.

Using the Snooze Setting

Pick up the phone in the morning when the smart alarm goes off to stop the alarm and use the 10-minute snooze. You can turn it off in the Settings.

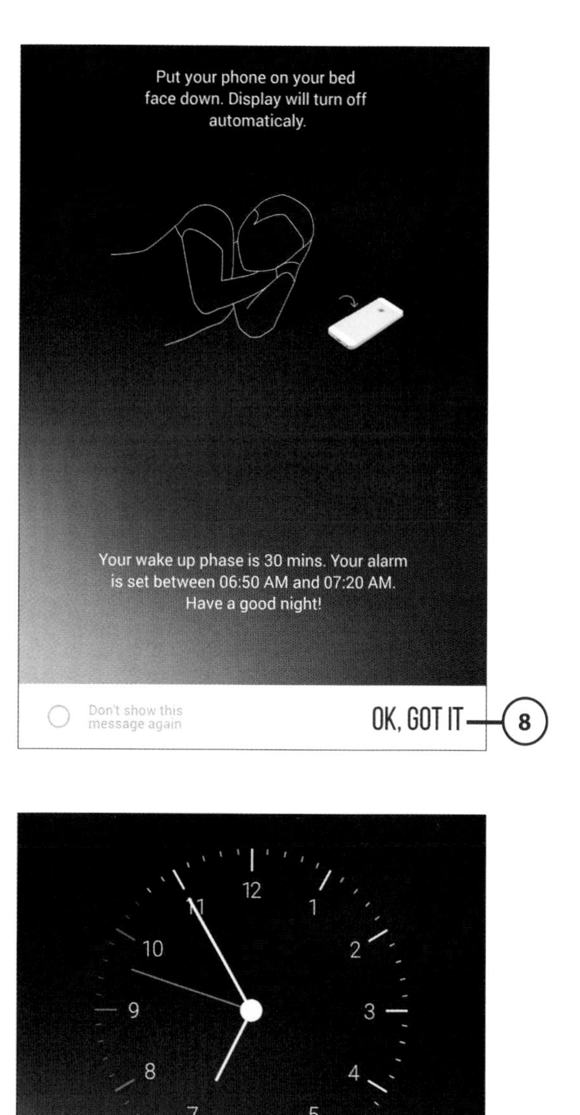

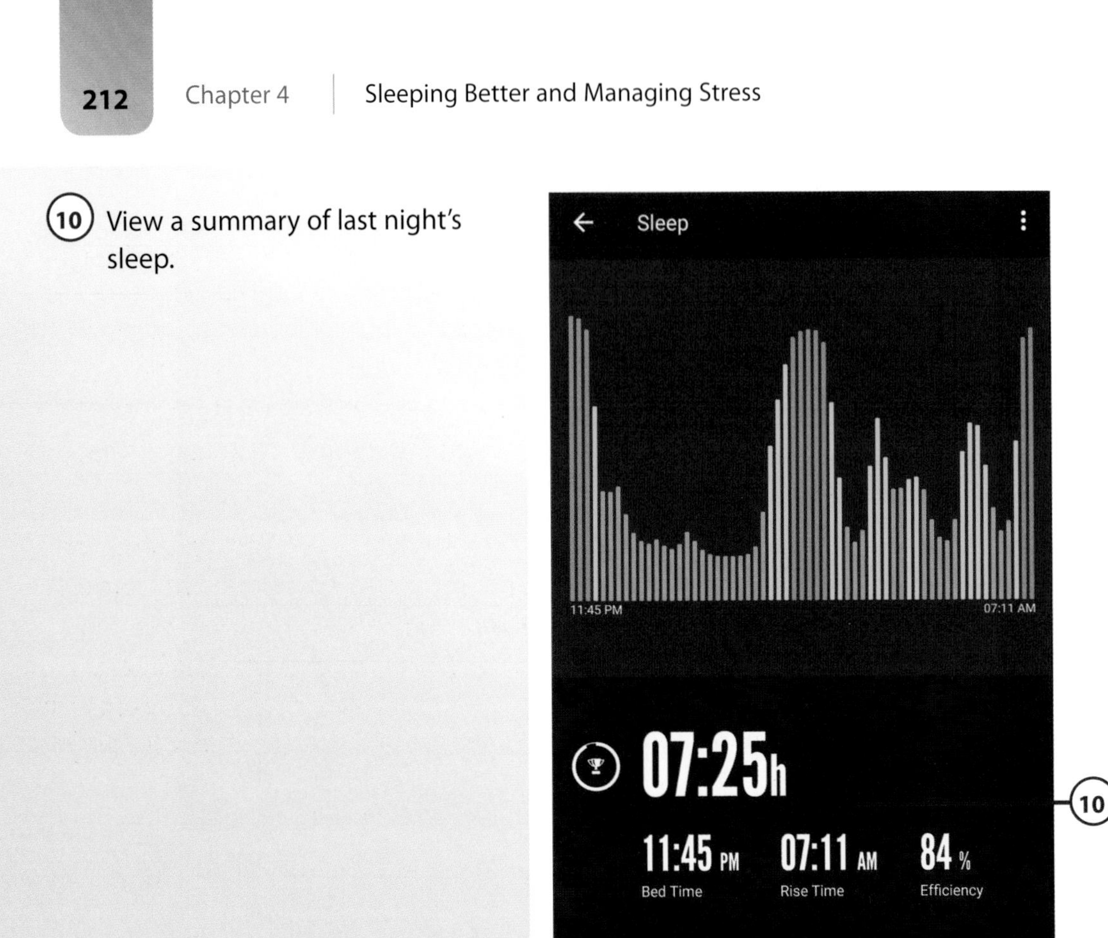

Using Apps to Help Relax and Fall Sleep

Bedtime is not the only time you might want to relax or have some peaceful time. Many apps for your smartphone are available that are large audio libraries for ambient sounds that help you to relax. You can choose from sounds such as soft rain, the ocean, calm stream, campfire, and many more. Sounds for meditation, yoga, and sleep can help promote a relaxing environment whether you are at work, reading a book in the living room, or decompressing for bed. This section introduces you to the Ambience, Relax Melodies, and Sleep Pillow Sounds apps, which can help you feel more positive and optimistic by showing you how to keep a gratitude journal, and use guided meditation, including techniques for mindfulness.

Use the Ambience App to Pick Relaxing Sounds

The Ambiance app offers a large library of soundscapes created for you to find the "perfect ambient atmosphere to focus, relax, and reminisce." It offers more than 3,500 free sounds to download, and you can create your own sound mixes as well as your own playlists. You can also set sounds as alarms so that you can wake to a pleasant soundscape such as Spring in the Countryside or Pacific Ocean Surf. You'll find sounds from an oscillating fan to French cafés, and binaural beats to Australian tree frogs.

The Ambience app is available for both Android and Apple (iOS) devices and for Mac and PC desktop computers. If you are an iPhone user, there is a paid version, and a free Lite version in the App Store. Try the Lite version to see whether you like the app. Only a paid version is currently offered for Android devices in the Google Play Store. As of this writing, the desktop version has a free two-week trial period, and then you must upgrade to continue to use Ambiance. The following examples are shown on an iPhone.

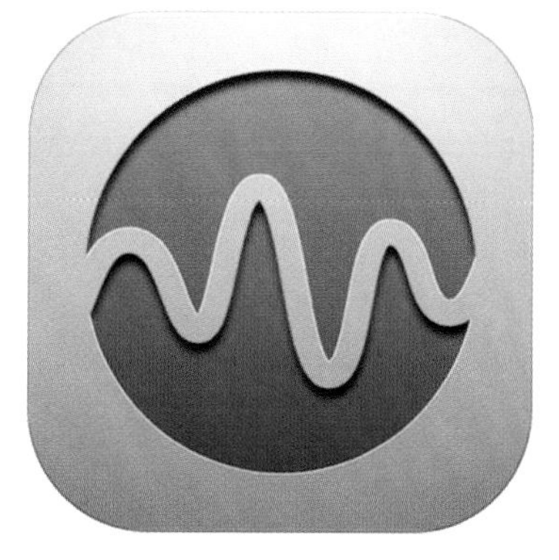

The Ambience Lite app

Selecting sounds from the Ambience Store in the app is easy, making it possible for you to incorporate relaxation time into your day when and where you can. You can preview sounds before you download them to your personal library so you know exactly what you're getting. All the soundscapes in Ambiance discretely loop, so there is no stop and start required after you download a file.

If you need a little extra help falling asleep at night, the Ambiance app is designed to help you do that. Browse the store, preview sounds, download sounds, and play sounds before you go to bed. You can even set a timer to let Ambiance know when to stop playback so you don't have to do it manually. Download the Ambience app, and then follow these instructions to pick relaxing sounds to help you get to sleep.

1. Open the Ambiance app, and tap Store on the main screen. The Store opens as a list of categories.
2. Scroll down the page and tap a category.

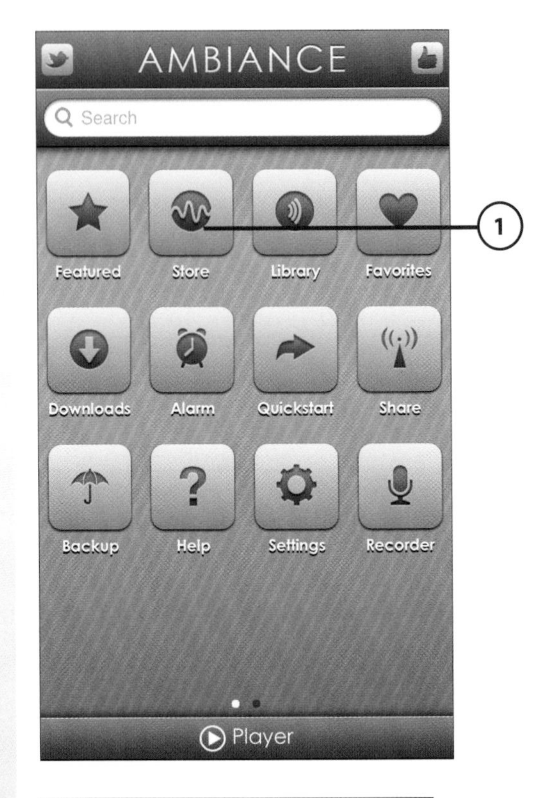

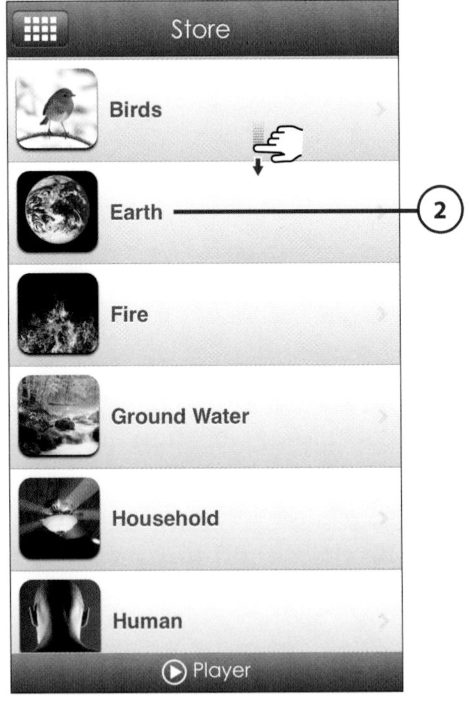

3. Filter the options by tapping a tab at the top of the screen.
4. Tap a sound.
5. Read the description, and then tap Preview to listen to a preview of the sound.
6. Tap Download to download the sound to your library. A message appears asking whether you are sure you want to download the sounds.
7. Tap Download again. The sound downloads to your library.

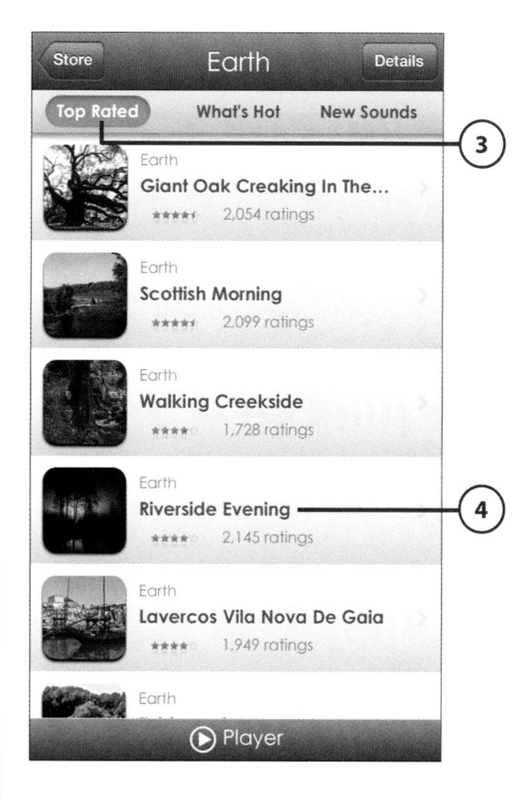

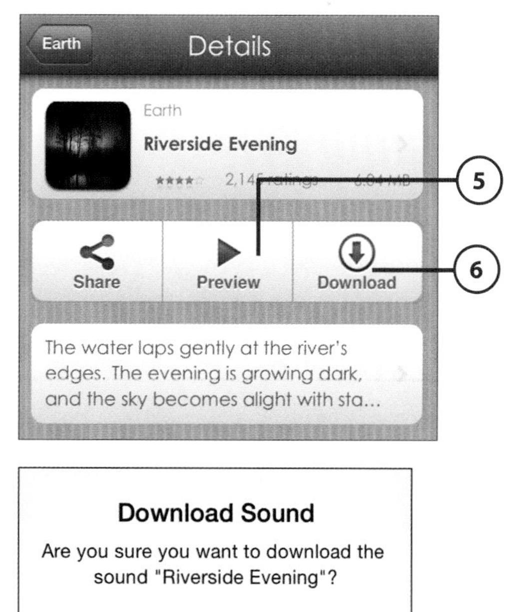

8. Keep tapping the buttons that appear in the upper-left corner to get back to the main screen.
9. Tap Library. The category from which you downloaded the sound now appears.
10. Tap the category.

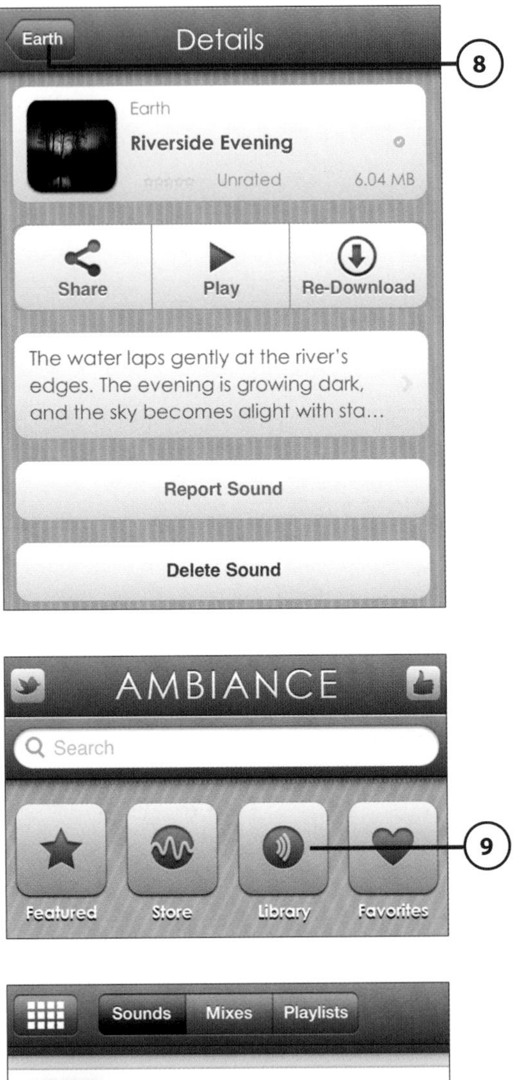

Re-Download
The water laps gently at the river's edges. The evening is growing dark, and the sky becomes alight with sta...
Report Sound
Delete Sound

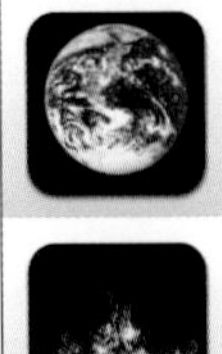
Sounds
Mixes
Playlists
Earth
Riverside Evening
1 Downloaded Sound
10
Fire
1 Downloaded Sound
Ocean
5 Downloaded Sounds

(11) Tap the Play button. The sound begins to play and opens full screen.

(12) Tap the Timer icon that looks like an alarm clock to set the duration for the sound to play.

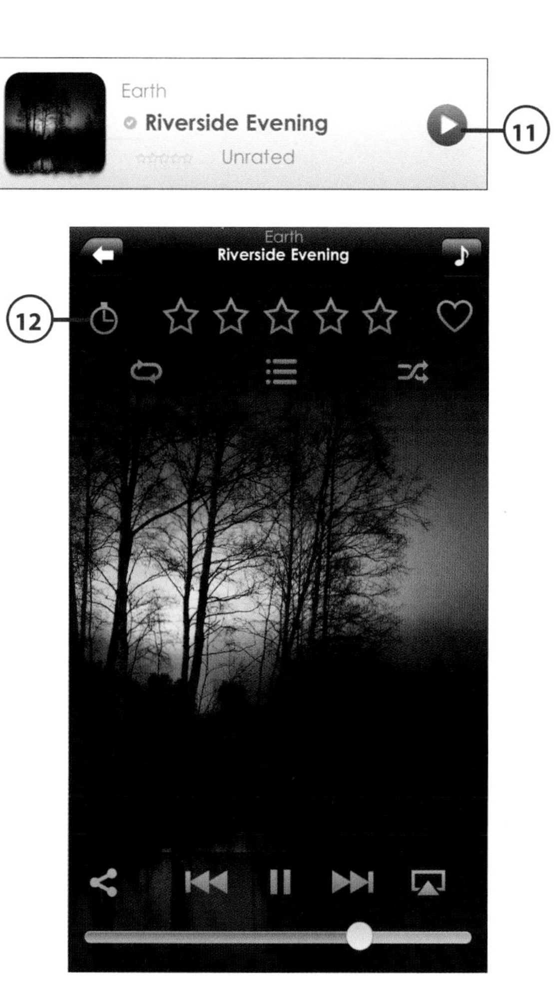

Get to Sleep Faster with the Relax Melodies App's Zen Sounds and Melodies

Relax Melodies is another great resource for sleep, yoga, meditation, and concentration. Its core benefit is to give you the power to mix your own sounds and music to personalize your experience. Here's how it works. Simply combine sounds and melodies to create a mix that you can use to fall asleep faster, use during a yoga session, and whenever you need to relax. The power of this app is in its customization. You can even combine music from your own music collection on your smartphone. If you like the thought of creating your own unique soundscape, give Relax Melodies a try.

As of this writing, this app is available in a free version and a Pro version for Android phones, the iPhone, and Windows Phones. Try out the free version just to see how you like the experience. The following examples are shown on an Android Phone.

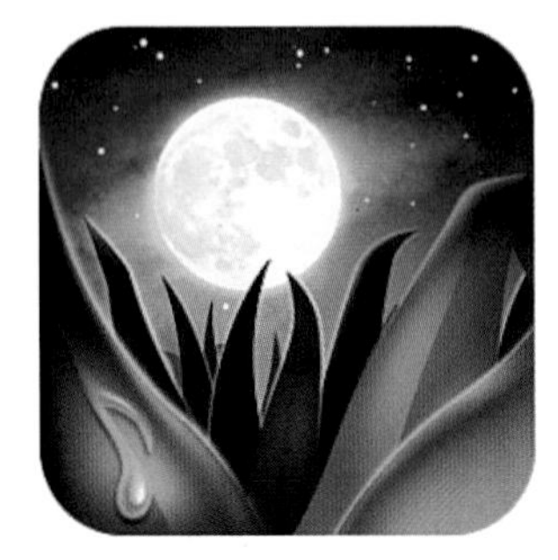

Relax Melodies

The Relax Melodies: Sleep and Yoga app offers 52 sounds and melodies that you can select one by one by tapping. Each sound gently intertwines with the next, creating a relaxing melody. Add your own music to create a playlist and save it for later. Selecting the sounds and melodies for your mix is a simple and cathartic process.

Download the app, and then follow these steps to create a truly unique relaxation experience.

1. Open the Relax Melodies app, and swipe the screen left or right to view collections of sounds and melodies. If you are using the free version, some tiles on a screen have a lock icon on them, so you have to upgrade to use them.
2. Tap a sound to hear it. The sound highlights as it begins to play, and the tile is highlighted while swaying from left to right.

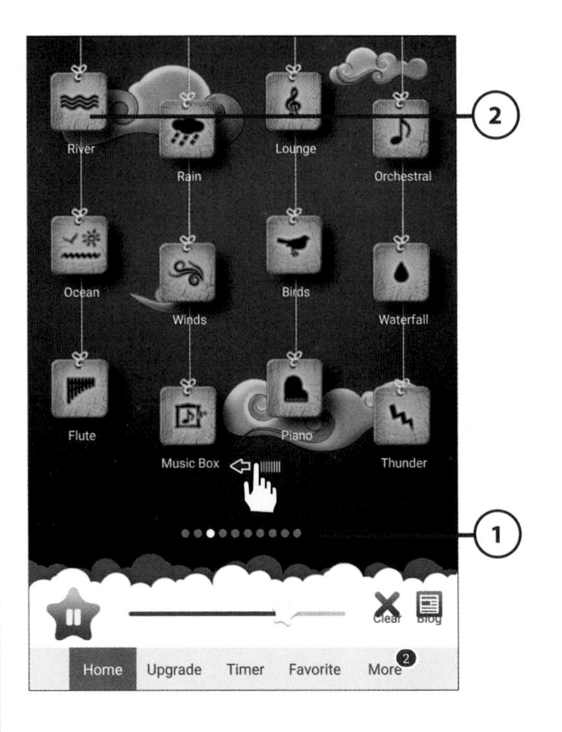

3. Tap another sound to add to the first sound.
4. Tap another sound to add to the previous two. All sounds mix together, creating a unique soundscape. If you don't like a particular mix, tap on a tile again to deselect the sound and end it.
5. Tap Timer to select the duration for the mix. If it typically takes you 30 minutes to fall asleep, you can set it to 30 minutes.
6. Tap Favorite to save this mix.
7. Tap the Add button that looks like a plus sign in the upper-right corner of the screen.

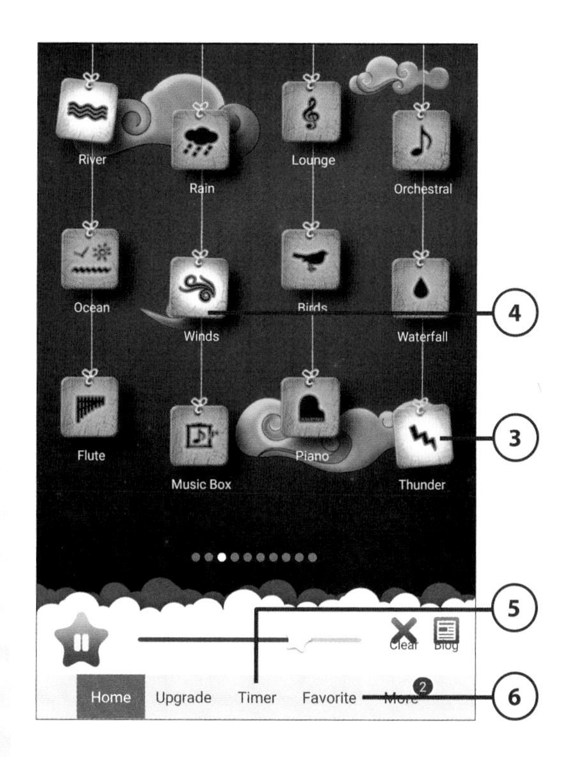

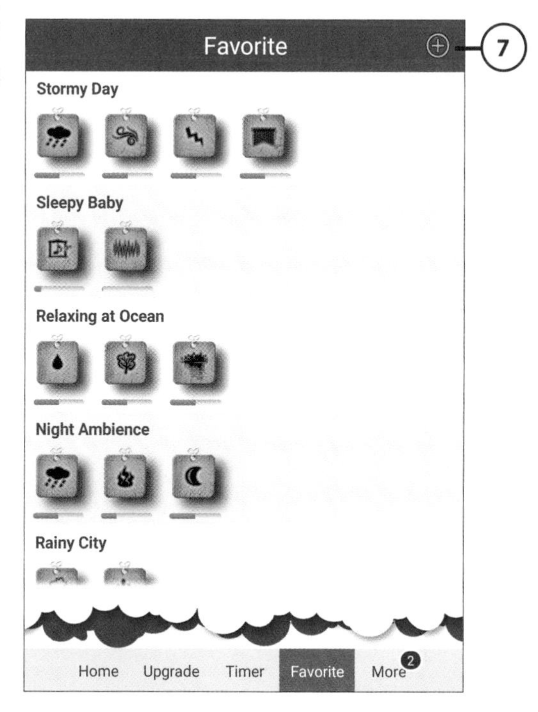

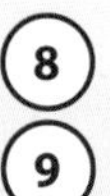

8. Type in the name for this mix.
9. Tap Save.
10. The soundscape you have created now appears in your list of favorites.

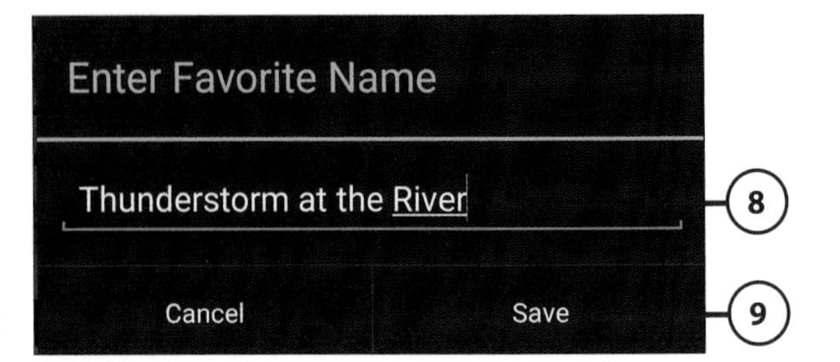

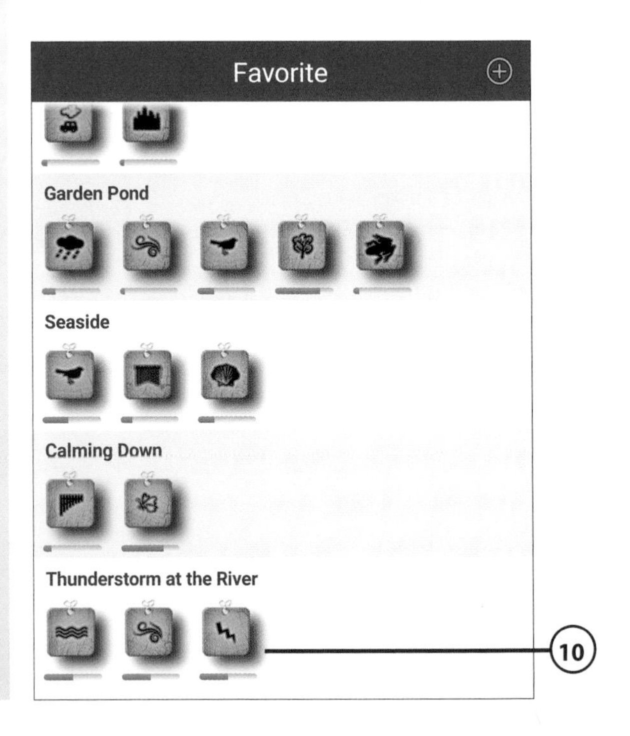

Make Relaxing Soundscapes with the Sleep Pillow Sounds App

If you like the idea of creating your own soundscapes, the Sleep Pillow Sounds app is another great option to consider. This app provides 70 naturally recorded sounds, each premastered and high quality, with up to 300,000 combinations of possible sound mixes. You'll find sounds ranging from beach waves and birds, to quiet city traffic; you can choose from whale songs to an outside bonfire. Sleep Pillow Sounds also has a sleep timer with a slow fade-out to get you to sleep and an alarm clock with a slow fade-in to get you up in the morning.

As of this writing, this app is available for the iPhone, iPod, and iPad. As of this writing, the version in the App Store is free, but you can use the upgrade option within the app to unlock all the app's features. The following examples are shown on an iPhone.

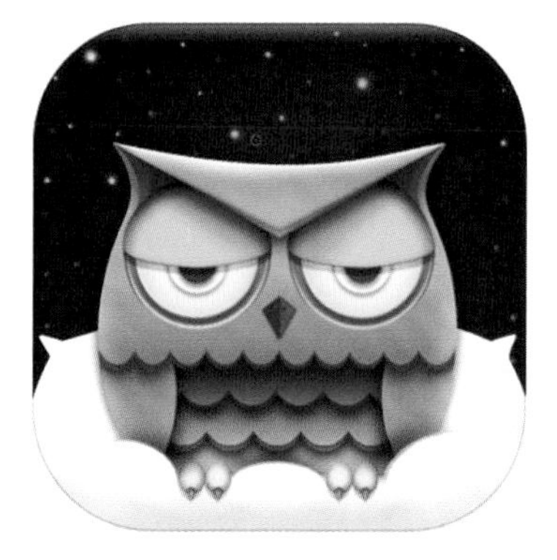

Sleep Pillow Sounds app

The Sleep Pillow Sounds app has an intuitive interface that lets you easily preview and select sounds and create mixes that can help you get to sleep faster. Creating a unique and relaxing soundscape takes only a few simple steps.

Follow these steps to select ambient sounds and create mixes.

1. Open the Sleep Pillow Sounds app, and swipe the screen to the left to see all the available sounds.
2. Tap a sound to play it. You can tap it again to end playback.
3. Tap the heart in the upper-right corner of a sound to add it to your favorites list.
4. Drag the slider to adjust the volume up or down.
5. Tap Mixes. The Mixes screen opens.
6. Tap the square icon that has a pencil in it to start creating a mix.

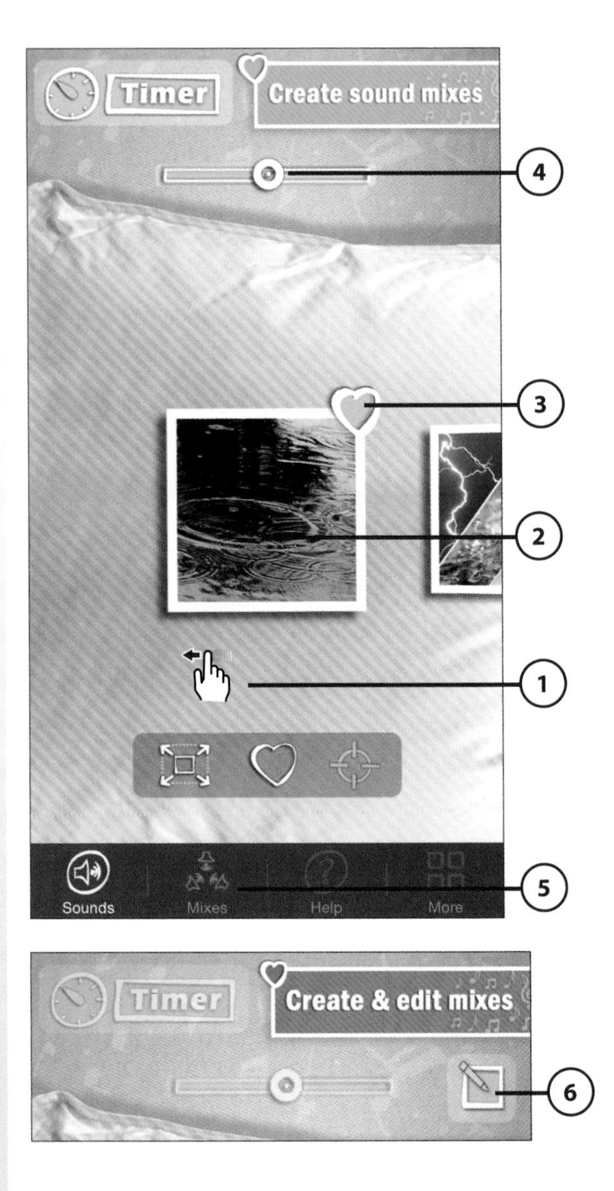

7. Swipe to scroll the rows of sound icons from the left and right to find the sounds you want, dragging the desired sounds over top of the volume sliders to hear them.
8. Tap the play button to hear your creation in real time.
9. Adjust the volume buttons under each sound until the levels are where you want them.
10. Tap a sound that you do not want to mute the sound.
11. Tap Save to save the mix.
12. Tap Timer to set a time for your natural soundscape to fade out as you fall to sleep.

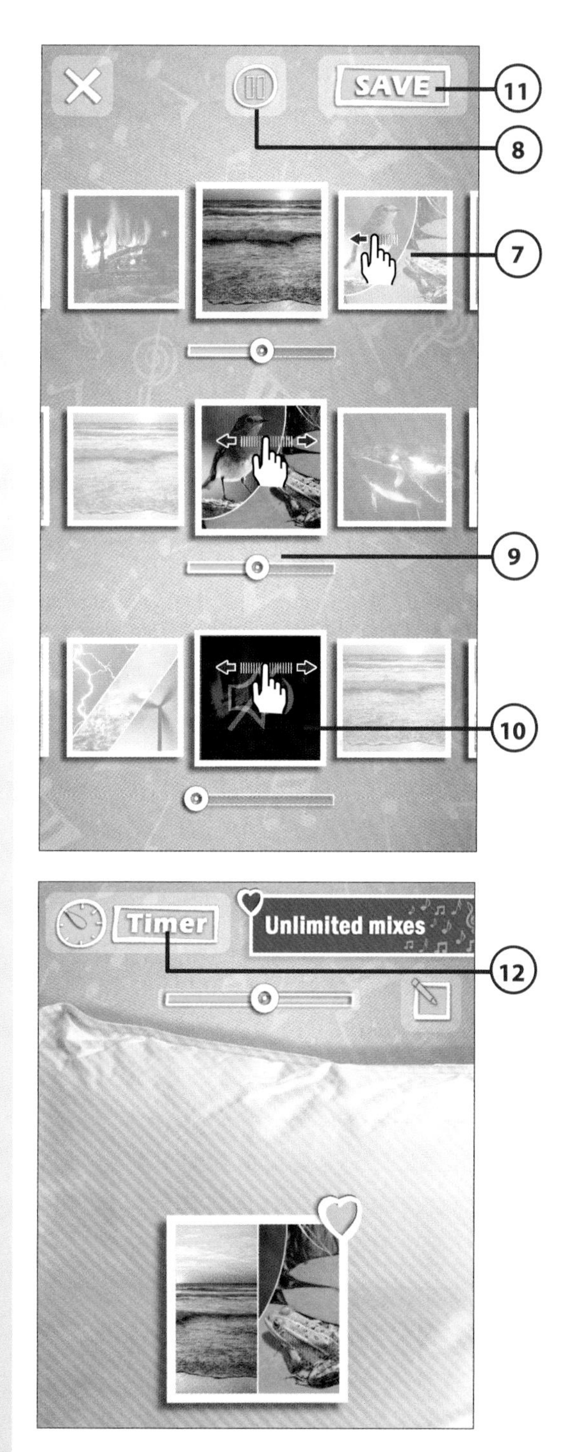

Upgrade the App for More Options

You can upgrade the app by tapping the Help button at the bottom of the main screen. Upgrading gives you access to more sounds, unlimited sound mixes, and more sleep timer and alarm clock options.

Exploring Meditation Apps

Incorporating relaxation techniques such as meditation and yoga into your lifestyle can help you manage your stress level. If you participate in these practices, then you already know the value of reducing stress responses in the body. You'll be happy to know that you can incorporate some quality meditation and yoga into your life, even if you can't make it to a formal class. There are apps that offer easy-to-follow guided meditation, including mindfulness techniques, for calming anxiety, anxiety release, and more. Many of these resources can be used on a lunch break with a pair of earbuds or headphones, in your living room, on your lawn, or any time or place where you can fit in an emotional boost.

Relax with the Calm App

If you need to add a little calm into your day, you can use the Calm app for meditation, sleep, relaxation, and more. This app allows you to easily incorporate meditation throughout your day by providing 7 guided meditation sessions, ranging from 2 to 30 minutes. If you're new to meditation, the Calm app also offers detailed meditation programs such as the 7 Days of Calm program where you learn how to meditate with guidance. As of this writing, the app is free for using the 7 Days of Calm program and Meditation Timer, in which you choose a time between 1 to 240 minutes to meditate. You also have access to the Calm, Body Scan, and Deep Sleep guided meditations for free. You'll need to subscribe to unlock all the features in the app. Subscribers gain access to the 21 Days of Calm program where you "deepen your meditation practice," and many more programs including 7 Days of Sleep, 7 Days of Happiness, and a total of 50 guided meditation practices. The Calm app is available for Android and the iPhone on the Google Play Store and the App Store.

The Calm app has a minimalist, intuitive interface that has 10 immersive nature scenes that you can easily access. In just a few taps, you can be on your way to being more relaxed. Download the Calm app, and then follow these steps to begin meditation with the Calm app. The following examples are shown on an Android phone.

1. Open the Calm app, and swipe the screen to the left or right to access the immersive nature scenes. As soon as you open the app, you should hear and see the default scene.
2. Tap Profile to track your meditation progress in regard to date, longest streak, total meditation, and total sessions.
3. Tap scenes to see a visual of all the immersive nature scenes available, all at once as tiles, and simply tap a scene.
4. Tap Meditate. The meditation options appear.

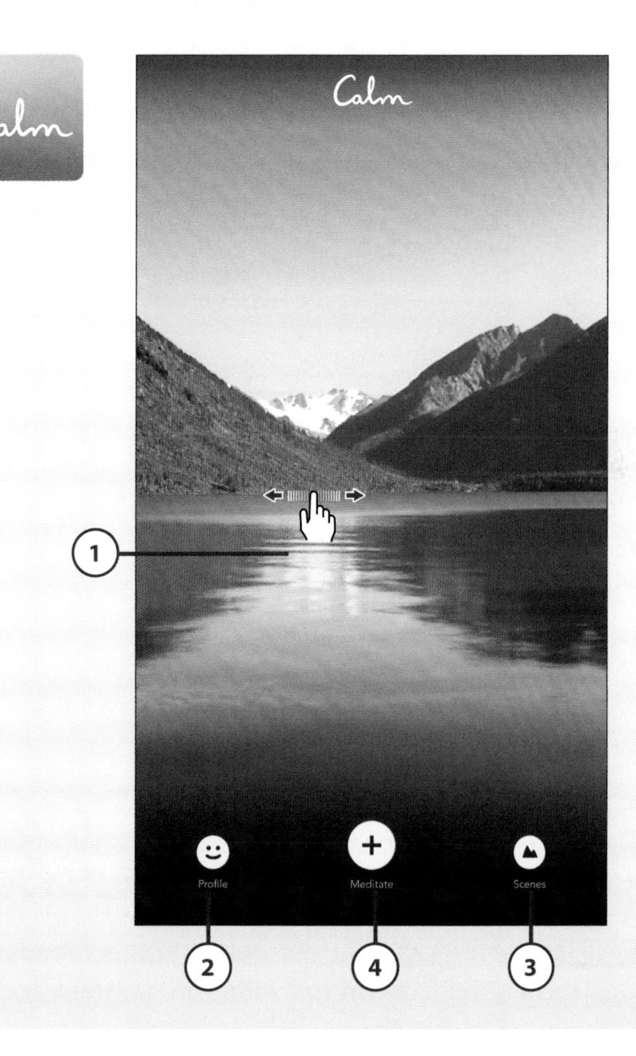

5. Swipe to scroll up and down the screen and tap an option to begin. Options available only to subscribers have a lock icon located at the end of the field. Tap a locked feature to get the option to upgrade.

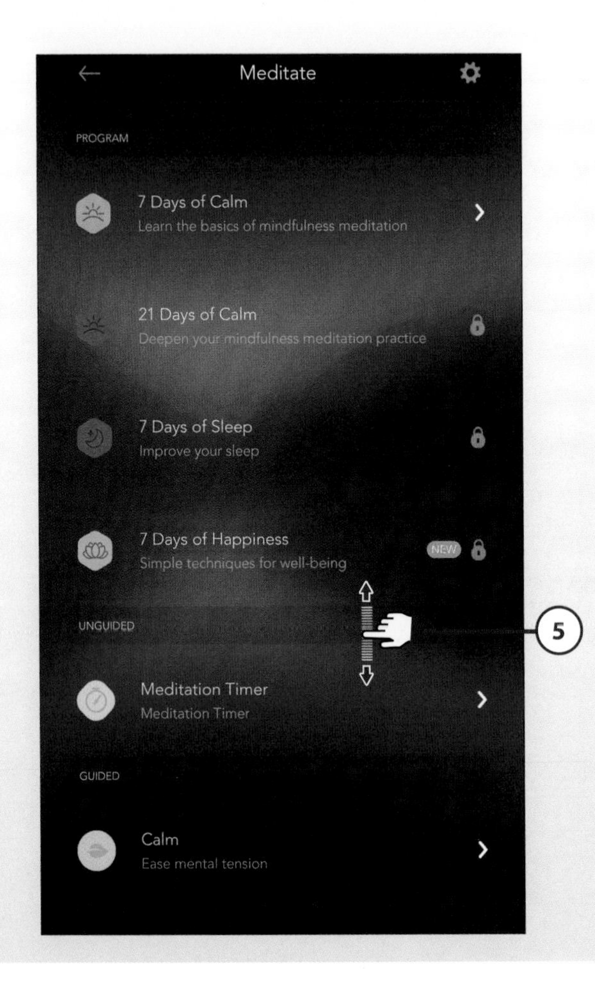

Find Your Happy Place with the Happier App

The mission of the developers of the Happier app is to make you happier in your everyday life. If you need to learn to live in the moment and stay positive, this may be just the app for you. Think of the Happier app as your personal mindfulness coach, an "on-the-go gratitude journal" where you can record happy moments, big and small. This app gives you access to short, expert-led courses to help you find pathways to joy, calm, and satisfaction in your everyday life and share those experiences with others. The app has both free and paid premium courses. Read inspiring quotes, take refreshing meditation breaks, and capture and share positive voice messages with others.

The Happier app is available for both Android and the iPhone. After you have downloaded the app and created an account, follow these steps to begin sharing your happy moments and become inspired by others. The following examples are shown on an iPhone.

1. Inside the Happier app, view the featured quotes and content.
2. Tap Share Quote to share a posted message on one of your existing social media accounts.
3. Tap in the field beneath a quote to comment on a post.
4. Tap to find and invite friends from your phone's Contact list to join Happier.
5. Tap to view some free courses on gratitude and meditation.
6. Tap Share Happy to share some happiness from your own life. You can type a message and add a photo from the photo library on your phone.

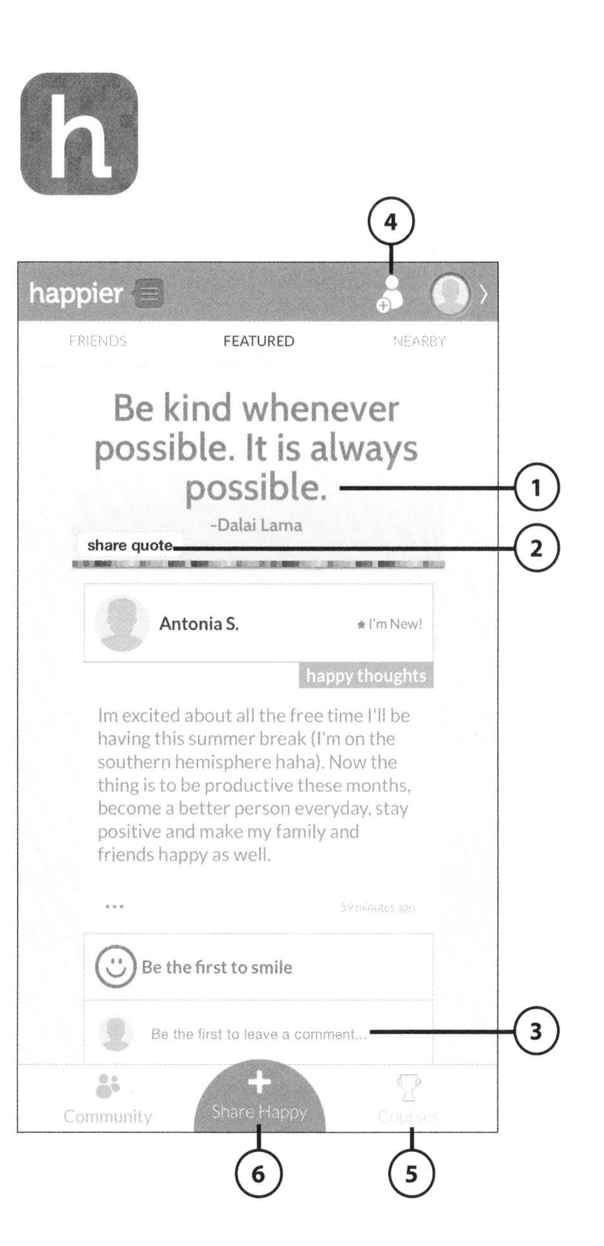

happier
FRIENDS
FEATURED
NEARBY
Be kind whenever possible. It is always possible.
-Dalai Lama
share quote
Antonia S.
I'm New!
happy thoughts
Im excited about all the free time I'll be having this summer break (I'm on the southern hemisphere haha). Now the thing is to be productive these months, become a better person everyday, stay positive and make my family and friends happy as well.
Be the first to smile
Be the first to leave a comment...
Community
Share Happy
1
2
3
4
5
6

Get in Touch with Your Inner Calm with Headspace

Headspace promotes its app as "a gym membership for your mind." The free Take10 program is a 10-day program that teaches you the basics of meditation in just 10 minutes a day. If the program makes you yearn for more calm and clarity that you can incorporate into your lifestyle, subscribe to unlock the entire Headspace collection including hundreds of hours of content. This includes guided and unguided content lasting from two minutes to an hour. Browse the collection and select what suits your current mood or lifestyle, choose your session length, and learn how you can apply mindfulness to your everyday activities. This service also includes special collections including Health, Performance, and Relationships. You can track your progress, team up with friends for motivation, and get rewards as you go.

Headspace is designed for you to use anywhere, at anytime. You can access programs online on your computer, on Android and Apple smartphones, and on tablets. Download the app from the Google Play Store and App Store and sign up for free, and then follow these steps to get started with Headspace. The following examples are shown on an Android phone.

1. Open the Headspace app, and tap Timeline to access your Take10 meditation sessions.

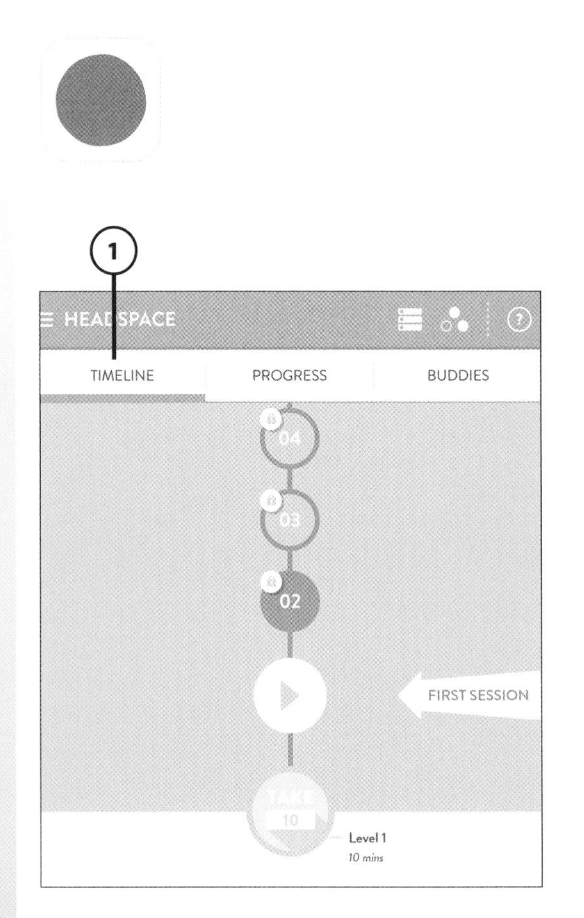

2. Tap Progress to view your stats, see how many users are meditating, and check your Run Streak—how many days you meditate in succession.
3. Tap Buddies to invite friends and track each other's progress.

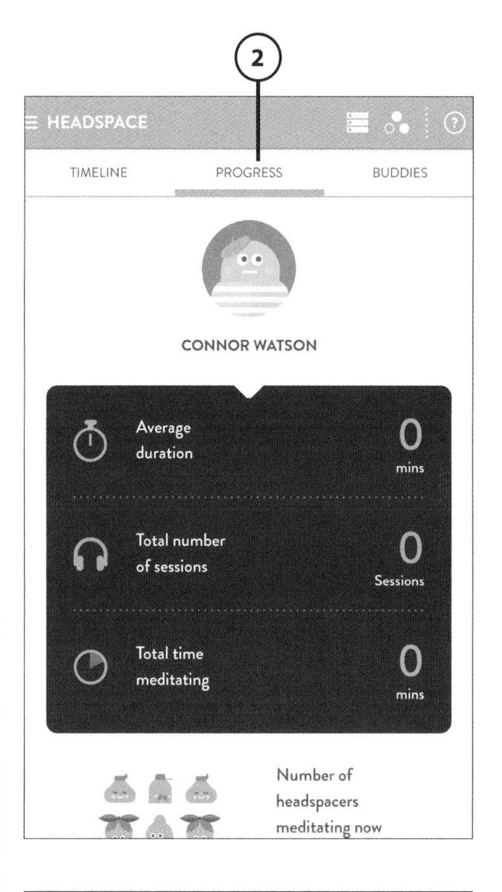

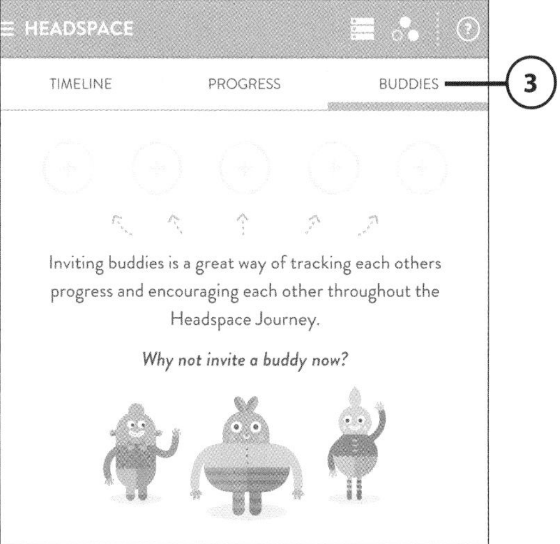

Use the Mindfulness Meditation App

The Mindfulness app is another great resource for reducing stress. This paid app is marketed to both beginners and those experienced in meditation and mindfulness. This app lets you choose which type of guided meditation you want to participate in, or if you simply want to meditate in silence. You also decide the duration of your session. Guided meditations range from 3 to 30 minutes. Personalize your session by including or excluding bells in your silent meditations. You can set reminders for when it's time to meditate. The app also includes a store of guided meditations led by some of the world's most influential meditation teachers. The seven different categories enable you to choose the kind of meditation you need at the moment. The Mindfulness app is available for Android and the iPhone.

If you are looking to increase your awareness in life, give the Mindfulness meditation app consideration. Download the app, and then use these steps to get started with the app. The following examples are shown on an iPhone.

1. Open the Mindfulness meditation app, and tap Meditate to choose your guided or silent meditation experience.
2. Tap Reminders to set reminders for when it's time to meditate.

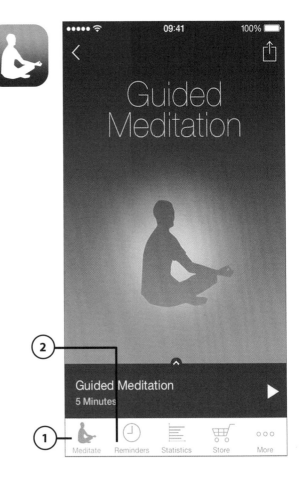

3. If you turn on reminders, you will receive a message asking you whether you want to meditate now. Click Yes or No based on your schedule.

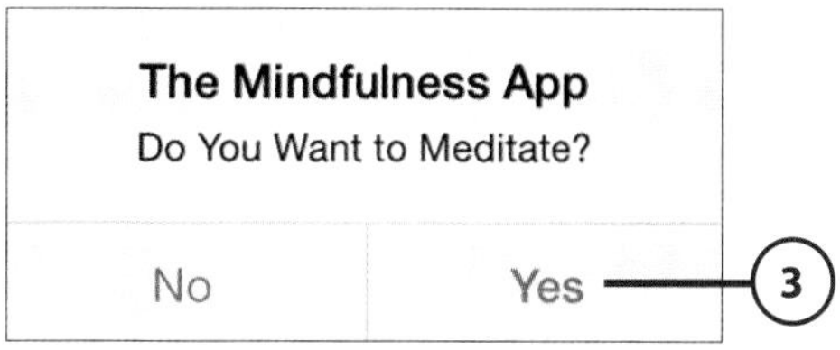

4. Tap Statistics so you can monitor how your meditation practice is progressing over time and motivate yourself.

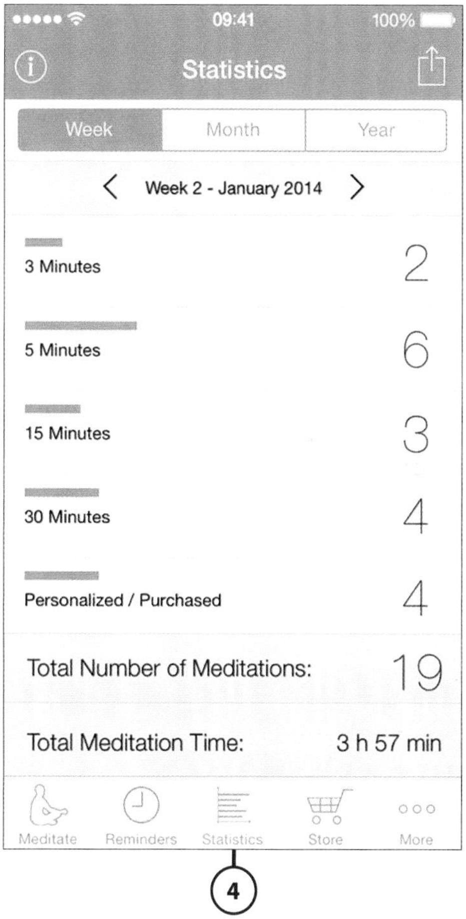

App Bundle for iPhone

The Mindfulness app is part of a four-app bundle for the iPhone: Mindfulness Complete. You can purchase all of these apps together at a discount at the App Store. As of this writing, it appears that this bundle is not available for Android devices.

The Mindfulness App
Do You Want to Meditate?
No
Yes
3

09:41
100%
Statistics
Week
Month
Year
Week 2 - January 2014
3 Minutes 2
5 Minutes 6
15 Minutes 3
30 Minutes 4
Personalized / Purchased 4
Total Number of Meditations: 19
Total Meditation Time: 3 h 57 min
Meditate
Reminders
Statistics
Store
More
4

(5) Tap Store to browse a variety of guided meditations by some of the most well-known teachers in the world.

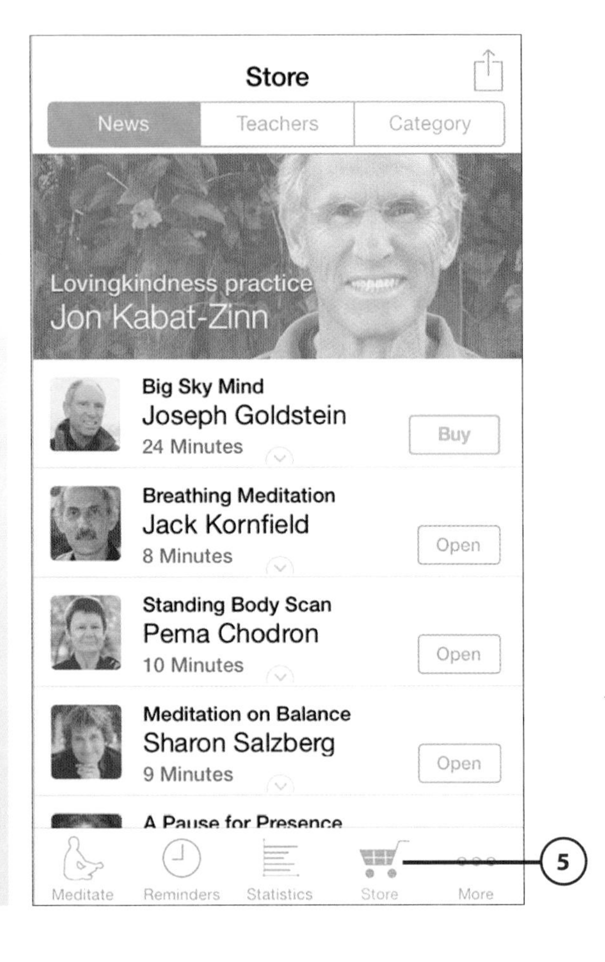

Release Stress with the Simply Being App

The Simply Being app enables you to enjoy stress relief through meditation via voice-guided, step-by-step sessions. You can choose between 5, 10, 15, or 20-minute durations where you can listen to the meditation with or without music or nature sounds. Or, simply listen to the music and nature sounds alone. The app offers separate volume controls for voice, music, and nature sounds so you can customize your experience. Read the supplied instructions to enhance your meditation sessions. The Simply Being app is marketed for both beginners and experienced meditators and is available for both Android and Apple devices. It is a paid app.

Download the app and follow these steps to begin meditating with the Simply Being app. The following examples are shown on an Android phone.

1. Open the Simply Being app, and tap Guided Meditation.
2. Choose the background you want to use for your session. Brook was chosen in this example.

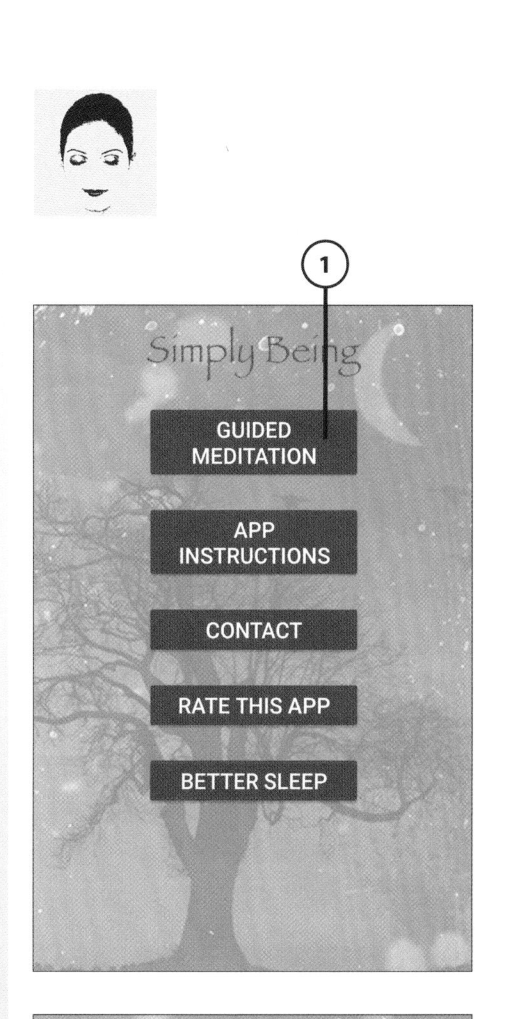

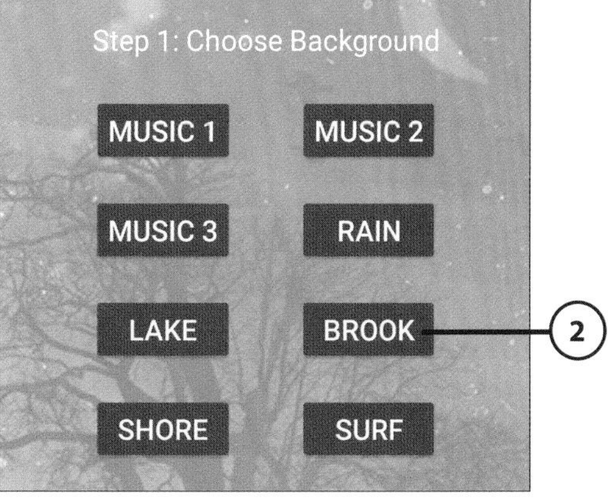

3. Choose the duration for your session. This example shows 10 minutes chosen.
4. Tap Start to begin your meditation.
5. Drag the sliders to change the volume for the voice for your guided meditation and the background sound (Brook).

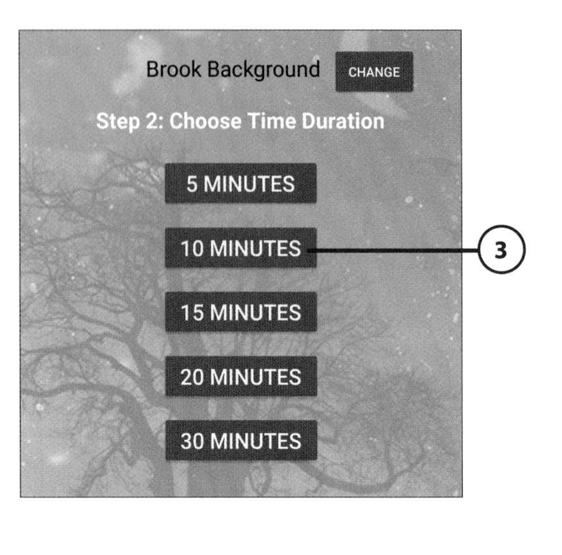

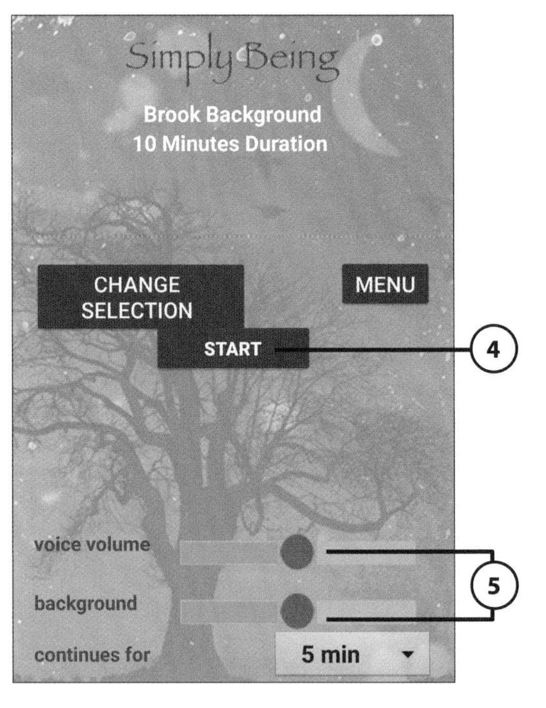

Break Up a Stressful Day with the Take a Break! App

The Take a Break! app and the Simply Being app icons look very similar. They are made by the same developer, and the objective of both is to lower your stress level through meditation. The Take a Break! app offers voice-guided step-by-step meditation sessions, and its feature set is more scaled backed than the paid Simply Being app. You can choose between two relaxing audio sessions: Work Break Relaxation (7 min) and Stress Relief Meditation (13 min). Choose to listen with or without music or nature sounds, or listen to the music and nature sounds alone. You can adjust the volume of the background sounds and the voice independently so that you find the perfect balance. This app is available for both Android and Apple devices.

Download the Take a Break! app and follow these steps to begin adding meditation to your day. The following examples are shown on an iPhone.

1. Open the Take a Break! app, and tap Listen.

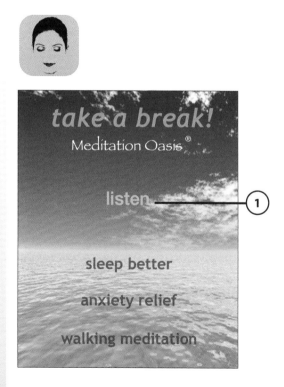

2. Tap to choose which session you want to do.
3. Tap to choose a background sound and theme.
4. Tap to choose how long the background continues or if you want to play any background sounds at all.
5. Tap the Play button to begin the session.
6. Adjust the volume sliders to find the perfect mix for you.

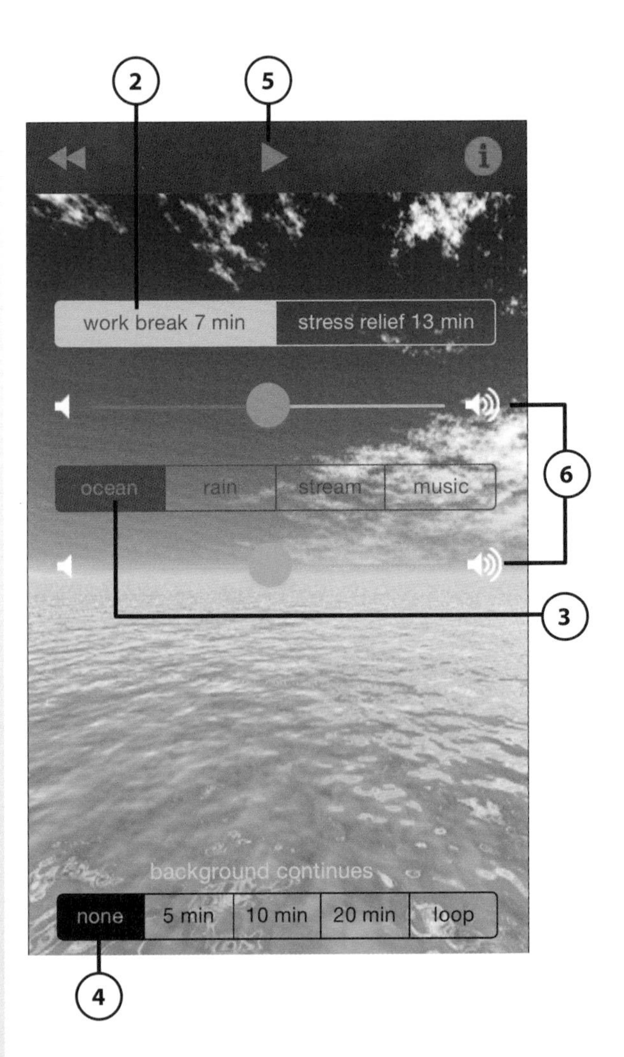

App Bundle for iPhone

The Take a Break app is part of an eight-app bundle for the iPhone called Meditation Oasis. You can purchase this eight-app bundle at a discount on the App Store. As of this writing, it appears that this bundle is not available for Android devices.

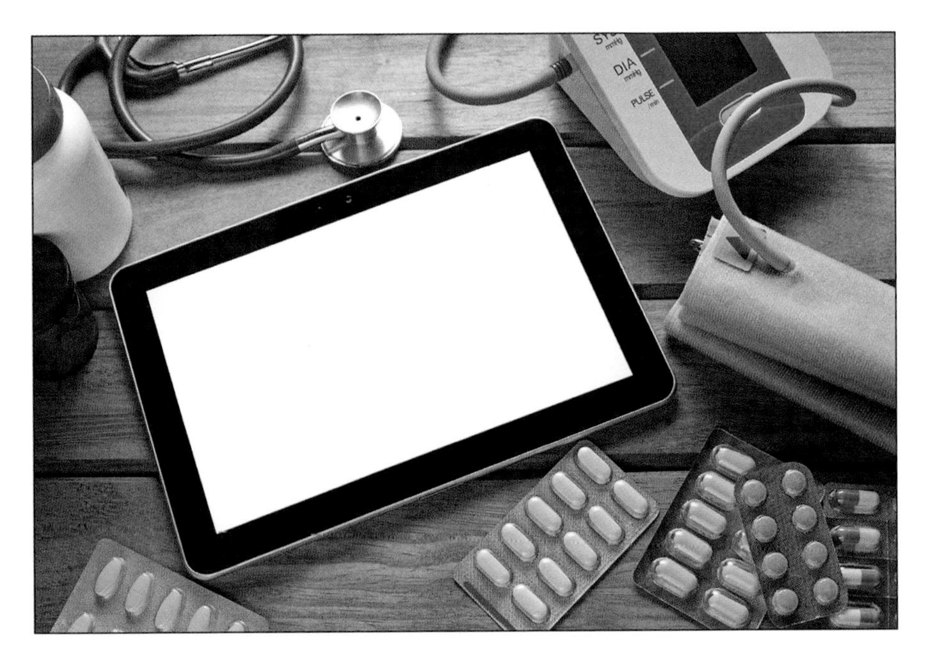

Credit: ©amenic181/Fotolia.com

Use apps, online resources, and medicine adherence devices to stay on top of your medicine regimen.

In this chapter, you explore options for medication management including scheduling and monitoring regimens online, receiving reminders when it's time to take your medicine, and adhering to the right dose.

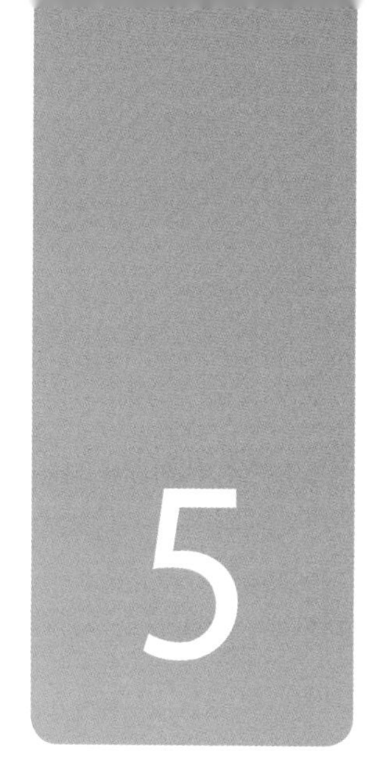

Staying on Top of Your Medicine

Not taking your drugs as advised by your physician can have dire consequences and can make the difference in quality of life, or even life and death. If you are not used to taking medication and have started a regimen, or have a lot going on in your life, taking your meds might slip your mind. If the regimen you're on is complex, involving a variety of medications spaced throughout the day or staggered throughout a week, keeping track of everything can be difficult. Fortunately, a variety of resources exist to choose from that help ensure you take your medication(s) at the right time and at the right dose. Some options are as simple as using a website or your local pharmacy's app to send reminders to your phone. Some tools can speak or play recorded reminders from a loved one, such as Reminder Rosie. A smart pill bottle cap device such as the CleverCap® can send audio and visual cues when it's time to take your medicine. This device can also send reminders to your phone, and allow for online monitoring. The CleverCap® can even dispense the proper dosage at the right time. These are only a few of the resources to get you started. This chapter offers a closer look so you can decide which of these apps and devices best fit your lifestyle and medicine-monitoring needs.

What to Do Concerning Missed Doses

Always consult your doctor on what you should do if you miss a dose.

Considering the Med Reminder App

If you have an iPhone, the Med Reminder app might be the perfect aid for reminding you to take your medicine at the right time. As of this writing, no Med Reminder app is available for Android devices. This app comes in two versions: Med Reminder Pro for $2.99 USD and Med Reminder for free. If you take one medicine daily, up to five times a day, the free app is for you. The Pro version is what you need if you take several medications daily, weekly, or monthly. Before purchasing the Pro version, try the free version to see whether you like the way Med Reminder works. Each version lets you set up your regimen, create reminders, and monitor your regimen.

Med Reminder Pro provides the added benefit of helping you understand the impact of your medicine on your body. You can input notes after each dose, including blood sugar levels, cholesterol, blood pressure, and any side effects you might be experiencing. You will need other resources to collect this data after each dose, such as a glucose monitor, in-home cholesterol monitoring kits, or blood pressure cuff. Med Reminder Pro works best the more information you enter in to the application.

Schedule and Monitor Regimens

The following examples are shown in the free version of Med Reminder. Whichever version you use, each lets you enter the medication(s) you are taking, the dosage, whether to take the med(s) with a meal or not, and set times for when to take the med(s). You can set reminders so that your phone vibrates or an audible alarm activates when it's time for you to take your medication. After you set up the app the way you want it, you don't need an Internet connection for the app to work. The app keeps a history of your medication adherence so you can see the times you went off schedule. After you download the app from the App Store, follow these examples to set up the Med Reminder app.

1. After you open the Med Reminder app, tap OK to allow the app to send you notifications. An Introduction box opens, giving you a succinct overview of how the app interface works.
2. Tap OK in the Introduction message. An Introduction message appears for each selection you tap onscreen. Read the introductions and simply tap OK for any of the remaining Introduction boxes, as they will not continue to be shown in this example. The Main screen is now visible.

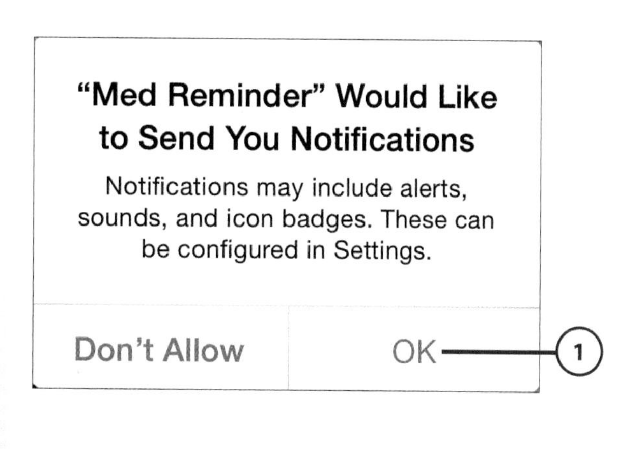

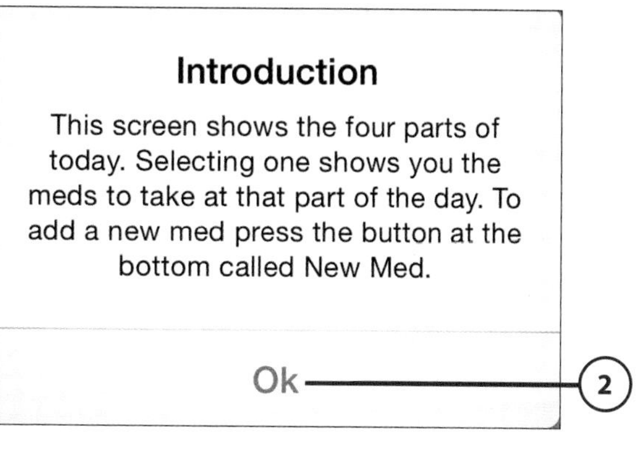

Introduction
This screen shows the four parts of today. Selecting one shows you the meds to take at that part of the day. To add a new med press the button at the bottom called New Med.
Ok
2

3. Tap New med to begin entering your medicine regimen into Med Reminder.
4. Tap in the Name of medicine field and enter the name of the medicine and the dosage via the keyboard.
5. Tap in a blank section of screen to hide the keyboard.
6. Tap if you are supposed to take the med with food, or if it's OK to take it without food.
7. Tap Frequency to select a Daily, Weekly, or Monthly regimen.
8. Tap Continue to add more detail to your regimen.

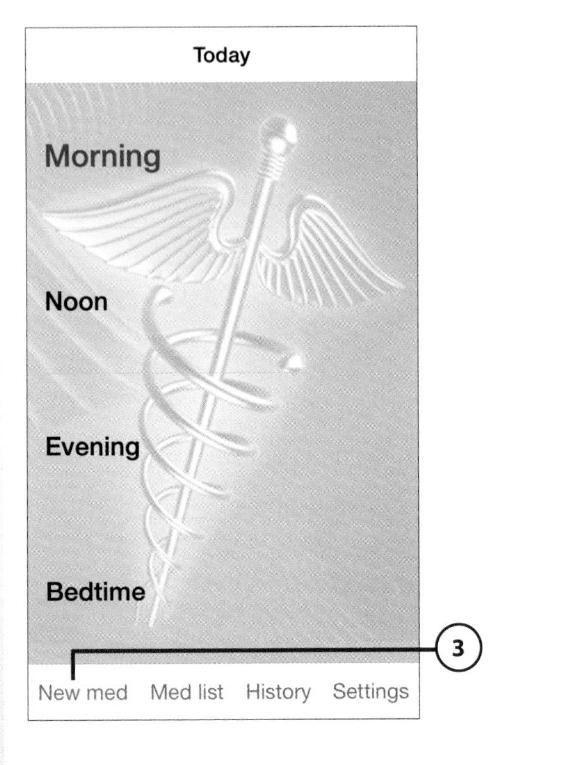

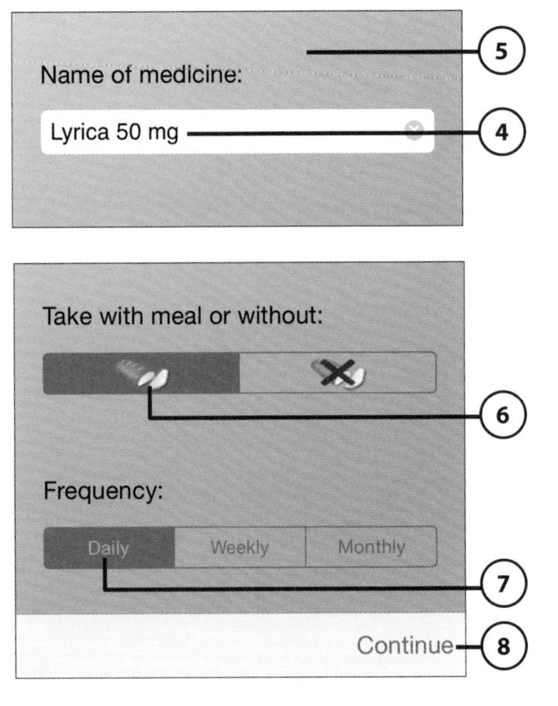

9. Tap the number of times you take the medicine each day. The Time of takings columns that appear at the bottom of the screen adjust to the number of times you take the med in a day.
10. Swipe up and down using the scroll wheels to designate the specific times you take the med throughout the day. The times in this example coincide with my breakfast, lunch, and dinner.
11. Tap Continue to add more detail to your regimen.
12. Tap in the Remark field to leave any notes you deem relevant for this med. For example, you can type the specific purpose for the drug along with the common side effects.
13. Tap OK. The Medicine is now added to your regimen. When it is time for you to take your med, an alarm will sound.

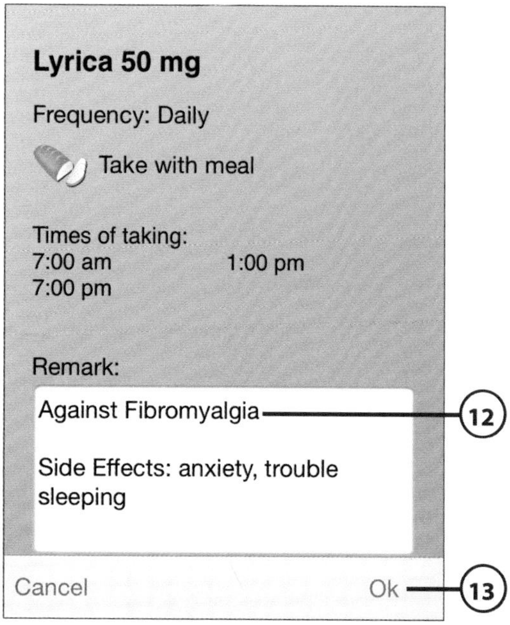

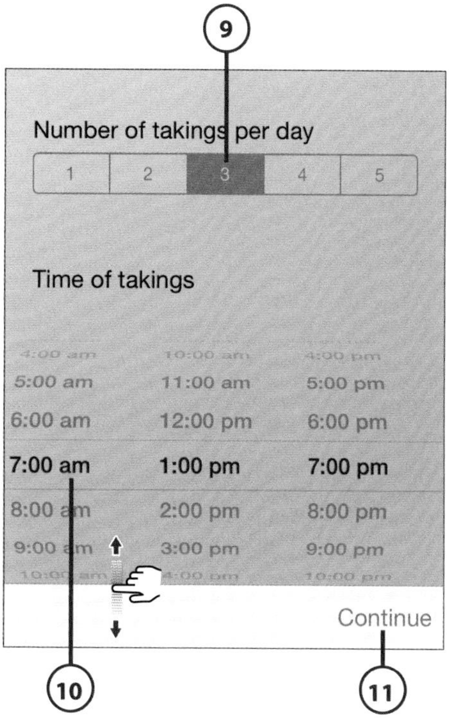

14. After you receive a notification on your phone and engage with it to open the app, tap on the time of the day for the current dose, which appears in a different color and is enlarged.
15. Tap Mark as Taken. Late intake is also shown if you don't take your medicine at the designated time.
16. Tap Today to go back to the previous page.
17. Tap Med list to view a detailed list of all the medicine you are taking. You can also delete medication through this option and edit the information you entered for a med.
18. Tap History to view a history of all taken doses by date or medicine.
19. Tap Settings to choose a different audible alarm or to not use an audible alarm. You can also choose alarm repetition intervals and get help about the app.

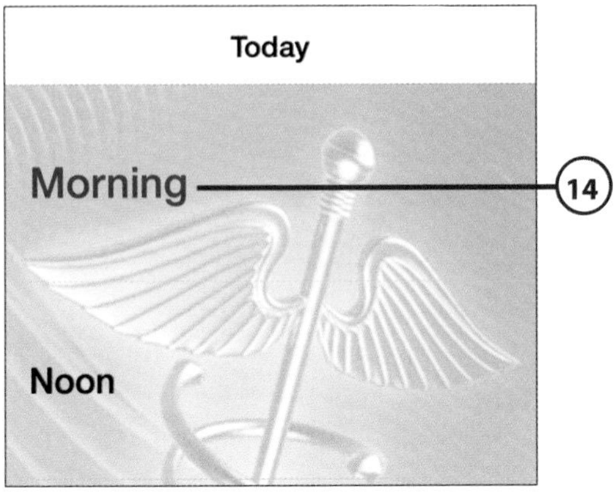

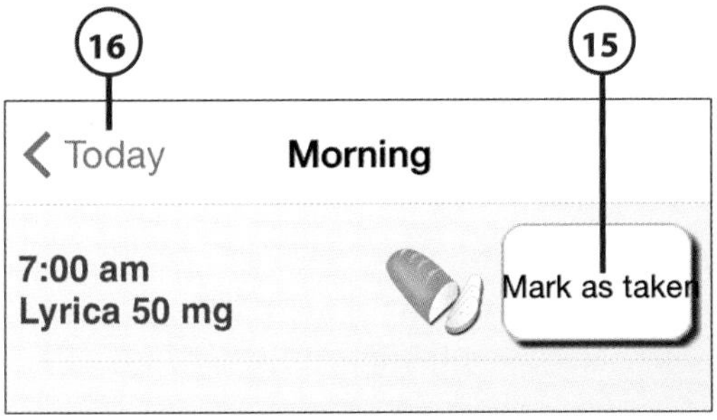

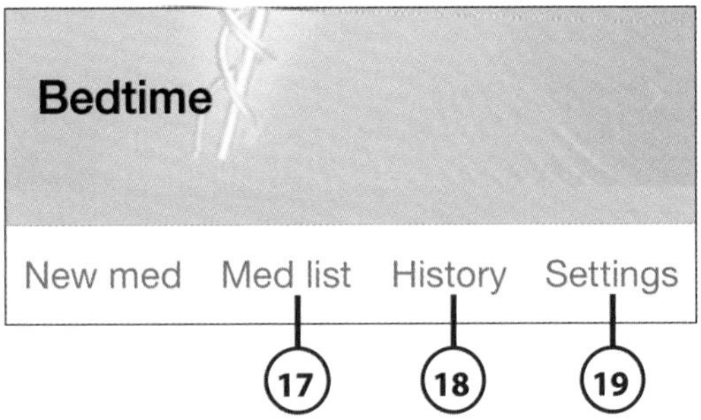

Responding to Notifications on Your Phone

Android phones and iPhones use different methods for engaging notifications from the lock screen, which is the screen you encounter after your phone falls asleep. On an iPhone you can slide the notification from left to right to engage it. On an Android phone you can double-tap the notification. Both of these methods open the app so you can respond to the notification.

Considering Reminder Rosie

Reminder Rosie is an advanced, voice-controlled, reminder system with an intuitive clock interface that can help you remember appointments and everyday tasks, including taking your medication. You don't need a smartphone; Rosie is a standalone device. Rosie is also a great companion for the visually impaired. One of the many strengths of Reminder Rosie is that the reminders can be played in the voice of a loved one. You, your family member, or a care provider can record a personal message as a reminder. For example, at a designated time set by you or someone else, Rosie speaks, "Hello, Mom. It's time to take 1 blue pill after breakfast. I love you." Rosie can remind you to take your medication throughout the day or week and help improve medical adherence and reduce complications due to medication disruptions. Reminder Rosie needs to be in a close enough vicinity for you to hear it, but the device does repeat reminder alarms every 5 seconds for 30 minutes. You can learn more about Reminder Rosie and purchase the device at www.reminder-rosie.com or by searching for the device on the Internet.

Let's take a look at how Reminder Rosie can assist you by providing personalized daily living voice reminders.

Set Up the Date and Time

Setting up Reminder Rosie is a simple process that you can do via voice commands or a series of buttons on the back of the unit. To begin using Rosie, you first need to set the correct time and date, as follows:

1. Plug in Rosie near where you, or the person Rosie will assist, spend the most time. As soon as you plug in Rosie, she begins to give you a brief introduction on how to set up the system. After the introduction finishes, you are ready to start using Rosie. The first step is to "wake up" or activate Rosie.

2. After Rosie says her introduction, activate Rosie by speaking the voice-activated trigger, "Hello Reminder Rosie" or by pressing down on the top of the unit. There is no set button to press; just press firmly on the top. Rosie replies, "Can I help you?" Always wait until Rosie finishes speaking. If you begin speaking before she is finished, she will not hear you. Now let's set the time and date.

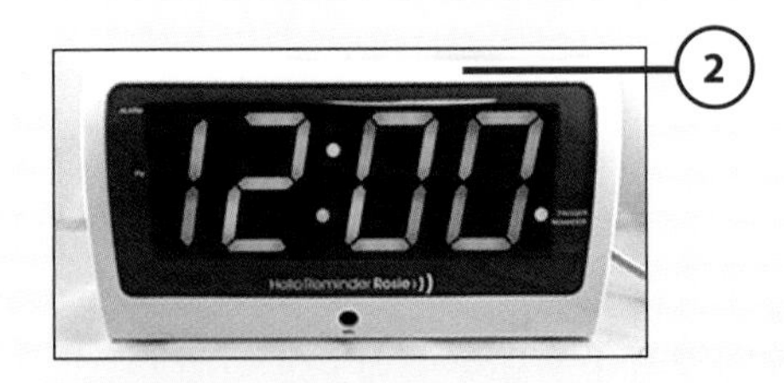

3. Say, "Hello Reminder Rosie." Rosie replies, "Can I help you?"
4. Say, "Set time." Rosie replies, "Please tell me the time including AM or PM."
5. Say the current time followed by AM or PM. For example, say, "2:47 PM." Rosie replies, "The time is set to 2:47 PM."

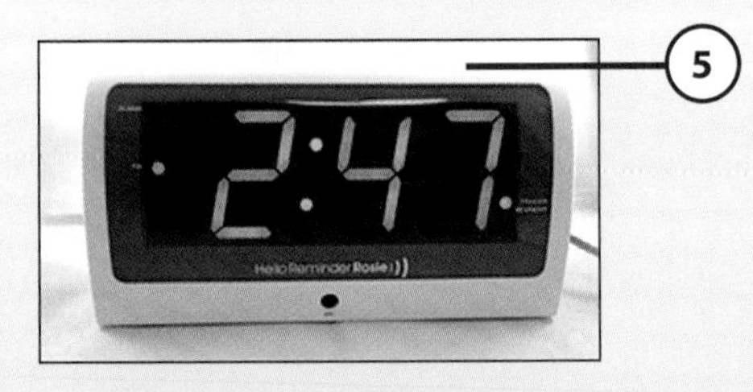

6. To set the date, say, "Hello Reminder Rosie." Rosie replies, "Can I help you?"
7. Say, "Set date." Rosie replies, "Please tell me the month."
8. Say the current month—for example, "March." Rosie replies "Please tell me the date.
9. Say the current date—for example, "15." Rosie replies, "Please tell me the year.
10. Say, for example, "2000 and 16." Rosie then tells you the current date. Now you are ready to start adding reminders.

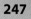

Use Batteries with Rosie

It's important to install three AAA batteries into Reminder Rosie in case of a power outage, or if you need to unplug the device and move it to another area. When Rosie is running strictly on battery power, the LED clock display is not displayed, and to wake up Rosie you must press on the top of the device.

Set Up Rosie's Activation Trigger and Create Reminders

By default, Rosie is constantly listening for the voice-activated trigger "Hello Reminder Rosie." In a noisy, communal setting, Rosie might hear similar phrases that cause her to activate. You can turn off Rosie's voice-activated feature to avoid confusion and just press the top of the device to "wake up" Rosie. Creating reminders that can help you or a loved one remember to take medication(s) is also a simple process.

1. Turn around the device so you can see the backside, and then press the Trigger On Off button. The voice-activated trigger "Hello Reminder Rosie" is now off. Rosie audibly confirms that trigger mode is off.

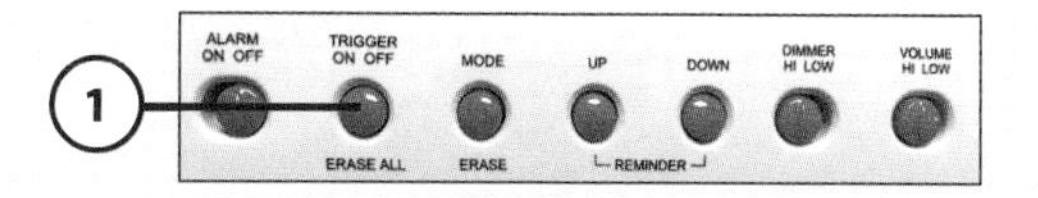

2. Press down on the top of the device to activate Rosie, and then wait for the beep. To cancel a command, simply press down the top of the device again. Now let's record a reminder. The remaining steps show how to record a reminder when the trigger is set to off.
3. Press down on Rosie to wake her up, and then wait for the beep.

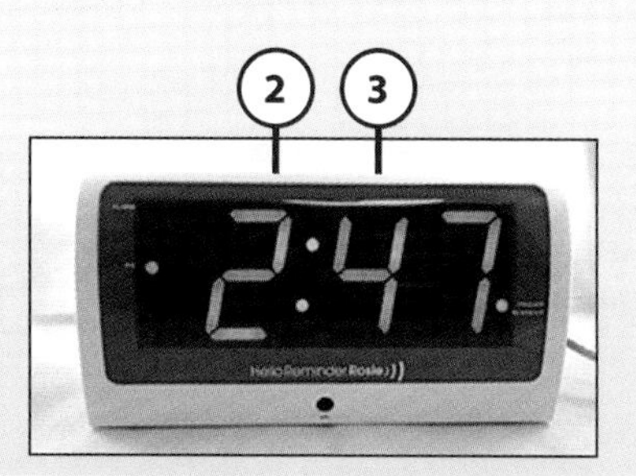

4. Say, "Record Reminder." Reminder Rosie says, "Please record a reminder," and then beeps.
5. Speak a reminder. For example, say, "Hi Mom. Be sure to take your blue pill after breakfast. I love you." Reminder Rosie plays the recorded message back for you, and then replies, "Say 'keep reminder' or 'record again.'"
6. Say "Keep reminder" if you like the recording. Reminder Rosie then says, "Please tell the time that the reminder should play, including AM or PM."
7. Say the time, including AM or PM. For example, say "8:30 AM." Rosie replies, "8:30 AM. Is this correct?"
8. Say, "Yes" if the time is correct. Rosie asks "Is this reminder for today only?"
9. Say, "No." Rosie replies, "Please say the day of the week, or say 'every day', or say calendar date."
10. Say, "Every day." Rosie replies, "The reminder will play every day at 8:30 AM. Is this correct?"
11. Say, "Yes." Rosie replies, "Reminder saved."

How Reminders Work

A reminder plays every 5 seconds until you turn it off. If you are not around, a reminder will repeat every 5 seconds for 30 minutes and then shut off automatically. These missed reminders will automatically go to the missed reminder queue, and an indicator light will blink on the LED screen. The next time you "wake up" Rosie, she will play all of your missed reminders.

---

12. To turn off a reminder, you simply need to wait until a reminder finishes playing, and then say, "Reminder Off" or press down on top of Rosie. Rosie will then verbally confirm that the reminder has been turned off.

Play and Erase Reminders

Reminder Rosie makes it easy for you to play back just today's schedule or all reminders. This feature makes it convenient for you or your caregiver to quickly review whether the day's tasks were completed. When reminders become no longer relevant, you can delete them with a simple voice command after the reminder has finished playing.

1. Press the top of the device to activate Rosie, and then wait for the beep.
2. Say, "Today's reminders." Rosie plays back the reminders for the day. Rosie also gives you the option to play back all reminders, regardless of day. When you choose to play back all reminders, you have the option to delete a reminder after it has finished playing.
3. Press the top of the device to activate Rosie, and then wait for the beep.

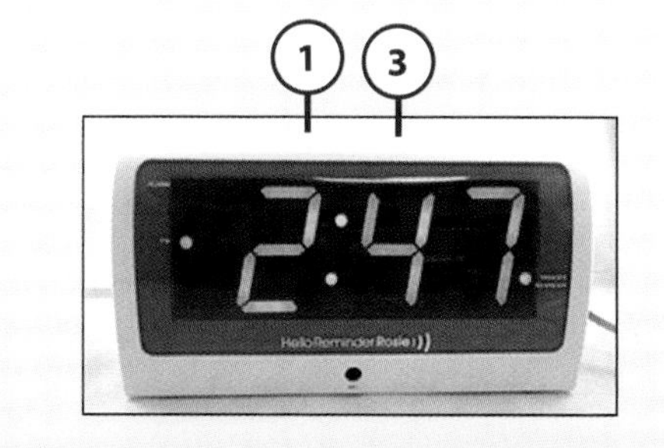

4. Say, "Play all reminders." Rosie provides some instructions on deleting reminders and then immediately begins to play back reminders.
5. After the reminder that you want to delete finishes playing, say, "Erase" to delete the reminder. Rosie verbally confirms the message has been erased and then proceeds to the next message.

Receiving Reminders from Pharmacies

One of the most basic precautions you can take to remind yourself to take your medications is to employ the help of your pharmacy. Many pharmacies have their own apps that function similar to the Med Reminder app and alert you when it is time to take your medication(s).

As of this writing, the CVS Pharmacy app for Android does not have a Med Remind function. This convenience will most likely will be added by the time you read this book, so be sure to check in the app description on the Google Play Store. Also as of this writing, the Walmart app does not include a reminder function for medicine adherence.

Consider one of these apps for a simplistic approach to medication adherence. Search the Google Play Store or the App Store to see whether your pharmacy offers an app.

Taking the Right Medication at the Right Time at the Right Dose with CleverCap®

CleverCap® is one of the most complete medication adherence and safety devices on the market. Not only does it help ensure that you take the right medication at the right time, but it also dispenses the prescribed number of pills and stays locked until the next time you need to take your medicine. (It can also be set to be unlocked depending on patient and therapy preferences.) Think of the CleverCap® as a smart pill-bottle cap that works seamlessly with standard pill bottles. Your doctor or pharmacist simply replaces the standard cap with the CleverCap® and then programs your medication regimen using the pharmacy management software. The information is then synced to the CleverCap®. Visual and sound alerts let you know when it's time for you to take your medicine. You can also receive alerts as phone calls, emails, and texts. CleverCap® dispenses the correct dosage, and activity sensors monitor what time you actually took your medicine. Your adherence history is stored in an encrypted online report that you and your doctor can review at any time, and you are actually given a score (CleverScore®) for how you've stayed on track. This way, you can easily monitor your progress and improve your medication adherence. You can ask your doctor or pharmacist for the CleverCap® the next time you are prescribed a medication.

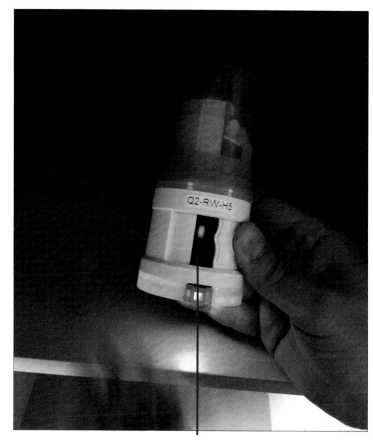

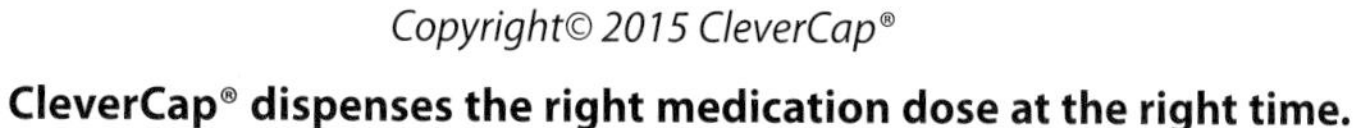

Copyright© 2015 CleverCap®

CleverCap® dispenses the right medication dose at the right time.

Sync Medication Regimens with the CleverCap®

The wonderful thing about the CleverCap® is that it doesn't require you to log in to a website to create an account or enter your own medication regimen. The enhanced prescription(s) are sent directly from your doctor's office to the pharmacist. The pharmacist programs CleverCap® according to your doctor's instructions, and you just pick up your medication as you normally would. To get a refill, simply take CleverCap® back to the pharmacist or prescribing doctor, mail it back when you receive a CleverCap® enhanced prescription refill via the mail, or reclose a refill with your existing CleverCap®.

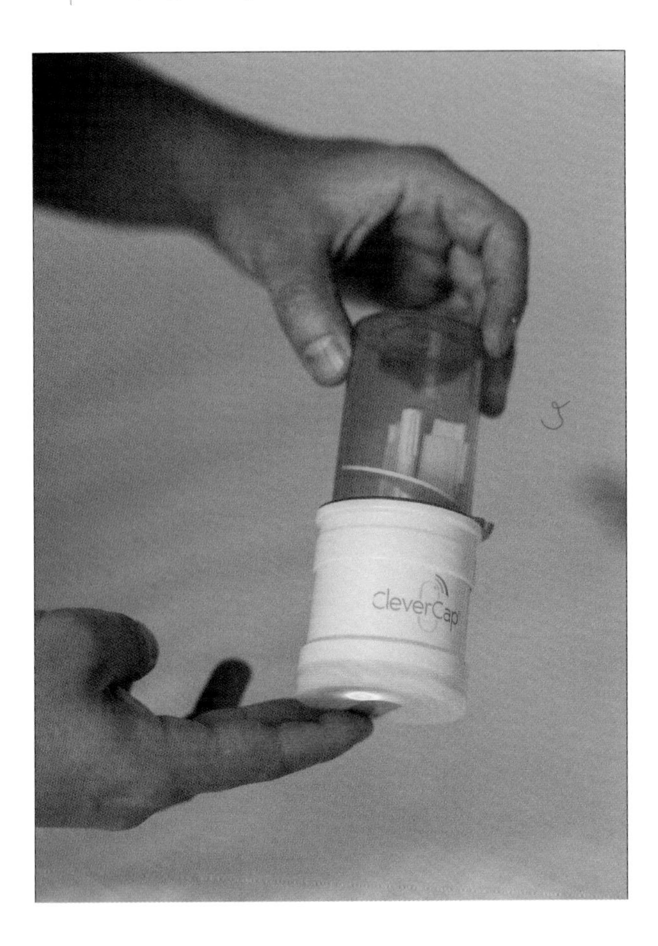

Use Visual, Sound, and Other Alerts for Medication Reminders

When it is time for you to take your medicine, CleverCap® uses multiple methods to remind you to take your medication as directed by a doctor. CleverCap® flashes a blue light and beeps when it's time for you to take your meds. It then dispenses the exact prescribed dose for the medication. If you are on the go, you can include other reminder methods such as text messaging, emails, and phone call follow-ups. After you have obtained your CleverCap®, contact CleverCap® to set up your login details so you can enter into the Customer Care Portal at CleverCap.org. From your profile you can then decide whether CleverCap® should use a flashing light or audible alert. You can also choose if you want to receive additional reminders via text messaging, emails, or phone call. You can add a relative or a health support team and grant them access to notifications, and help you keep a high adherence score.

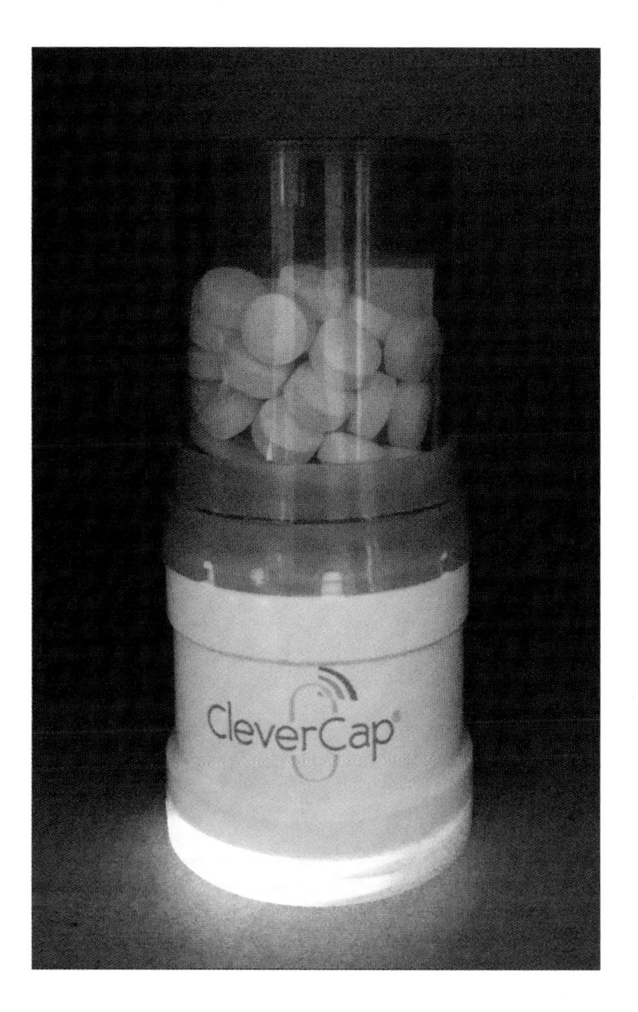

CleverCap® and Safety

CleverCap® has several optional features. One of them uses a tamperproof lid so your medication doesn't end up in the wrong hands. It also dispenses the correct dose during an allocated window of time, and dispensing is child resistant. These safeguards not only make the CleverCap® childproof, but also provide an extra level of protection against abuse of drugs that might be highly potent and addictive.

Access Medicine Regimen Online Reports

CleverCap® uses special activity sensors to record when you take a pill out of the bottle after it has been dispensed. If you forget, CleverCap® can send a notification to you, your support system, your family, and/or your clinician. Each pill is recorded by time and date, and whether it is taken on schedule, off schedule, or missed. That information is stored securely in CleverCap's® databanks and is web accessible by signing into the Customer Care Portal at clevercap.org.

Some of the information you can view includes the following:

- Dose-by-dose adherence results
- Summary reports detailing changes and trends
- Your CleverScore® measures medication use versus the prescribed regimen

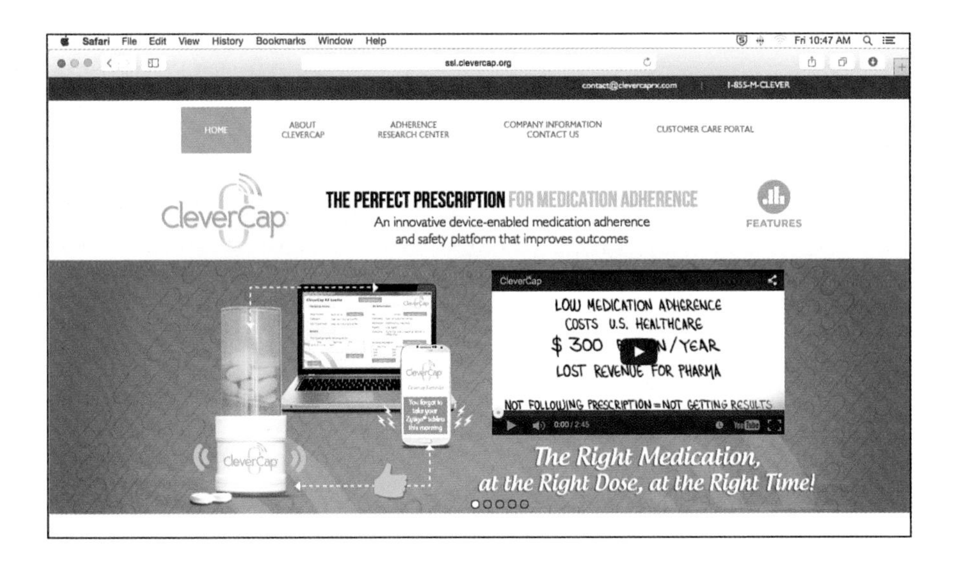
Safari File Edit View History Bookmarks Window Help
Fri 10:47 AM
ssl.clevercap.org
contact@clevercaprx.com
1-855-M-CLEVER
HOME
ABOUT CLEVERCAP
ADHERENCE RESEARCH CENTER
COMPANY INFORMATION CONTACT US
CUSTOMER CARE PORTAL
CleverCap
THE PERFECT PRESCRIPTION FOR MEDICATION ADHERENCE
An innovative device-enabled medication adherence and safety platform that improves outcomes
FEATURES
LOW MEDICATION ADHERENCE COSTS U.S. HEALTHCARE
LOST REVENUE FOR PHARMA
NOT FOLLOWING PRESCRIPTION = NOT GETTING RESULTS
The Right Medication, at the Right Dose, at the Right Time!

What If I Miss Taking My Medicine as Directed?

Always consult your doctor about what you should do if you are late taking a medication or miss a dose. CleverCap® can be set to stay locked until the instructed time for you to take your med(s). If you miss your scheduled time, you can initiate an off-schedule dose by manually overriding the locking mechanism. Refer to your dispensing doctor or pharmacist about how to off schedule doses.

Staying on Top of Your Medications with Medisafe

The Medisafe app is a visually oriented, easy-to-use app that helps remind you to take your medication and manage your pill usage. Medisafe presents times of day—Morning, Afternoon, Evening, and Night—split as a pie chart. Each part of the day, or slice, of the pie chart shows how many medications you need to take. At a glance, you can watch how your medication regimen progresses throughout the day. As each part of the day reaches an end, that segment of the chart turns blue. The medicine in that slice either has a green check mark or a red exclamation point next to it signifying if a dose has been taken on time or missed.

Medisafe sends a notification to your device(s), including your Apple Watch and Android Wear watch, when it's time to take your medication. You can even have notifications and your medication adherence data sent to a doctor, family member, friend, or caregiver for support. Medisafe also curates coupons and special offers just for you. This flexible app allows for multiple medications taken up to 12 times a day or in intervals of every 12 hours, 8 hours, or 6 hours.

To learn more about Medisafe and download the free app, visit medisafe.com. As of this writing, the Medisafe app is available for Android devices, the iPhone and iPad, and is also available in the Amazon App Store. You do not have to register for an account to use Medisafe on your phone.

After you have downloaded the app, you can set up your virtual pillbox as described in the following section. You use the Medisafe app without an account. The following steps are shown on an Android phone.

Set Up Your Virtual Pillbox

Medisafe provides an intuitive interface for you to set up your virtual pillbox. As you add in your medication regimen, Medisafe supplies tools so that you can properly identify each pill. As an extra level of support, Medisafe makes it possible for you to designate friends and family members as Med-Friends who can help you remember to take your meds in case you forget. You can even send your medication adherence information to your doctor.

1. After you have downloaded the Medisafe app, open it and tap Start Now.

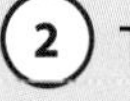
2. Tap Add Med.

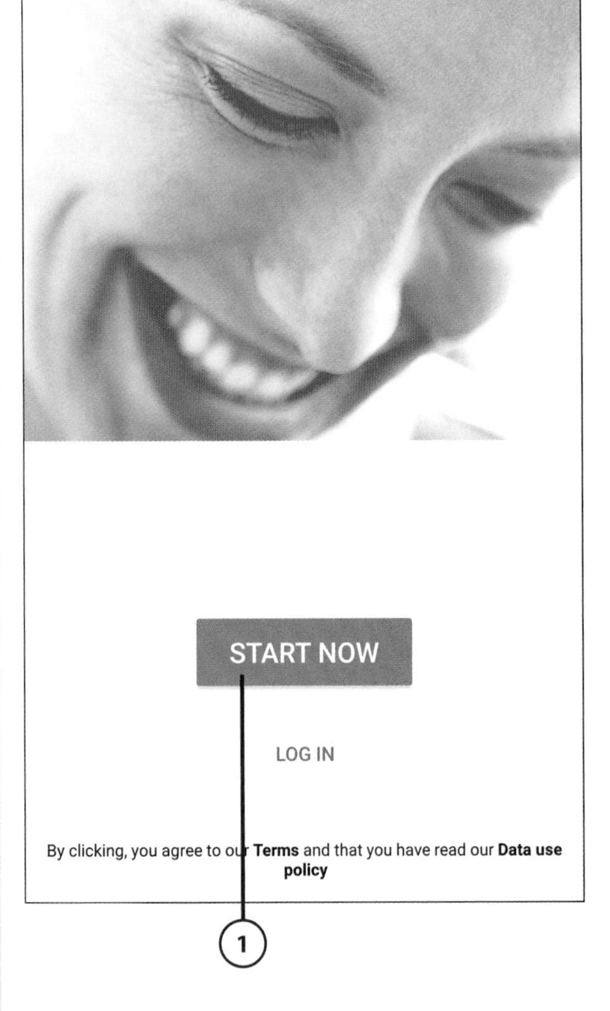

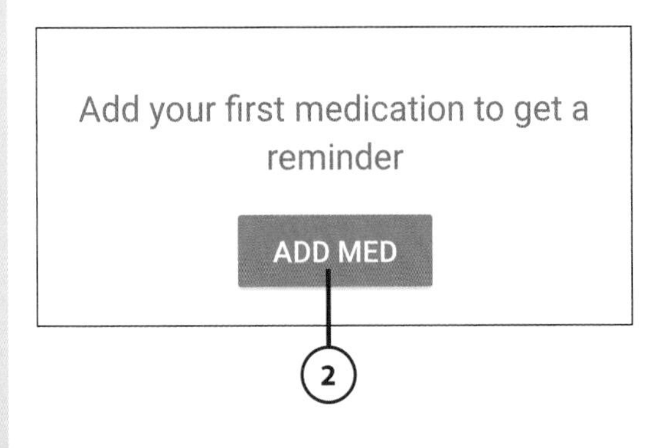
Add your first medication to get a reminder
ADD MED
2

3. Begin typing the name of the medication, and then tap the correct medication in the list of possible results that appear under the field. Multiple results may appear for the medicine you are entering. Choose the one with the proper dose.
4. Tap the downward arrow in the Reminder Times field, and choose the Frequency (Once a day, Twice a day, 3 times a day) and an interval (Every 12 hours, Every 8 hours, Every 6 hours).
5. Tap the arrow in the Schedule field to specify the duration you need to take the med (continuous, number of days), and which days (every day, specified days of week, days interval, birth control cycle).

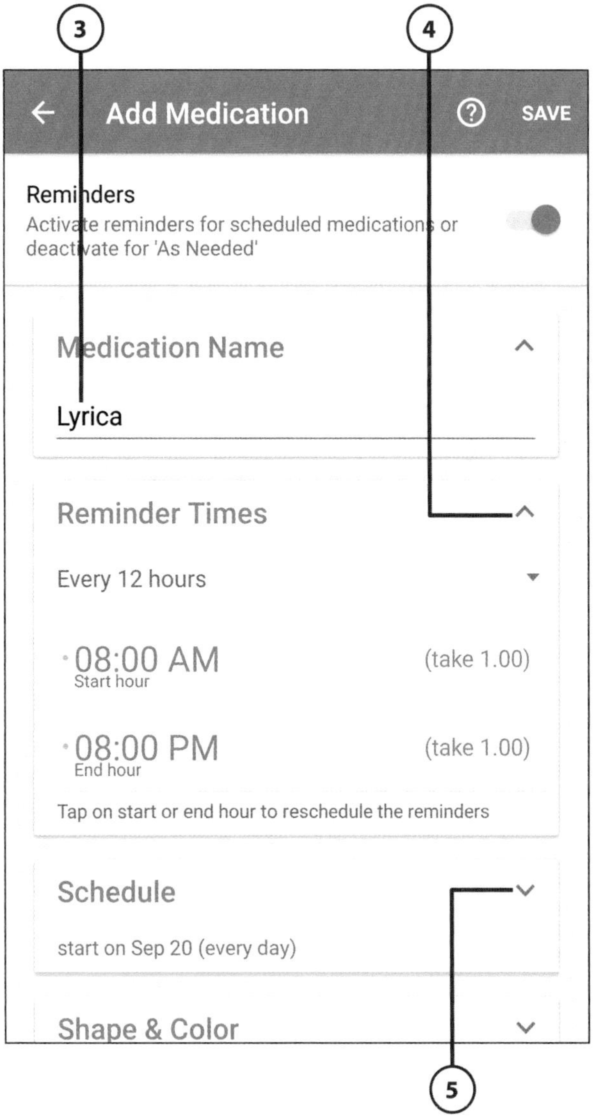

6. Swipe down and tap the downward arrow in the Shape & Color field and tap on an illustration that looks like your medicine. You can choose the color of the medication. This step is usually completed automatically at the point of entering the name of the medication along with dosage.
7. Tap Med-Friend to designate another person to help you remember to take your meds in case you forget.
8. Tap More Options to specify dosage, special instructions, and refill information.

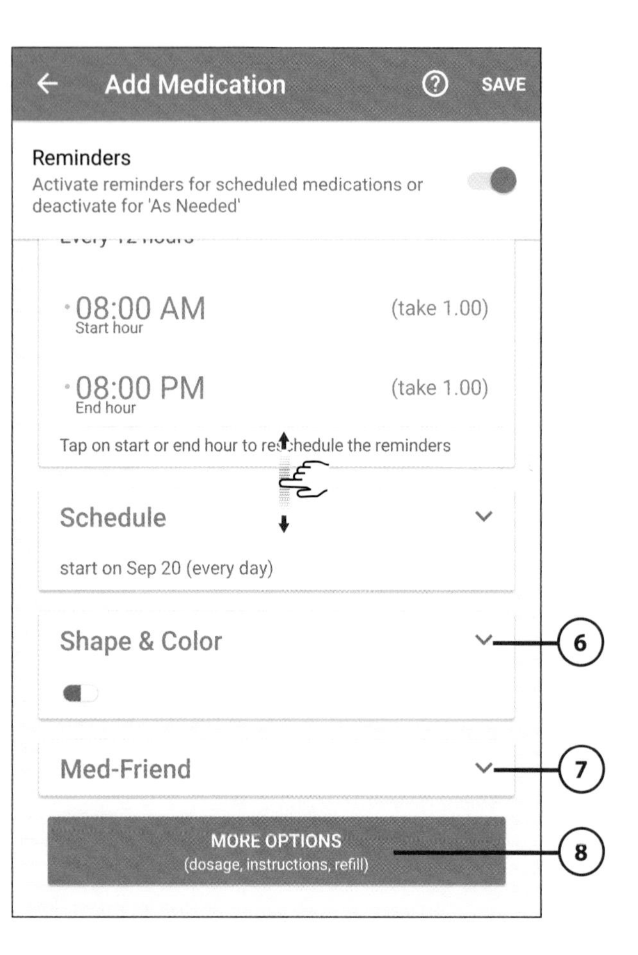

9. If the doctor changes your dose, tap Dosage to change the dose.
10. Tap Instructions to specify special instructions for taking this medication, including before food, with food, after food, or no food instructions. You can even type in your own personalized instructions.
11. Tap RX Refill Reminder to set reminders to refill your prescription. In this option you can set reminders to remind you to refill in days or number of pills left.
12. Tap Doctor to add the prescribing doctor's information so that she can have a record of your medication adherence. Before entering your doctor's information, discuss with her if she would like to receive, or have a system to receive, updates on your medication adherence.
13. Tap Save after you have entered all the information for this med. A visual representation of your medication regimen appears. You are now ready to receive notifications. When it is time to take your medication, an alert sounds, your phone vibrates, and the Medisafe app opens. You can then choose to tap Taken, Skip, or Snooze.

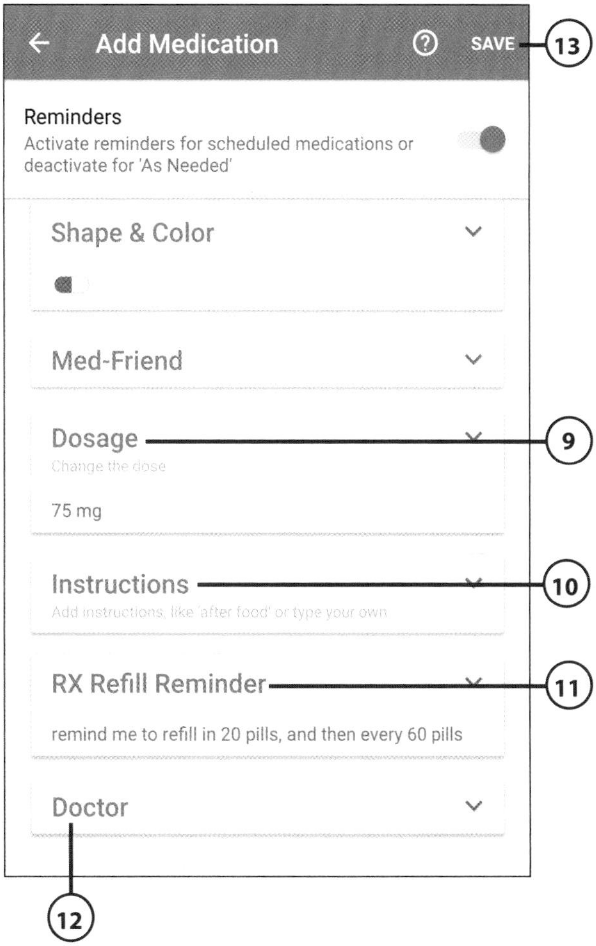

14. On the Pillbox screen, tap the Add (the plus sign) button to add a dose, add a measurement (including blood glucose, calories consumed, calories expended, blood pressure, and more), invite a Med-Friend, add a doctor's appointment, and add a medication.
15. Tap the Main menu that looks like three horizontal lines to navigate the entire Medisafe app.
16. Tap Medications to edit drug information, suspend notifications for specific meds, and delete drugs from your pillbox. You can also get available coupons for your meds.
17. Tap Report to review your medication adherence progress and view your weekly adherence score.

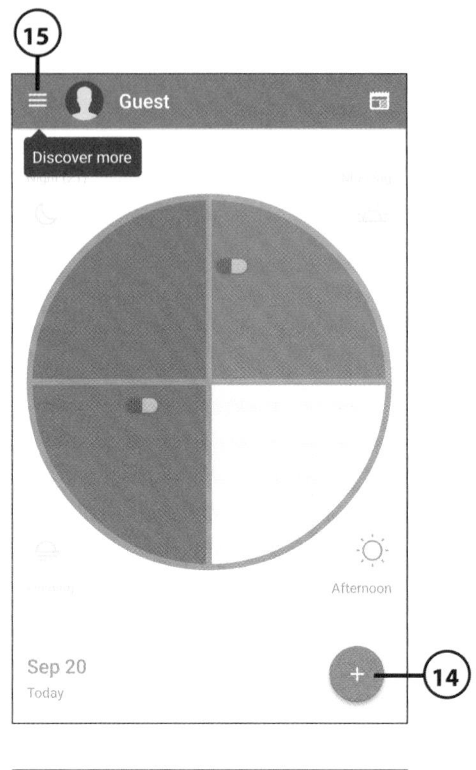

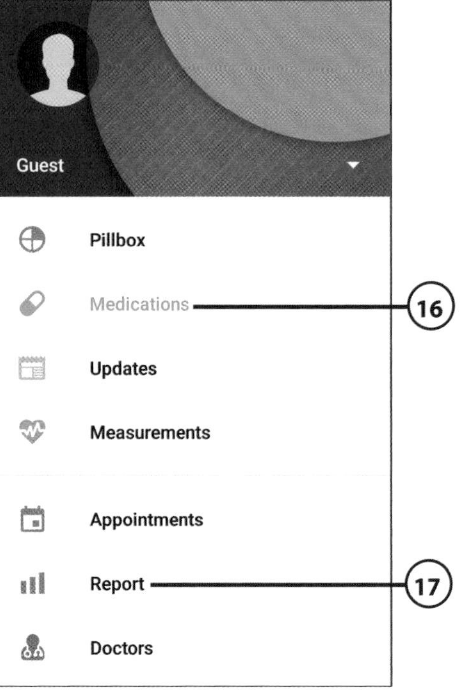

Taking Care of Your Medications with the Mango Health App

The Mango Health app provides reliable medication reminders and drug interaction warnings. Before taking a new drug, always consult your doctor directly about drug interactions. This app also has a points and reward system just for taking your medication. As you stay on track, you earn points toward a chance to win gift cards to your favorite stores, donations to leading charities, and a whole lot more. The app also includes a daily health diary where your medication adherence is automatically tracked. In addition, you can edit the history for better accuracy and record information like symptoms and side effects so that you can monitor how you feel over time. The Mango Health app counts how many pills you have left and provides notice when it's time to get a refill. This app can track multiple medicines taken up to six times a day and push notifications to your Apple Watch.

As of this writing, the Mango health app is available for Android devices and the iPhone and iPad, and can be purchased on the Google Play Store and the App Store. You can begin using the app without creating an account. After downloading the app, follow the steps (shown on an iPhone) in the next section to create a medication regimen and check for drug interactions.

Create a Medication Regimen

You can enter your medication regimen into the Mango Health app in just a couple of minutes. Some of the information you enter includes medication identifiers such as form (tablet, capsule, and so on) and color for added security. There is even an option for medicines you take as needed.

1. Open the Mango Health app, read the Terms of Service, and then tap I Accept.
2. Tap Start Without Code. Mango Health uses activation codes for certain programs it runs through health care programs, or when it distributes the app through certain events such as charity runs.

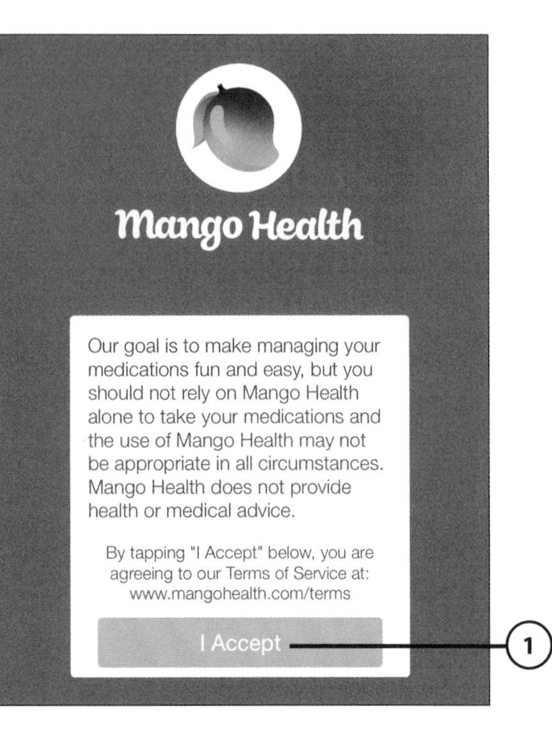
Mango Health
Our goal is to make managing your medications fun and easy, but you should not rely on Mango Health alone to take your medications and the use of Mango Health may not be appropriate in all circumstances. Mango Health does not provide health or medical advice.
By tapping "I Accept" below, you are agreeing to our Terms of Service at: www.mangohealth.com/terms
I Accept
1
Have an activation code?
Enter code
Submit
Start Without Code
2
No activation code? No problem.

3. Tap Let's Get Started to create your medication regimen. A cursor appears in the Medication Name field.

4. Begin typing the name of the medication into the Medication Name Field, and then tap the correct medication in the list of possible results that appear under the field.

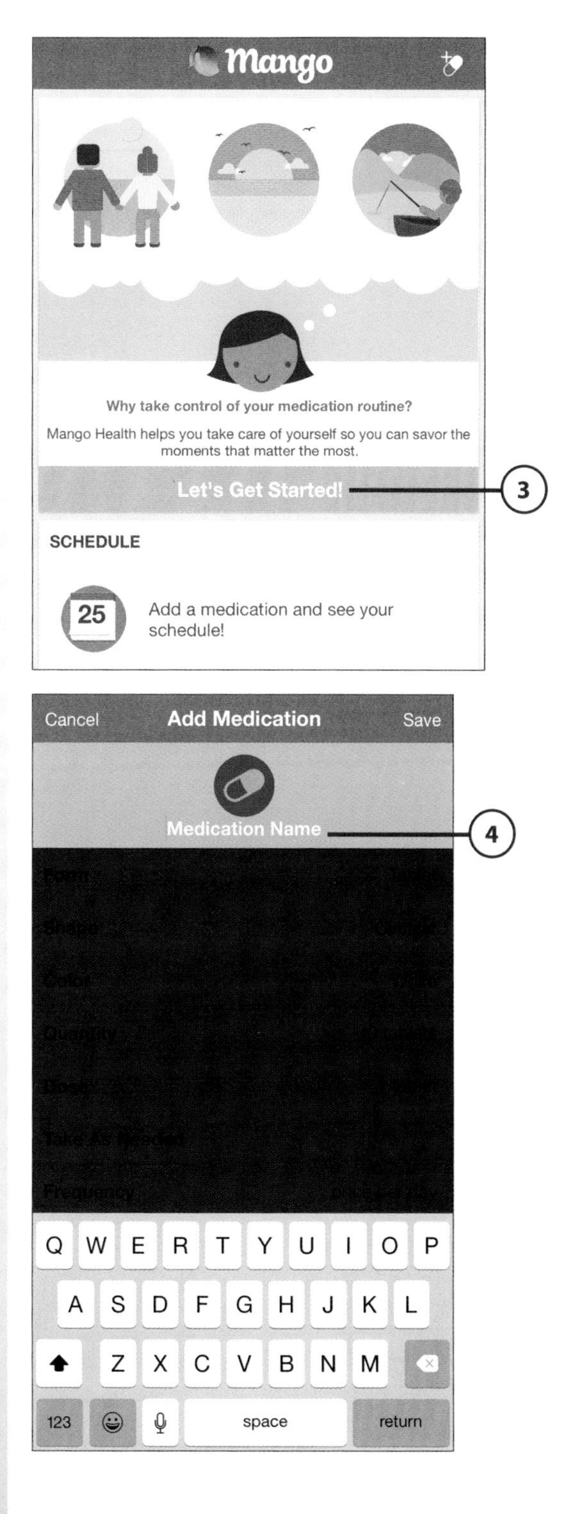

5. Tap Form to specify the form of pill.
6. Tap Color to properly describe the color of the pill.
7. Tap Quantity to enter the exact number of pills prescribed to you per bottle.
8. Tap Dose to enter the proper dose.
9. Slide the Take As Needed option to On if you only take the drug at your own discretion.
10. Slide the Advanced Schedule option to the On position for options related to Frequency and to reveal an option for a specified Start Date.
11. Tap Frequency to enter how many times a day you take the medication. Under this field, the number of Reminder fields changes according to the frequency you enter.
12. Tap each Reminder to set the times you are supposed to take your medication.
13. Tap Save. An app message appears informing you that Mango Health will notify you when it is time to take your medication.

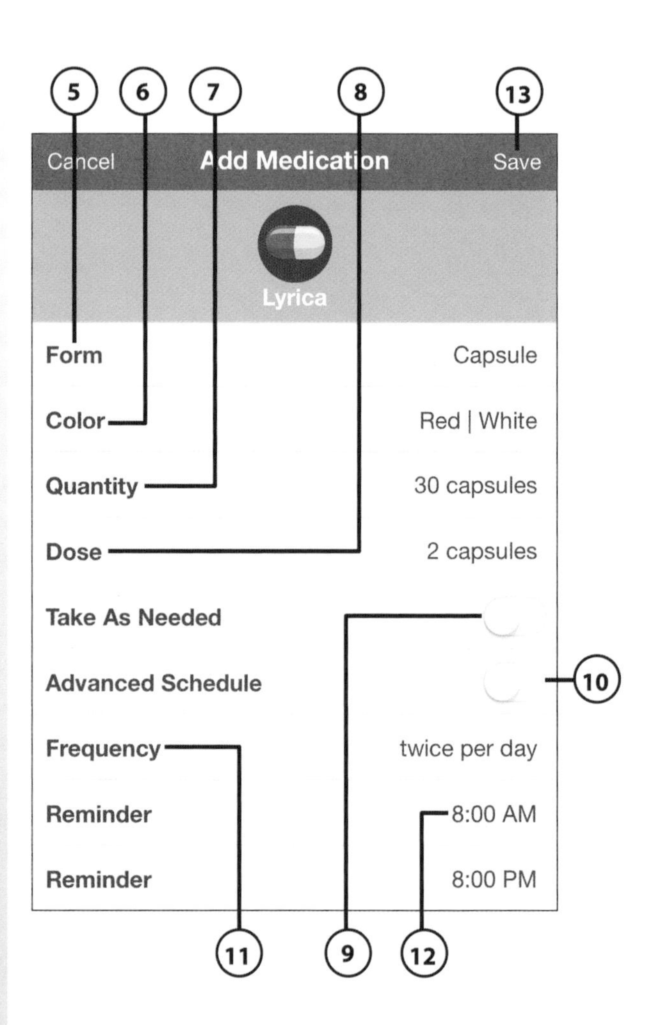

14. Tap OK to receive notification for when it's time to take a dose. Another message appears asking whether it is OK for the app to send alerts to your phone. Choose OK.
15. Tap OK. Now you are ready to receive notifications when it is time to take your medication(s). The Mango Home screen appears again. When you respond to a notification, it opens the Mango Health app where you can tap one of these three options: I Took It, Snooze It, Skip It. Use the Mango Home screen to view a list of all your medications, see how many points you've earned, view your medical adherence history, check your inbox for helpful messages from Mango Health, and keep a mood log as you take the drug.
16. Tap a drug in the list to use charts to track your medication adherence over time, edit a medication or its schedule and alerts, and view important information you need to know about your medication. You can also simply finish/delete the medication.

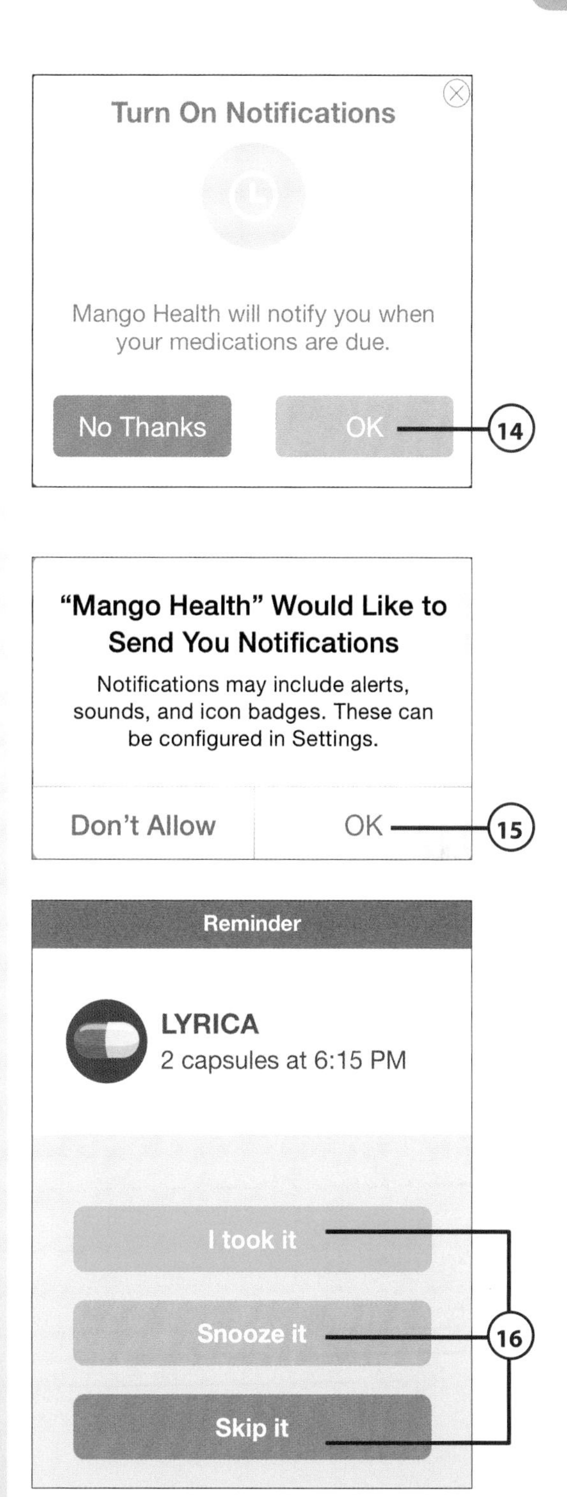
Turn On Notifications
Mango Health will notify you when your medications are due.
No Thanks
OK
14
"Mango Health" Would Like to Send You Notifications
Notifications may include alerts, sounds, and icon badges. These can be configured in Settings.
Don't Allow
OK
15
Reminder
LYRICA
2 capsules at 6:15 PM
I took it
Snooze it
Skip it
16

Check for Drug Interactions

The Mango Health app also provides important information about each drug you take, including food interactions, such as whether you can drink alcohol while using this drug. You also find help general information and instructions regarding specific medications. The app provides alerts for known drug interactions. Although all this information is convenient and at your fingertips, always consult your doctor regarding proper use of medications, possible drug interactions, and other details.

1. From the Mango Health Home screen, tap a medication.
2. Tap Alerts.
3. Tap Food to learn more about food interactions. If there are no known food interactions, none will appear.
4. Tap Information to view detailed information about the drug, including "What do I need to tell my doctor BEFORE I take this drug," and "What are some things I need to know or do while I take this drug?"
5. Tap OTC Interactions to view a list of over-the-counter drugs that react poorly with a particular medication. Always consult your doctor first and foremost concerning drug interactions.

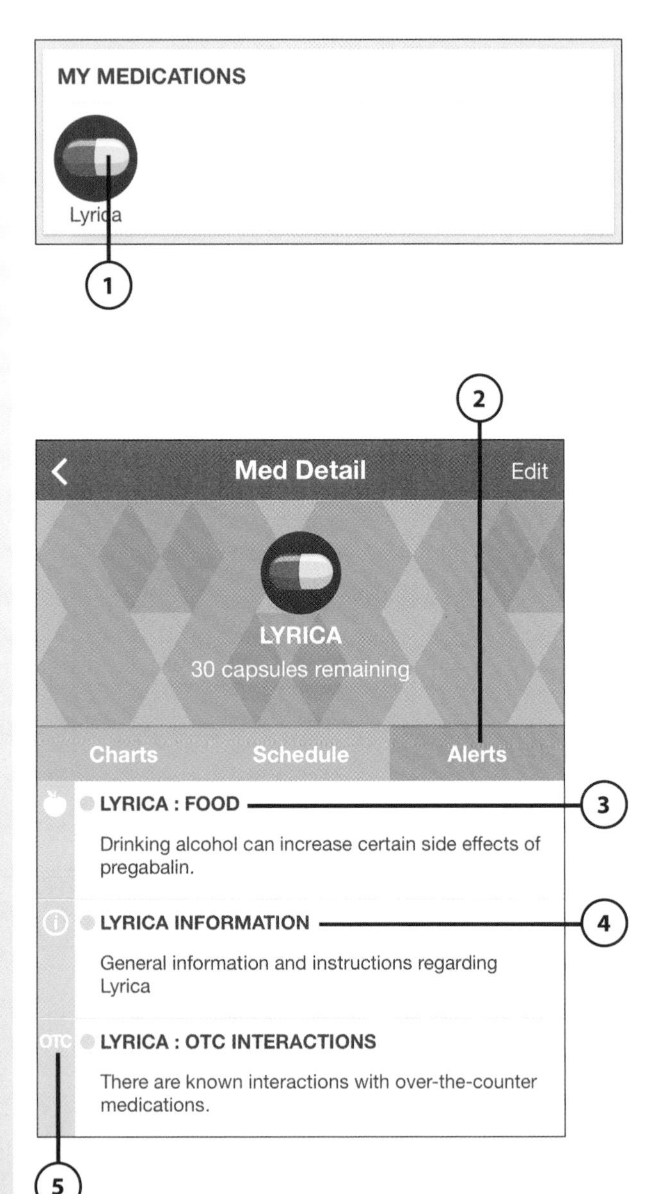

Managing Your Medications with PillPack

PillPack is a full-service, mail-order pharmacy that delivers your medications right to your door, sorted into individual packages that contain your medications organized by date and time. PillPack also has an app that can provide helpful medication reminders. Don't worry if you're not a PillPack member; the PillPack app can automatically import your medications from any pharmacist. If you're already a member, just log in to your PillPack account, and your medications and dose times will already be up to date and waiting. You don't need to be a PillPack member or receive shipments to use the app to remember to take your current medications.

The PillPack app organizes your meds based on the dose time you designate. You can then create a regimen with flexible reminders based on time of day, day of week, and even location. Go to PillPack.com to check out all this app has to offer and see whether it is right for you. As of this writing, the PillPack app only works with the iPhone and Apple Watch and can be downloaded from the App Store. After downloading the app on your iPhone, use the following steps to sign up for PillPack services on pillpack.com, and then add your medications and set up flexible reminders on your phone.

Sign Up for PillPack

Creating a PillPack account is a very easy process. After you create an account, you can begin building your PillPack. Here's how it works after you become a member: PillPack transfers your medications from your current pharmacy, confirms the medications and start dates, delivers your shipments, and contacts your doctor for refills. Your medications arrive pre-sorted, shipping is free, and there is no extra cost, just your monthly co-pays. With PillPack, your co-pay stays the same as with your insurance plan. PillPack accepts most major insurance plans, including most forms of Medicare part D, Aetna, CVS Caremark, and Express Scripts. Visit pillpack.com to see whether your insurance is accepted.

If you are prescribed a new medication that is urgent and you need to start it immediately, such as an antibiotic, PillPack recommends that you fill that prescription at your local pharmacy. For non-urgent medications that you need to start right away, PillPack ships an interim supply that lasts until your next PillPack arrives. New PillPacks are shipped every two weeks.

Remember that you don't need to be a PillPack member to use the app. After you have gone to pillpack.com and vetted the information for yourself, and you decide it's the right move for you, here is how you sign up.

1. Go to pillpack.com, and then click Get Started.
2. Enter and read the information required for your profile, and then click Create My Account.

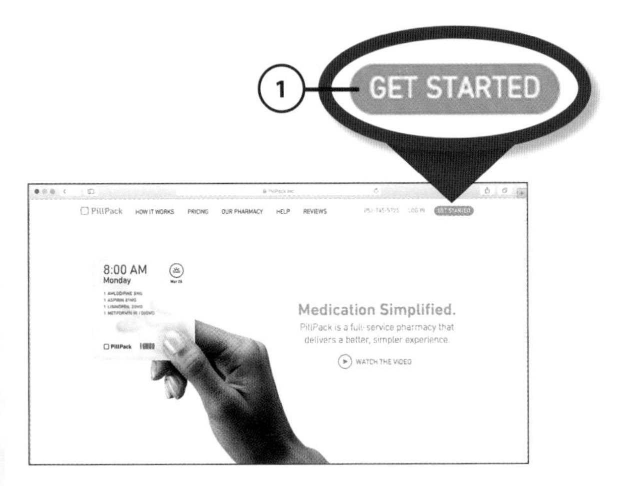

PillPack

Create A Secure Account
Once you do, you'll be able to complete your profile and build your PillPack.

First Name
Last Name
Email Address
Phone Number
Create Password (at least 8 characters)
Confirm Password

Check this button to agree to the PillPack Terms of Use, Child Safety Waiver, Billing Disclosure, HIPAA privacy policy, PillPack Privacy Policy.

CREATE MY ACCOUNT

2

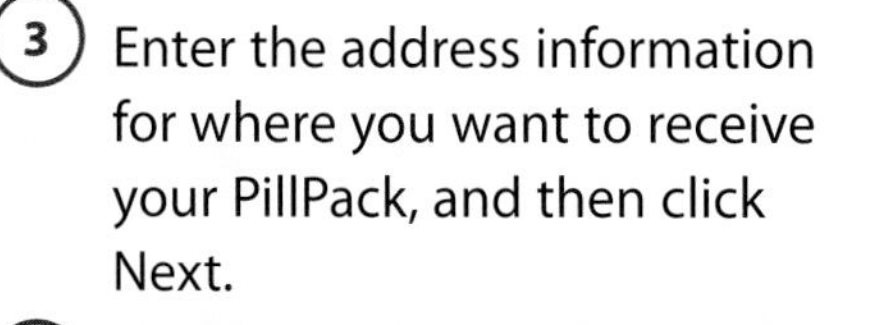

3. Enter the address information for where you want to receive your PillPack, and then click Next.
4. Fill out your personal information, and then click Complete My Profile.
5. Click Enter Medications Manually.

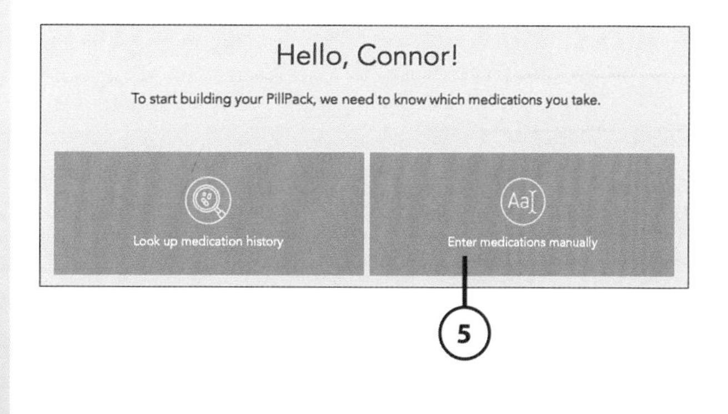
Hello, Connor!
To start building your PillPack, we need to know which medications you take.
Look up medication history
Enter medications manually
5

6. Click Add a Prescription Medication.
7. Enter the information for a medication, and then click Save.
8. Click Add Another Prescription Medication if needed. Keep choosing this option until you have added all of your medications.
9. Click Next: Add Vitamins/OTCs.

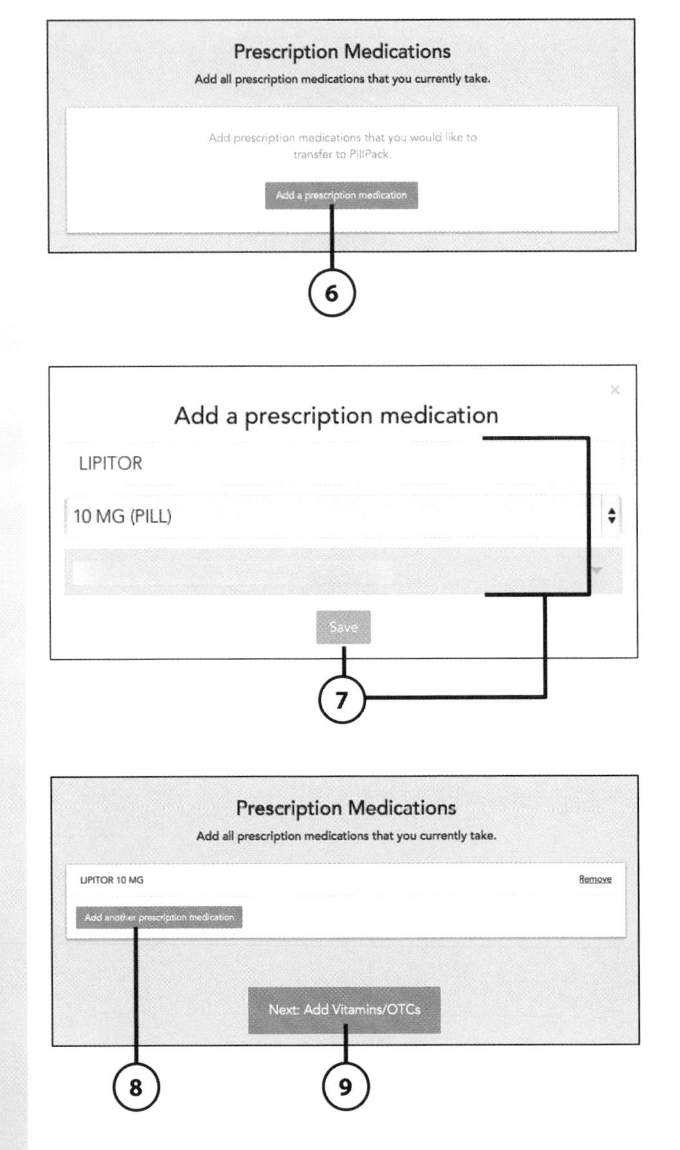

(10) Click Add a Vitamin/OTC, if applicable to your regimen, or skip to step 12.

(11) Enter the information for your over-the-counter medication and supplements, and then click Save. Note that you will be purchasing these medications through PillPack, as you can see by the price estimate onscreen.

(12) Click Add another Vitamin/OTC or click Next: Billing.

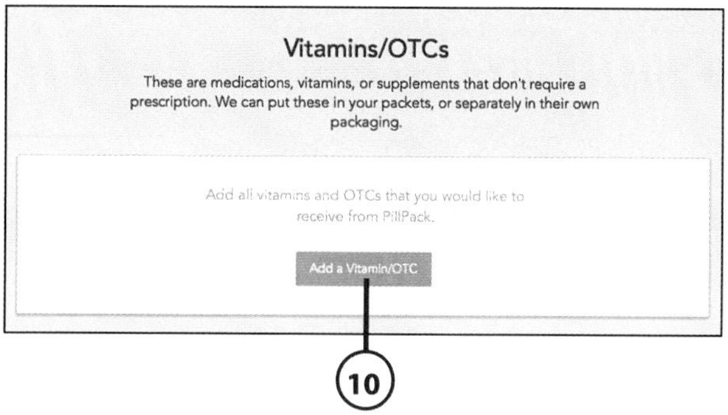

Vitamins/OTCs

These are medications, vitamins, or supplements that don't require a prescription. We can put these in your packets, or separately in their own packaging.

Add all vitamins and OTCs that you would like to receive from PillPack.

Add a Vitamin/OTC

(10)

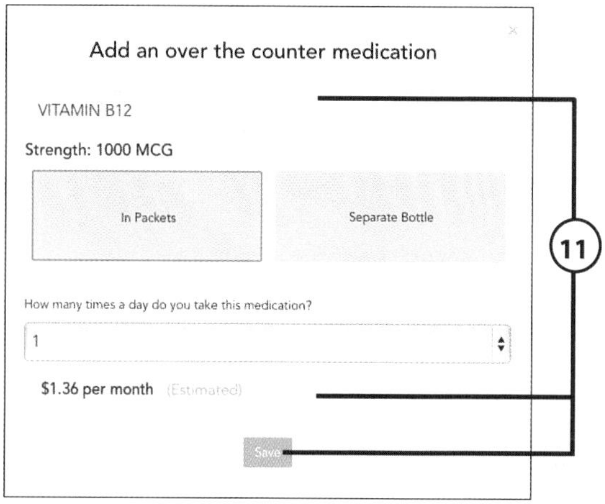

Add an over the counter medication

VITAMIN B12

Strength: 1000 MCG

In Packets

Separate Bottle

How many times a day do you take this medication?

1

$1.36 per month (Estimated)

Save

(11)

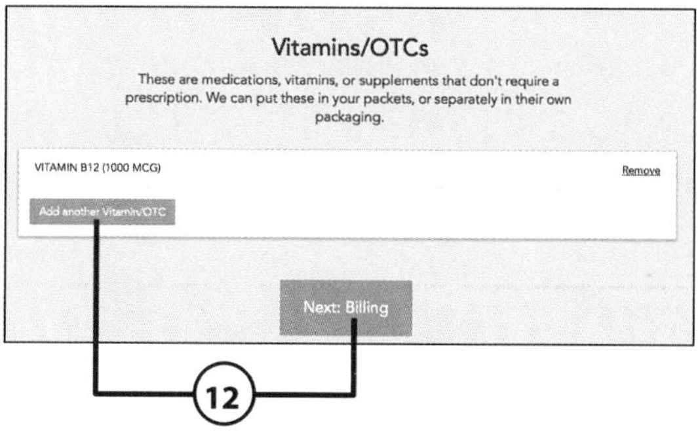

Vitamins/OTCs

These are medications, vitamins, or supplements that don't require a prescription. We can put these in your packets, or separately in their own packaging.

VITAMIN B12 (1000 MCG)

Remove

Add another Vitamin/OTC

Next: Billing

(12)

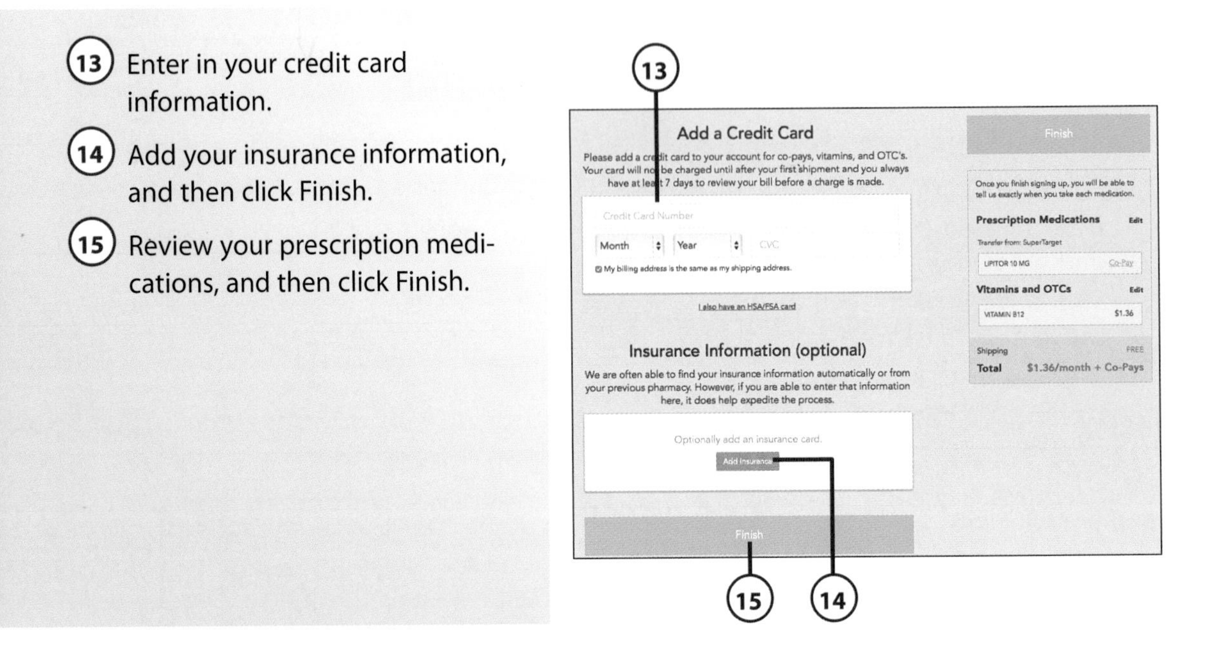

13. Enter in your credit card information.
14. Add your insurance information, and then click Finish.
15. Review your prescription medications, and then click Finish.

Add Medications and Set Reminders

You can input a medication regimen using the PillPack app without being a member. The PillPack app can automatically import your medication list using your pharmacy information or your insurance, or you can enter your medication manually. After your medication has been imported, you can create flexible reminders based on time of day, day of week, and even location.

If you take a medication more than once a day, you simply create a new PillPack for a different time, and then place that medication inside the new pack. You can also create a new pack for new medication or put multiple pills in a single pack.

Staying On Track with Your Daily Medicines Using the MedCoach App

The MedCoach app from the GreatCall company makes it easier for you to stay on track with your prescribed medication and vitamin schedule. A glance at the main screen lets you quickly access your list of medications, set up a pill reminder, access your pharmacy's website to order refills, and more. You can set multiple daily alarms, multiple doses, and automatic refill reminders. MedCoach also supplies detailed information about the medication you are taking, but be sure to consult your doctor if you have questions about your meds.

As of this writing, the MedCoach app is available for Android phones and the iPhone and can be downloaded from the Google Play Store and the App Store. After you download the app on your phone, use the following directions to register, add your medications, set up pill reminders, and order refills from your pharmacy. The following steps are shown on an Android phone.

Register and Add Your Medications

To use the MedCoach app, you first must register or sign in using an existing login. Registering only takes a few steps, and if you do not use an existing GreatCall device, you must register through the app. When you're finished, you can begin entering your medications and move on to create helpful reminders.

1. Open the MedCoach app, and tap Sign Up. If you are already a GreatCall subscriber, tap Log In and enter a valid email address and password.
2. Enter your information into the fields, and then tap Sign Up.

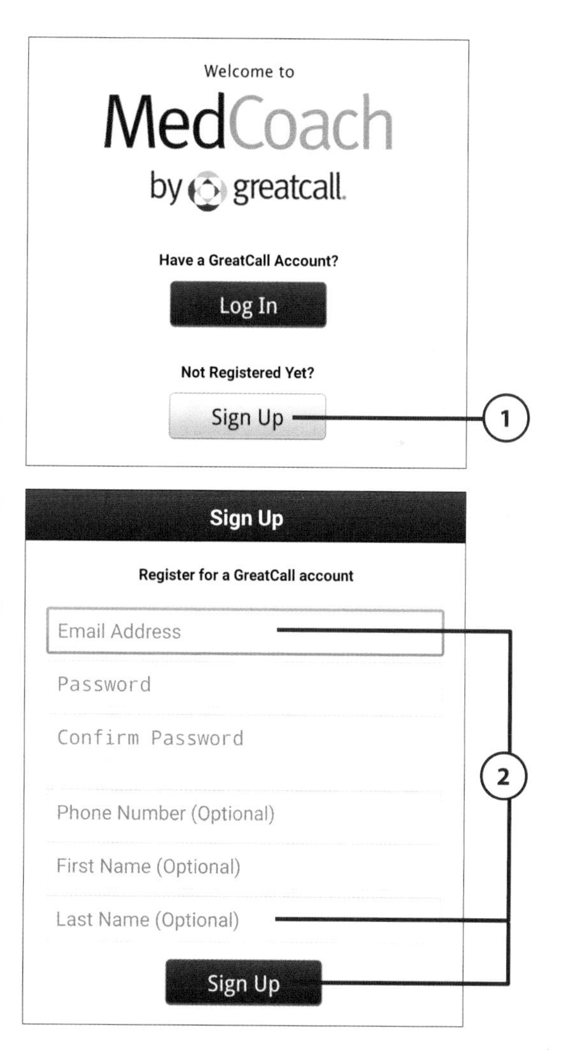

3. Read the Terms and Conditions, and then tap Accept. The main screen opens.
4. Tap Medications to get started. If you're ever unclear about what an icon does on the main screen, simply tap and continue to hold down an icon until a description appears in a little box onscreen.
5. Tap the plus icon to begin adding your medications.

Terms and Conditions

Welcome to the GreatCall MedCoach Service (the "Service"). By subscribing to the Service, you accept, without limitation or qualification, these terms and conditions of use ("Terms and Conditions"). GreatCall may change these Terms and Conditions periodically without notice, and you agree to be bound by any such changes. The Service is designed to offer you general health information for educational purposes only. GreatCall is not a healthcare provider and does not provide health care services. We do not prescribe, disperse, or refill prescriptions. As used in these Terms and Conditions, "we" refers to GreatCall, its content providers, affiliates, suppliers and any third parties mentioned on the GreatCall website. The Service is not intended to be professional advice and is not a substitute for professional medical advice, diagnosis, or treatment. You must always seek the advice of your physician or other qualified healthcare provider with any questions you may have regarding a medical condition and/or medical treatment. If you have or suspect that you have a medical problem or condition, please contact a qualified healthcare provider immediately. You should never disregard medical advice or delay in seeking it because of something you have read on this site. We do not recommend or endorse any vendor, physician, pharmacy, tests, products, drugs, or device manufacturers. The clinical information contained in the information is intended as a supplement to, and not a substitute for, the knowledge, expertise, skill, and judgment of physicians, pharmacists, or other healthcare professionals in patient care. The absence of a warning for a given drug or drug combination should not be construed to indicate that the drug or drug combination is safe, appropriate, or effective in any given patient.

We do not make any warranty that the content in this Service

Decline Accept (3)

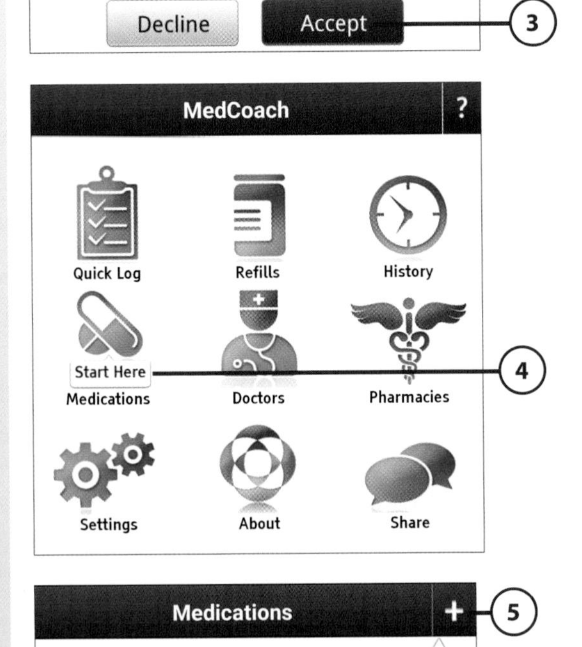

6. Enter the name of the medicine into the Select Medication field, and then tap the relevant search result that appears beneath the field.

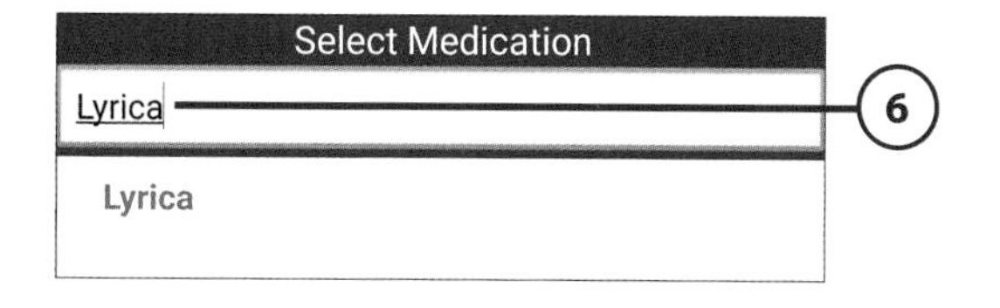

7. Tap to choose the correct dose of the medicine.
8. Tap OK.
9. Tap in the Amount I Take field and enter the amount of the medication you consume at each dose. Continue to the next section to see how to create detailed pill reminders. After you finish filling out all the information for a medication (pill information, pill reminders, refill information), you can add more medications.

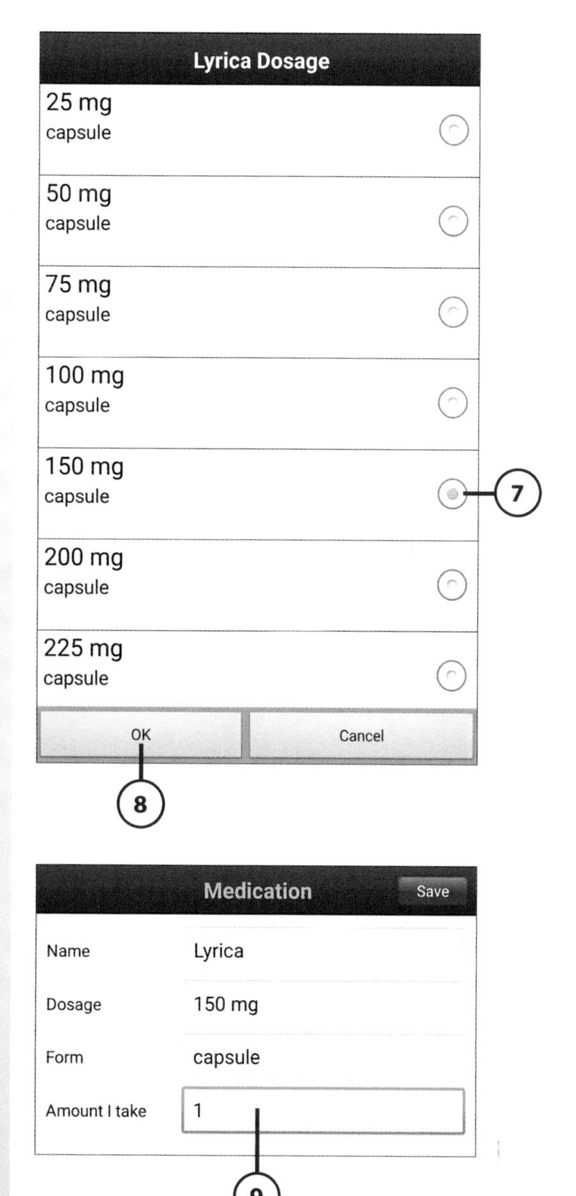

Set Up Pill Reminders

After you have added a medication, setting up a medication regimen is easy. You can set a medication for multiple doses throughout a day, an entire week, or just on specific days. Add the time you take your meds, and you're nearly ready to take full advantage of MedCoach as a medication manager.

1. On the Medication screen, tap Days I Take This to choose a specific day of the week or Select All to signify you take the drug on a daily basis.
2. Tap OK.

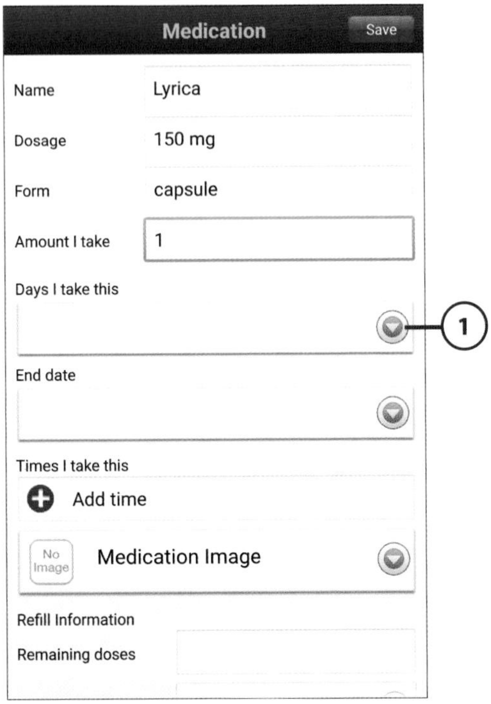

Medication Save
Name Lyrica
Dosage 150 mg
Form capsule
Amount I take 1
Days I take this
End date
Times I take this
Add time
No Image Medication Image
Refill Information
Remaining doses

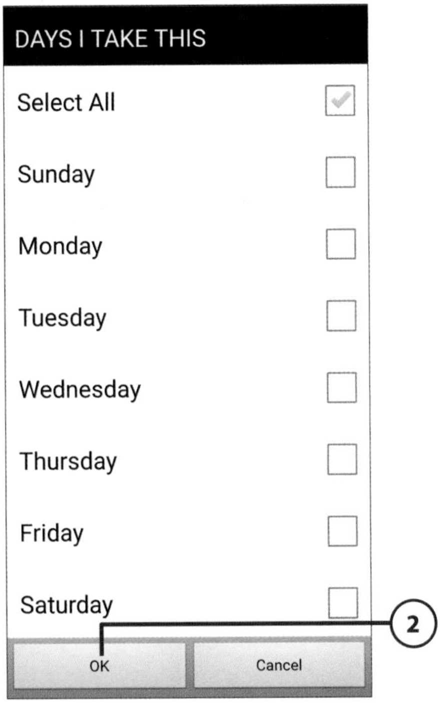

DAYS I TAKE THIS
Select All
Sunday
Monday
Tuesday
Wednesday
Thursday
Friday
Saturday
OK Cancel

3. Tap the End date drop-down arrow to specify when you can stop taking your medicine.
4. Tap plus or minus to move forward or backward through the months, days, and years. Tap OK when you are done.
5. Tap Clear if your intake will be ongoing. This option leaves the field blank.
6. Tap Add Time.
7. Tap plus or minus to move forward or backward through hours and minutes, and tap AM to switch to PM. Tap OK when you are done.

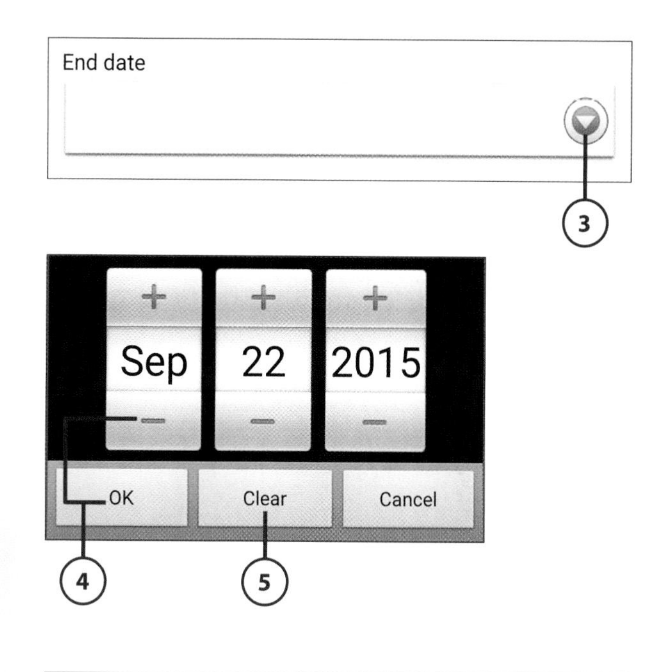

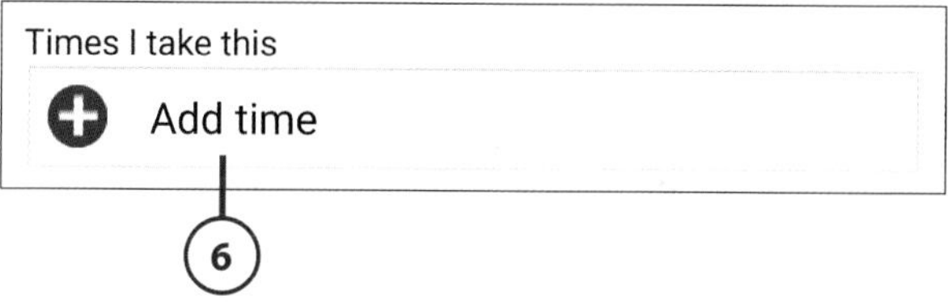

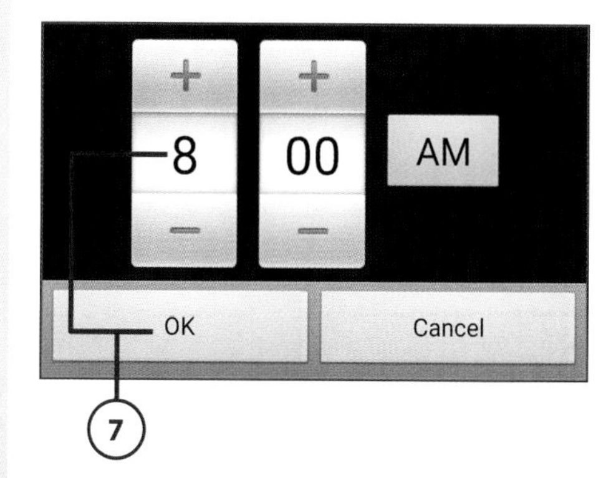

8. Tap Add Time again, if you take the med more than once a day.
9. Enter a time for your second dose, and then tap OK. Notice that you can add more times on the Medication screen.
10. Tap Medication Image so you can properly identify the medication.
11. Tap a method of adding a picture of your medication to your medication profile. For this example, Take a Photo was chosen. As soon as you take the photo it appears in the profile. Now you are ready to make getting refills easy by entering your refill information in the next section.

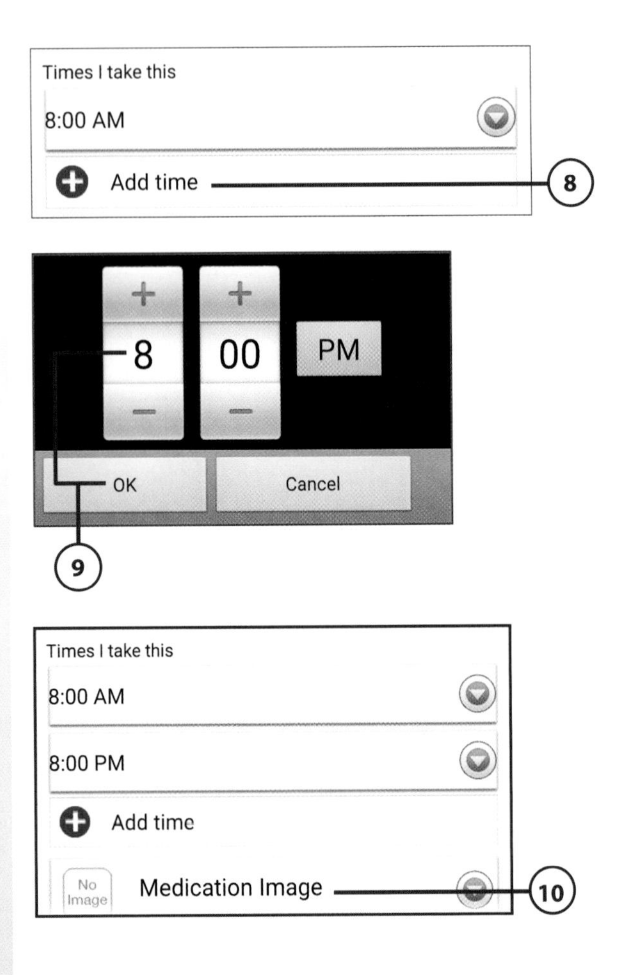

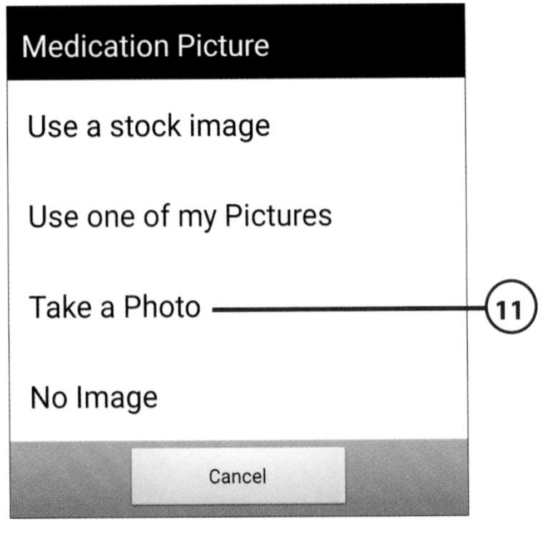

Order Refills from Your Pharmacy

MedCoach makes getting refills easy just by your entering a bit of information about your meds, the pharmacy you use, and the prescribing doctor. You can set a reminder to alert you that you are low on a medication and it's time to get a refill.

1. Swipe to scroll to the bottom of the medication screen, and then tap in the Remaining doses field and add how many doses you have left of your current prescription.
2. Tap Last refill and enter the date you last had your prescription filled.
3. Tap in the Rx Number field to enter the prescription number.
4. Tap Reminder and choose when you would like to be reminded when it's time for a refill. Your options are: 1, 2, 3 days before, or No need.
5. Tap Pharmacy to add a pharmacy to your list.
6. Tap Add Pharmacy.

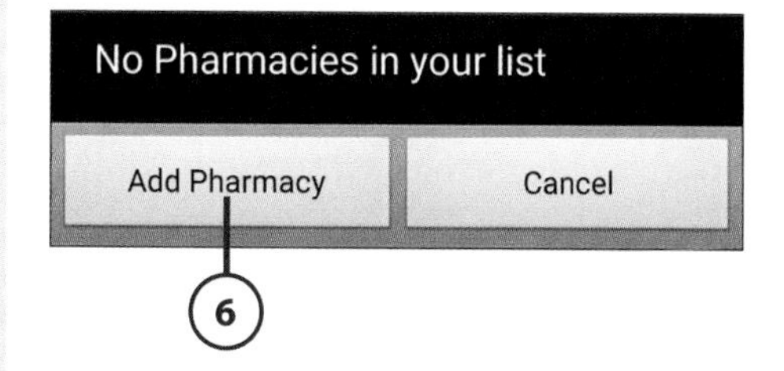

7. Enter the information for your dispensing pharmacy, and then tap Save. If your pharmacy contact information is already in your address book, you can tap Import from Address Book, and then follow the instructions to add this information.
8. Tap Prescribing Doctor.
9. Tap Add Doctor.

Add Pharmacy
Save
Name
Phone
Address
Address 2
City
State
ZIP
Import from Address Book

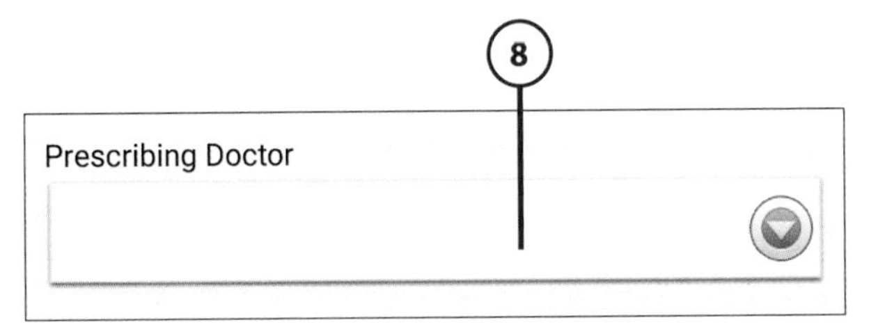

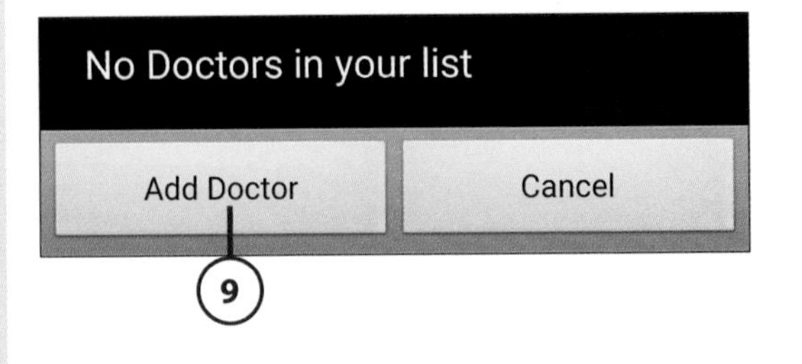

10. Enter the information for your prescribing doctor, and then tap Save. If your doctor's contact information is already in your address book, you can tap Import from Address Book, and then follow the instructions to add this information.
11. Tap in the Instructions field to leave any specific instructions for the pharmacist who is filling this prescription.
12. Tap Save to save all of your information for this medication. Now you are set up to receive reminders both for when to take your medication and when you need to refill a prescription.

Add Doctor
Save
10
Name
Phone
Speciality
Address
Address 2
City
State
ZIP
Import from Address Book

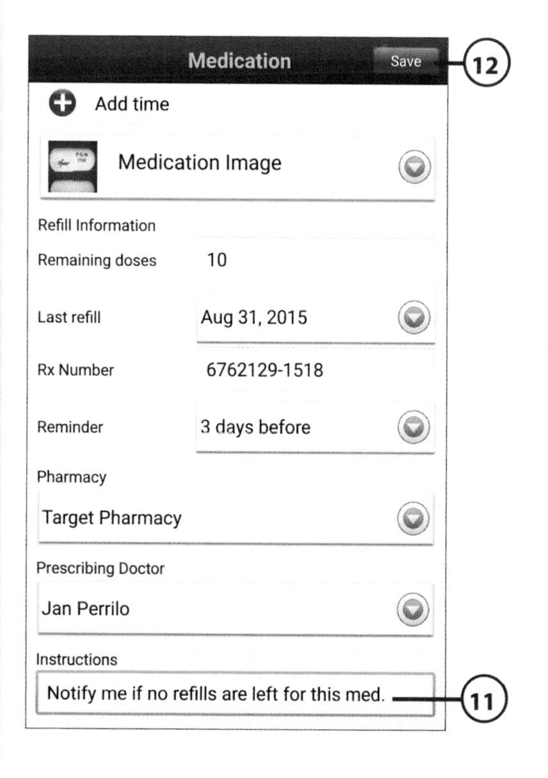

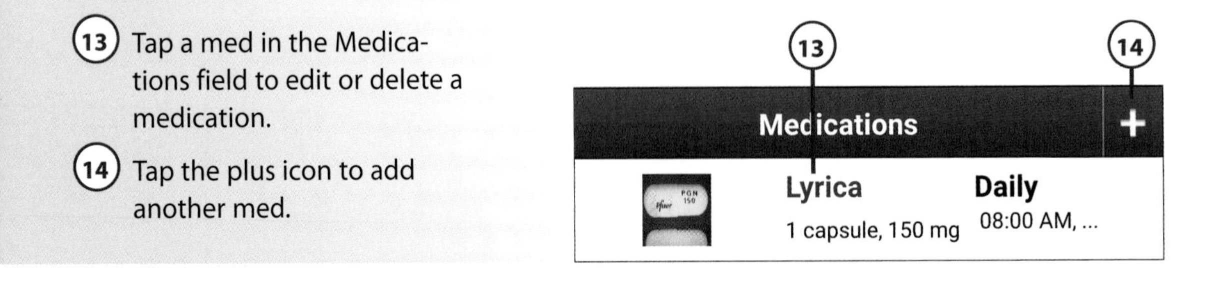

13. Tap a med in the Medications field to edit or delete a medication.
14. Tap the plus icon to add another med.

>>>Go Further

THE AARP RX APP

Another medication management resource for you to consider is the AARP Rx app, available for Android phones and the iPhone. AARP Rx lets you organize all your important information into one place. Carry a list of your medications in your pocket so that the next time a nurse asks which medications you're taking, you can simply hand her your phone.

AARP Rx makes it easy for you to enter all your medication into the app by using the camera on your phone to scan labels; no typing is necessary. Stay on track with your medication regimen by receiving reminders when it is time to take your medication or refill a prescription. You can even track when you take your medications and monitor your progress. AARP Rx organizes personal, medical, and safety information such as symptoms, medical contacts, and insurance information.

Access AARP expert advice on staying healthy, understanding your benefits and insurance, and planning for the future. Unlimited storage and priority customer support is offered for free for AARP members. Download the AARP Rx app for free from the Google Play Store and the App Store.

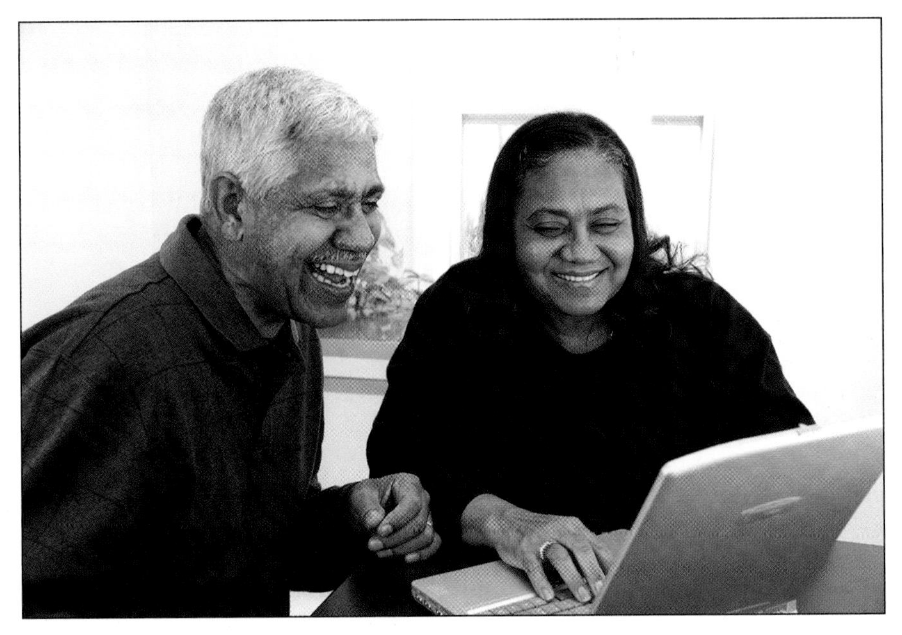

Credit: © Rob/Fotolia.com

Use online communities, web services, apps, consumer electronics, and ride-hailing services to stay engaged.

In this chapter, you explore options for staying socially engaged through online support communities and using ride-sharing services and electronic devices to help you stay in contact with family, friends, and coworkers.

6

Using Social Engagement as Health Support Systems

Social engagement can be a big part of living a healthy lifestyle—a life filled with vitality. In fact, studies show that being isolated is bad for your health. People who are older and isolated have much higher rates of mortality from breast cancer, high blood pressure, heart disease, and other chronic diseases. The National Science Foundation has found that chronic loneliness has also been shown to lead to depression. Online communities such as AARP and Ben's Friends can help you connect with people with common interests and concerns. Advancements in consumer technology, including smartphones and tablets, have made it increasingly easy to stay in contact with family, friends, and coworkers. If distance, a busy schedule, or mobility is keeping you from staying socially engaged, these advancements can help you stay connected. Ride-hailing services including Lyft and Uber can also conveniently get you around town. Whatever your situation might be, consider the options in this chapter for staying socially active, because maintaining healthy social connections can improve well-being.

Joining the AARP Online Community

AARP says it best: "You never know what (or who) you might discover in the AARP.org Online Community." That's a quote from their website. The AARP Online Community offers a great way to connect with others on similar interests, experiences, and needs, and it's free. All you need to do is register to create a personal profile, share photos, publish a blog, join groups, subscribe to e-newsletters, and start sharing in some good conversation. Get in on the conversation by joining groups for people with special interests. For example, you can join the "Rock 'N' Roll" group to chat with a group of fun people and share your memories and interest in music. There is even a group for new users to meet and get help navigating the community. Within the AARP community you can find discussions on Health that are as specific as Brain Health, Diet & Exercise, Health Care Reform, Healthy Eating, and much more. Start a dialogue of your own in other areas, including Work & Retirement, Money, Travel, or Home & Relationships for light or serious conversation.

To join the AARP online community, simply go to community.aarp.org and click Register in the upper-right corner.

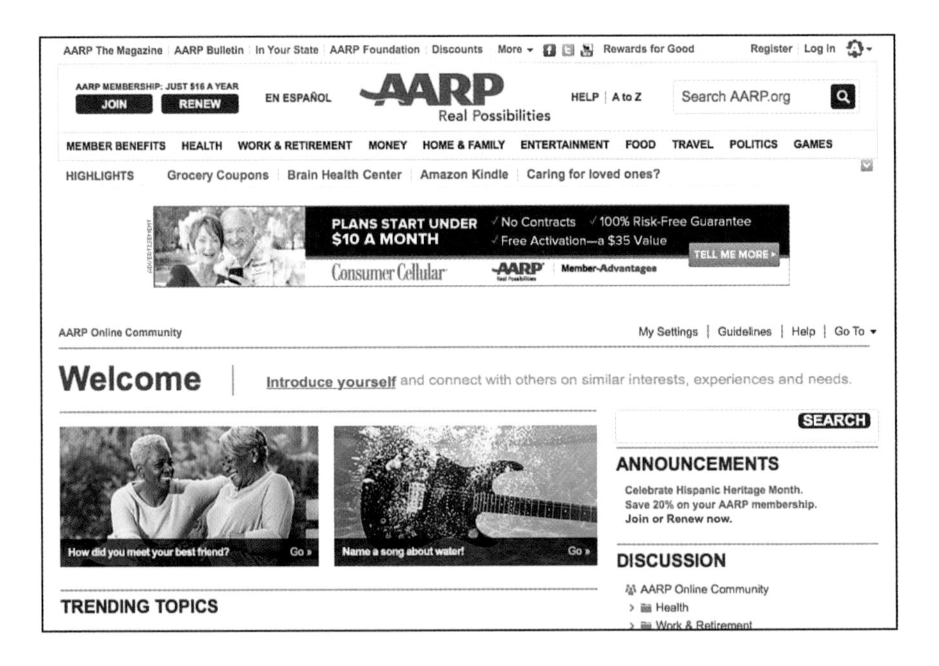

Exploring Transportation Services for Getting Around Town

Cabs aren't the only game in town anymore. Lyft and Uber are popular transportation alternatives to the traditional taxi service. Have you ever seen a car with a large, fuzzy, pink mustache on its front bumper in your city? That's Lyft. Ride-sharing services like Uber and Lyft arose from a desire to have an alternative to calling a taxi or raising a hand trying to hail one. People also wanted the rates to be cheaper and wait times to be shorter. Now all you have to do is take out your smartphone, make a few taps on an app, and then wait for your ride. Think of this new type of service like a ride-for-hire, or a tap- or click-to-book service. Unlike a taxi, you can get an up-front estimate of how much the trip will cost. You can also track your driver online instead of having to call back the taxi service and endure the uncertainty of when your ride might actually show up.

These are two popular transportation options available to you. These services might not be offered in your area, so be sure to check the service area for the option you pick. Now let's dive deeper into these services and see how they work.

Getting a Ride Using Lyft

Getting a ride with Lyft is simple. First, download the app for your Android phone or iPhone, and then sign up. Now you just open the app and request a ride. Lyft matches you with a driver that is closest to your area so you don't have a long wait to get picked up. Visit lyft.com to see whether Lyft is available in your city.

Sign Up, Request a Ride, and Choose a Payment Method

Signing up with Lyft is a short process that you can do easily online or on the phone. This example is shown in the app for Android devices. If you require a larger viewing area, visit Lyft.com on your computer and click Sign Up Now. After completing the sign-up process, you can request a ride with the click of a button, and then easily choose a payment method.

1. Open the Lyft app, and Tap Sign Up.
2. Enter your first and last names and the email you want associated with your Lyft account, and then tap Next. You can also sign up using your existing Facebook account. Keep in mind that logging in via Facebook can pose privacy issues by giving the app access to your social media data.

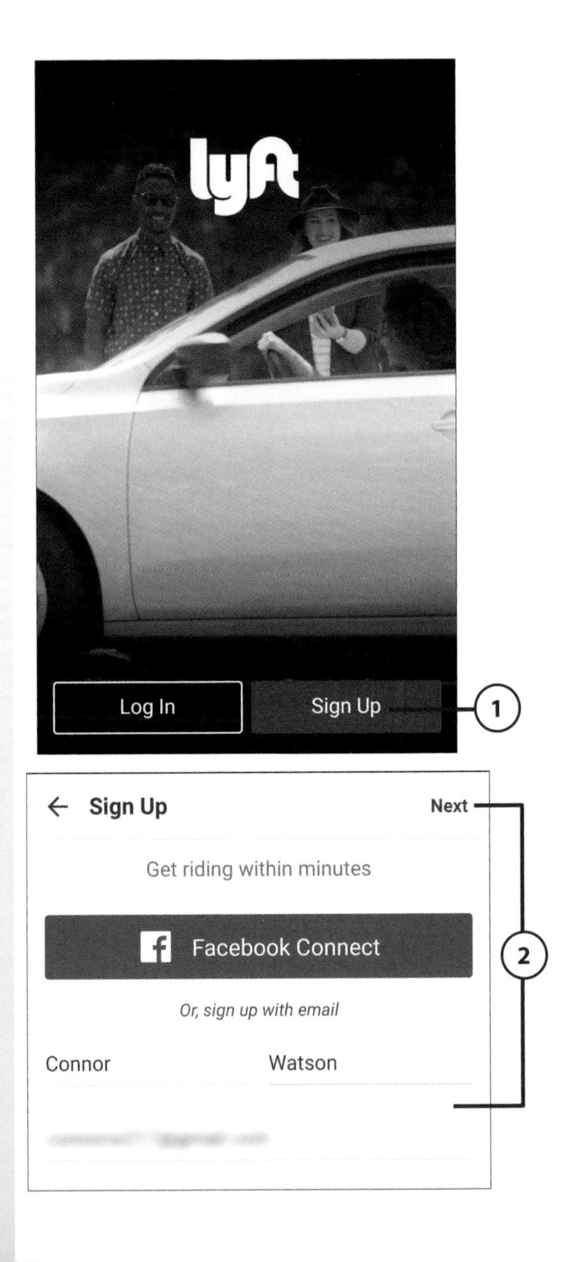

3. Enter your phone number, and then tap Next. The Lyft app sends you a code.
4. The code should already appear in the proper field, so tap Next. Lyft automatically detects your current location on a map and lists the services available in your area.

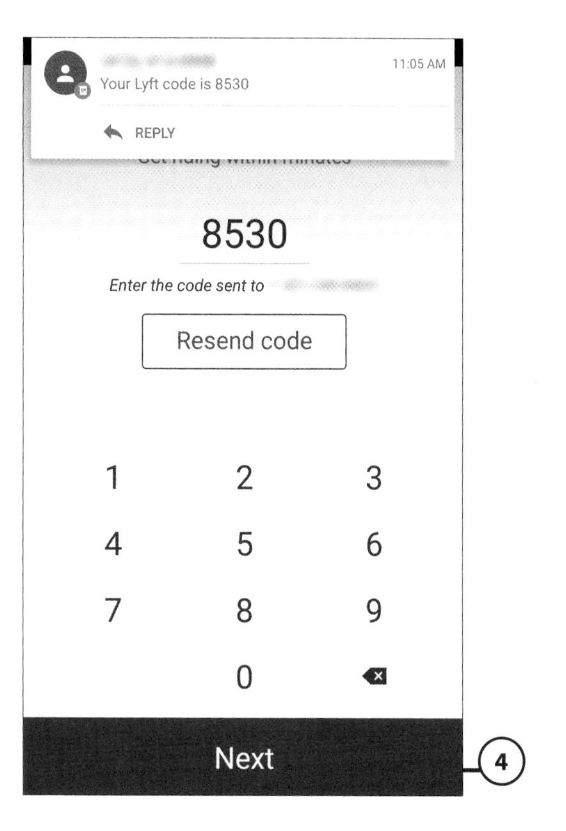

Moving Around in the Map

You can view different locations in the map by dragging your finger across the map. Pinch your fingers in or outward to zoom in and out of the map.

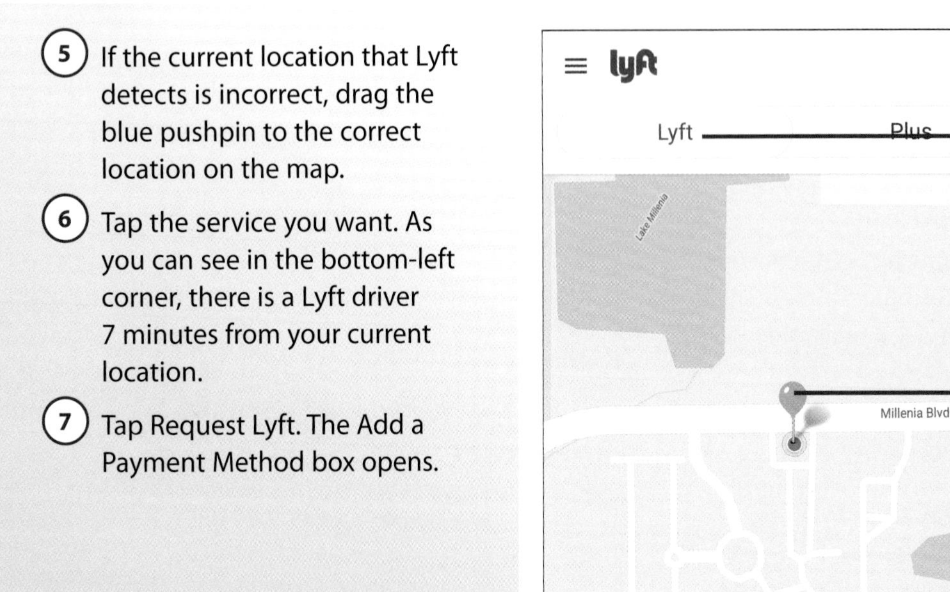

5. If the current location that Lyft detects is incorrect, drag the blue pushpin to the correct location on the map.
6. Tap the service you want. As you can see in the bottom-left corner, there is a Lyft driver 7 minutes from your current location.
7. Tap Request Lyft. The Add a Payment Method box opens.

>>>Go Further

THREE WAYS TO RIDE WITH LYFT

You can choose from three services depending on which city you live in.

Lyft: This is the original service where you can ride solo or with up to three friends.

Lyft Plus: This service accommodates a six-passenger ride.

Lyft Line: This option lets you share a ride with others who are going the same way for a lower price.

8. Enter your payment method and information, and then tap Save. A credit card number was used in this example. After the payment box goes away, your driver appears at the bottom of the screen with the car he or she will be driving. You can tap Add Photo to add a photo of yourself. View the estimated time of pickup at the top of the screen and watch the driver's travel on the map in the center of the screen.

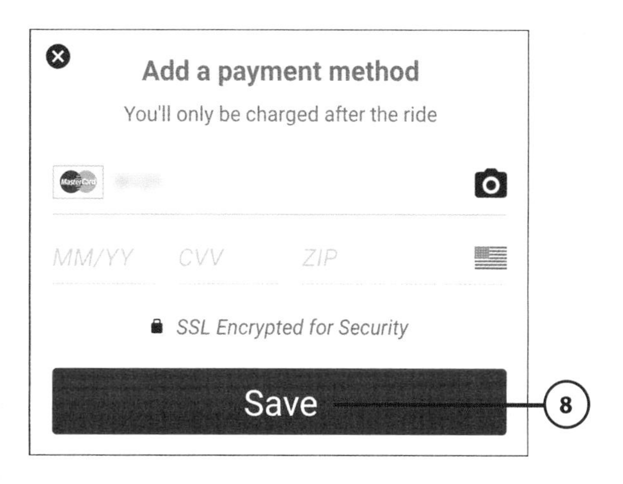

9. Tap Add Destination (the pink pushpin) to enter where you want to go.
10. Tap the three vertical dots if you need to cancel the ride.
11. Tap the main menu to split a payment among several people or to edit your method of payment.

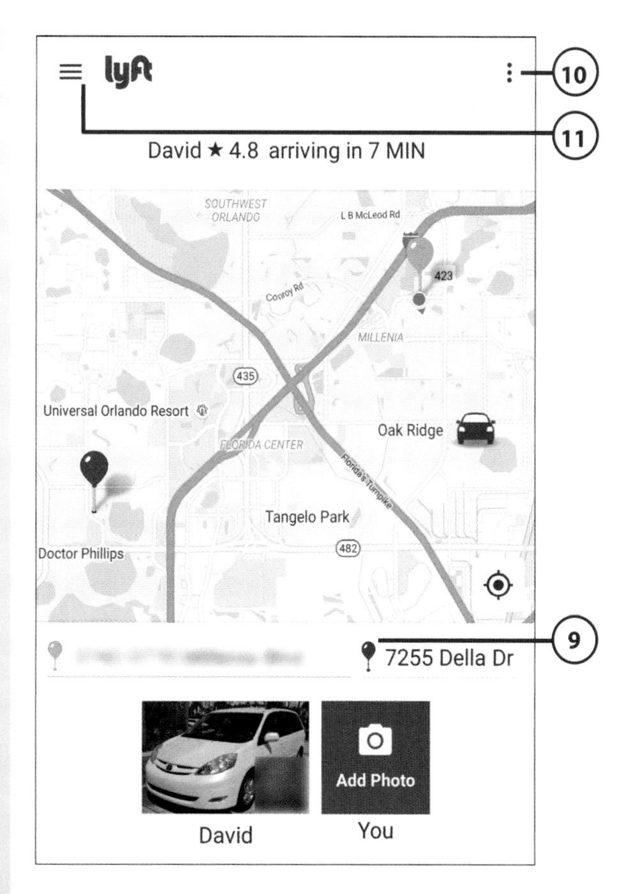

Cancellation Policy

A cancellation fee might be applied in certain cases to compensate the driver for time and gas spent. You're charged $5 ($10 if you live in New York or Boston) if you cancel 5 minutes after you request the ride or if the driver is within 5 minutes of the estimated time of arrival. In regard to the Lyft Line service, if you make multiple cancellations within a short amount of time, you might be charged $1 ($2 in New York City). Because Lyft Line is a ride-sharing service, two or more of those requests must be matched with another passenger for you to be charged.

Get a Fare Estimate

If you live in a Lyft Line–enabled area such as New York City, you can estimate the cost of a trip in Lyft Line mode by using the estimator built in to the Lyft app. After entering your pickup and drop-off locations, you see a guaranteed price for your ride. If you live in a city without Lyft Line, estimates are only available by going to lyft.com. Final calculations of Lyft charges are done and made available in the app when you have completed your ride, based on traffic, weather, or other conditions. If you want to see an estimate of your ride, go to lyft.com and perform the calculation by selecting your city, if it appears in the list.

1. Open your Internet browser and go to lyft.com.
2. Click Cities. A list of cities appears.

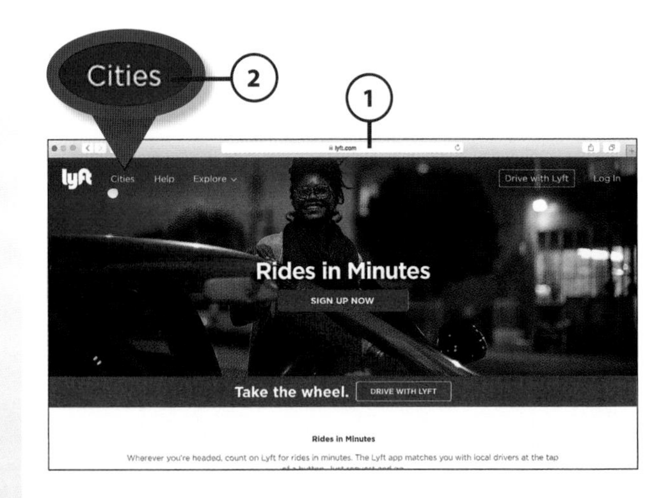

3. Click on your city.
4. Scroll down the page and enter the addresses in the Add pickup location and Add destination fields, and then click Get Estimate.
5. View the results beneath the From and To addresses. The total price for this 5.8-mile example is $10 dollars for the basic Lyft service, or $18 for Lyft Plus service.
6. Scroll down the page to see how Lyft calculates its pricing for various services.

Available Lyft Cities

Arizona
Oro Valley
Phoenix
Scottsdale
Surprise
Tempe
Tucson

California
Alameda
Antioch
Bakersfield
Berkeley
Burbank

Florida
Boca Raton
Boynton/Delray Beach
Clearwater
Fort Lauderdale
Homestead
Jacksonville
Kissimmee
Miami
Orlando
Sanford
St Petersburg
Tampa Bay
West Palm Beach

New York
New York City

North Carolina
Cary
Chapel Hill
Charlotte
Concord
Durham
Huntersville
Matthews
Raleigh

Ohio

3

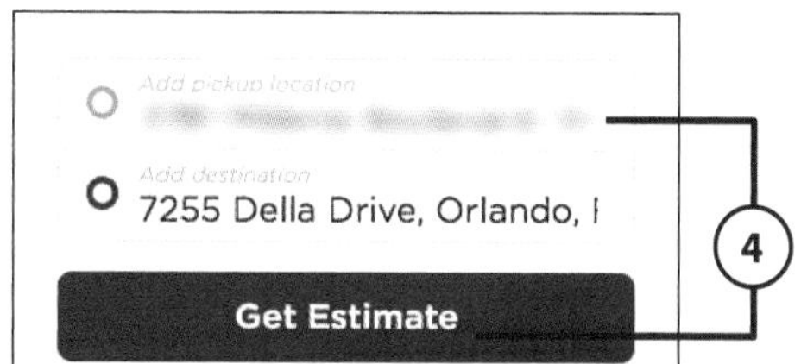

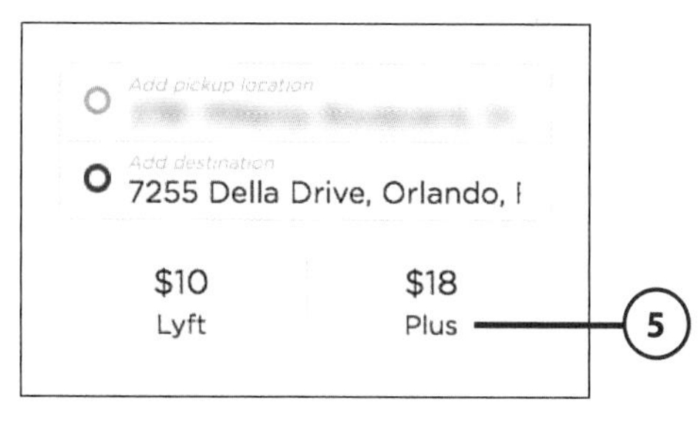

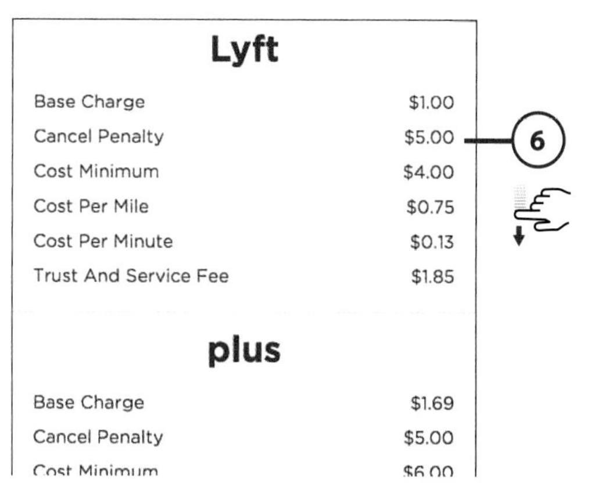

Lyft
Base Charge $1.00
Cancel Penalty $5.00
Cost Minimum $4.00
Cost Per Mile $0.75
Cost Per Minute $0.13
Trust And Service Fee $1.85
plus
Base Charge $1.69
Cancel Penalty $5.00
Cost Minimum $6.00
6

Getting to Know Uber

Uber is a ride-sharing service similar to Lyft where you can tap to book a ride from your Android phone or iPhone. The Uber app is also available for Windows Phones and can be downloaded from the Windows Store. With a single tap from you, Uber uses the GPS in your phone and Wi-Fi to pinpoint your location and connect you with the nearest available driver for a fast pickup. Uber is available in many cities, but before booking, go to uber.com and see whether your city is on the list. Let's get signed up to use Uber.

Sign Up and Designate a Payment Plan

The sign-up process also includes designating a payment method. For this reason, I recommend signing up on the Uber website so you can use a bigger screen and a full-size keyboard, and then you can just log in to the app on an iPhone. You can complete the entire process in the app, but you might find it more convenient to do it via computer.

1. From your computer's browser, go to uber.com, and then click Sign Up.
2. Click Allow for Uber to use your current location, and then proceed to sign up to ride. This example shows the Safari browser on an iMac being used to visit the Uber website. Your browser might also ask whether it's okay to use your current location. If it does ask, click OK.

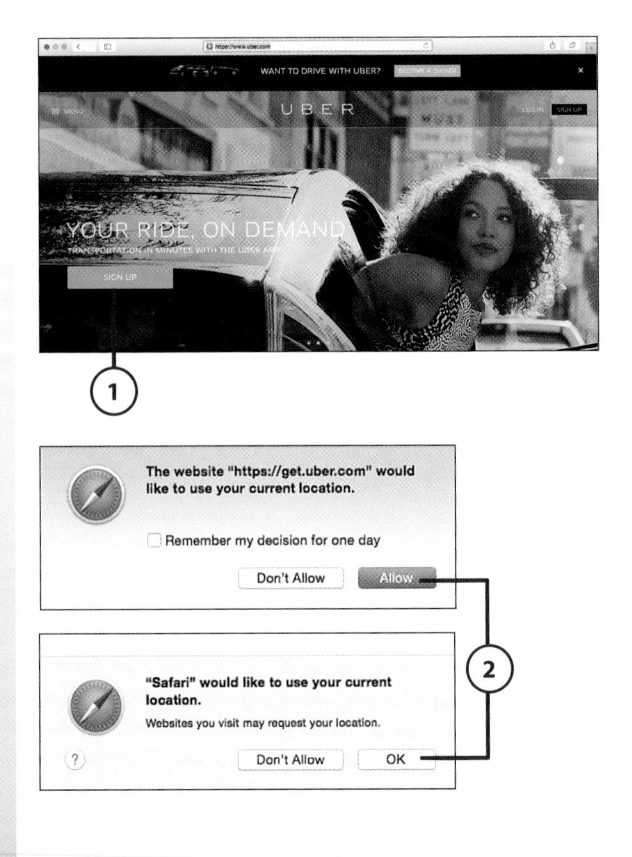

3. Enter your Account information.
4. Enter your Profile information.
5. Scroll down to the bottom of the page, and then enter your Payment information.
6. Click Create Account. A verification number is sent to your phone by text message. Write down the number because later you will be asked to enter it into the Uber app to confirm your account. Now let's switch to the Uber app.

Account
Required
EMAIL
name@example.com
PASSWORD
At least 5 characters

Profile
NAME
First Name
Last Name
MOBILE NUMBER
'+1'
(201) 555-5555
LANGUAGE
English (United States)

Payment
CREDIT CARD NUMBER
1234 5678 9012 3456
CVV
123
EXPIRATION DATE
month
year
POSTAL CODE
94103
PROMOTION CODE
Promotion Code

Please fill out all required (*) fields.

By clicking "Create Account", you agree to Uber's Terms and Conditions and Privacy Policy.

Request a Ride and Get a Fare Estimate

Requesting a ride from the Uber app is as simple as selecting your pickup location on a map. Uber provides you the convenience of getting an estimate of your trip before you go. You can compare a range of fares for your trip after you enter a pickup location and the destination. Keep in mind that traffic, weather, and other factors affect fare estimates. Download the Uber app and let's get started. The following example is shown on an iPhone.

1. Open the Uber app, and tap Sign In. A message appears asking whether it is okay for Uber to access your location while you use the app.
2. Tap Allow in the message box.

Modifying Notification Settings

You can always change your mind and edit the settings to not allow notifications and receive your trip info by text messaging.

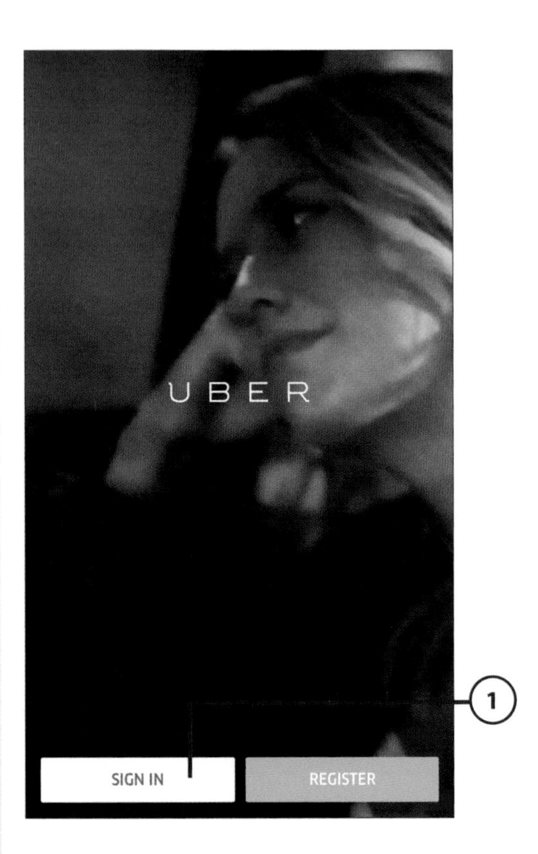

Allow "Uber" to access your location while you use the app?

We use this to set your pickup location and improve our services. Learn more in our Privacy Statement.

Don't Allow | Allow

2

3. Enter your credentials, and then tap Done. Note that you could have also signed in using an existing Facebook account. Keep in mind that logging in via Facebook can pose privacy issues by giving the app access to your social media data.
4. Enter the verification code that was sent to you by text message. The next screen appears as soon as you finish typing the four digits. This informs you that Uber can now send you trip notifications instead of using text messaging.
5. Tap Continue.

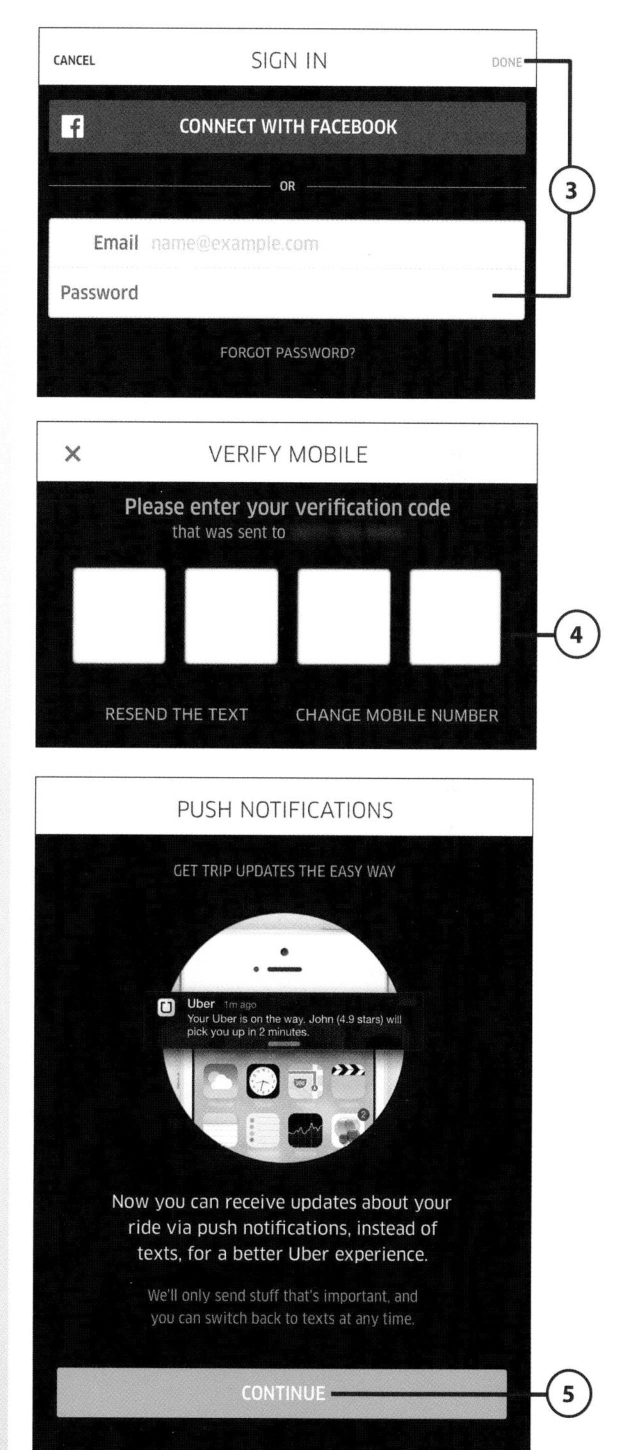

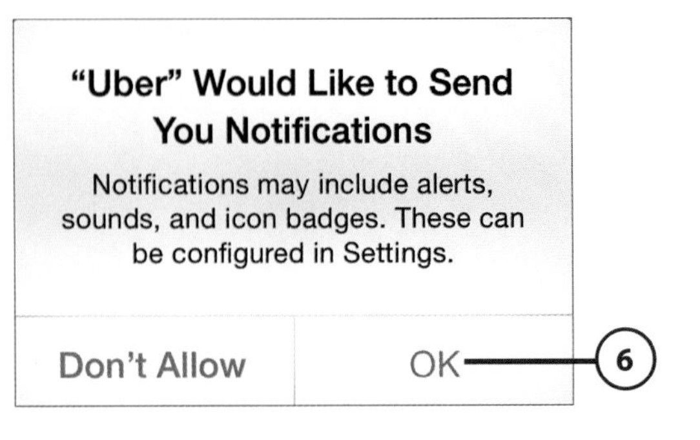

6. Tap OK. Uber uses GPS and Wi-Fi to automatically detect your location and places a blue dot on top of the location.
7. If the area that the app detects is incorrect, you can drag the Set Pickup Location black overlay to another location on the map where you want to be picked up. You can also tap Go To Pin to enter the exact address.

Moving Around the App

You can view different locations in the map by simply dragging your finger across the map. Pinch your fingers in or outward to zoom in and out of the map.

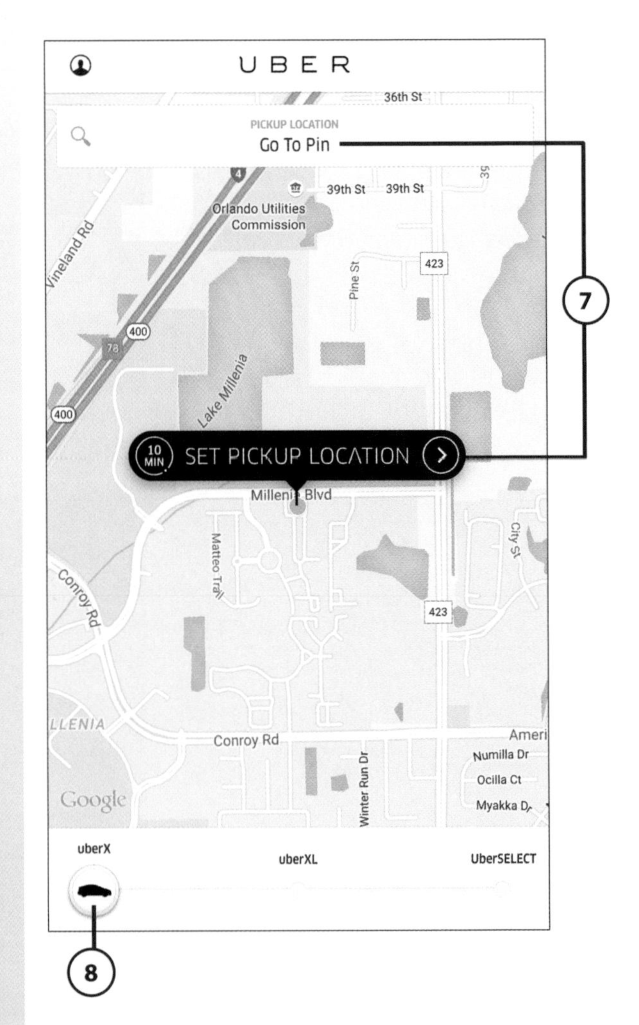

8. Drag the car icon at the bottom of the screen to select the Uber service that is right for you. All services might not be available in your area. This example shows UberX selected.

>>>Go Further

THREE WAYS TO RIDE WITH UBER

You can choose from a number of Uber vehicles for different occasions or for how many people will be riding along.

UberX: This is the everyday, non-luxury Uber car. For example, this could be a Toyota Camry, Prius, Honda Accord, and so on. This option is the least expensive of the group.

UberXL: This option is a non-luxury SUV such as a Toyota Highlander, Nissan Pathfinder, and more. Think spacious when considering this option.

UberSelect: This is a higher-end option to UberX with sometimes double the rates. Cars can include a BMW 7 Series, Mercedes S-Class, and more.

These options might have different names depending on where you live. Go to uber.com to review the entire line.

9. After you choose a service, tap the car icon to review more details about that particular service. In this example, an UberX car can accommodate four passengers and is 8 minutes away. The minimum fare is $4 USD. Tap the icon again to collapse the window.
10. Tap Set Pickup Location to designate the pickup spot.

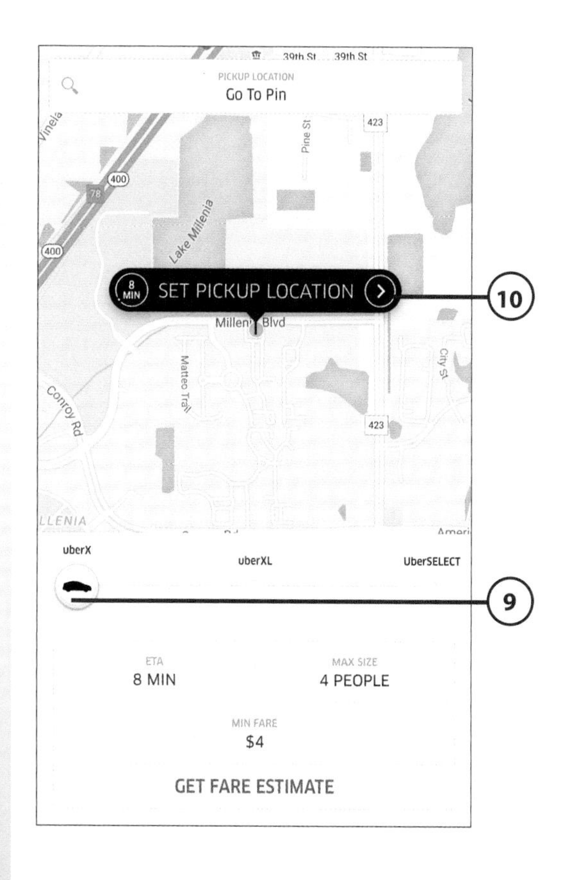

11. Tap Fare Estimate to enter a location and see how much the ride will cost.
12. Enter the destination, and then tap the correct result that appears under the search field. A fare estimate is shown.

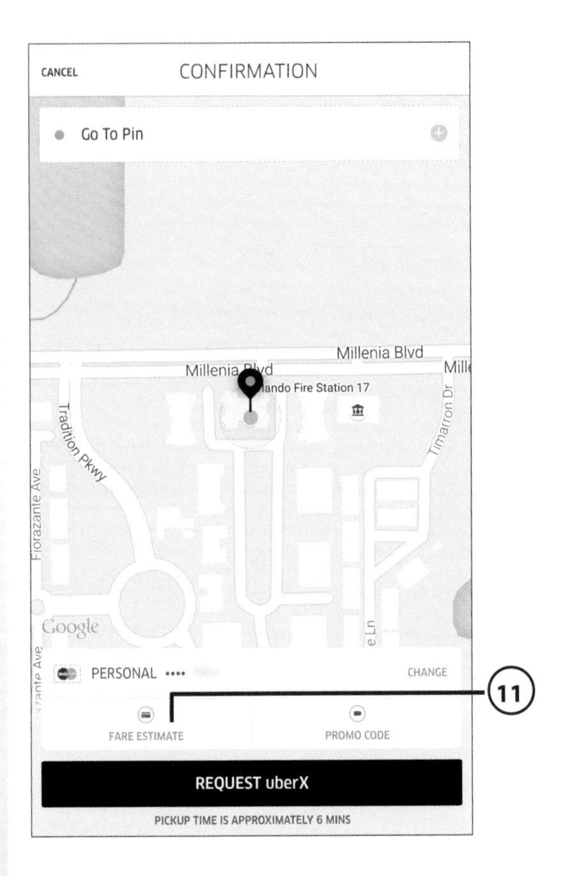

FARE ESTIMATE
7468 Sand Lake
12
7468 Sand Lake Commons Boulevard
Orlando, FL
7468 Sand Lake Road
Sky Lake, FL
7468 Sand Lake Rd
Orlando, FL
7468 Sand Lake Road
Altamonte Springs, FL
7468 Sand Lake Pointe Loop
Pine Castle, FL
Search for "7468 Sand Lake"

13. Tap the X to return to the previous screen. Your pickup point and destination now appear at the top of the screen. The route appears on the map and the pickup time appears at the very bottom of the screen.
14. Tap Request uberX at the bottom of the screen.

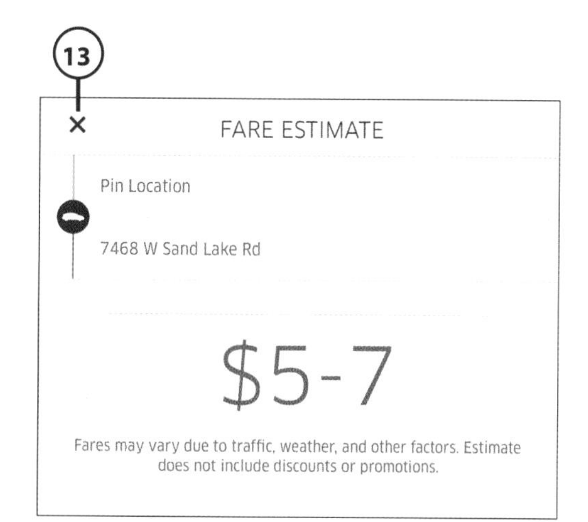

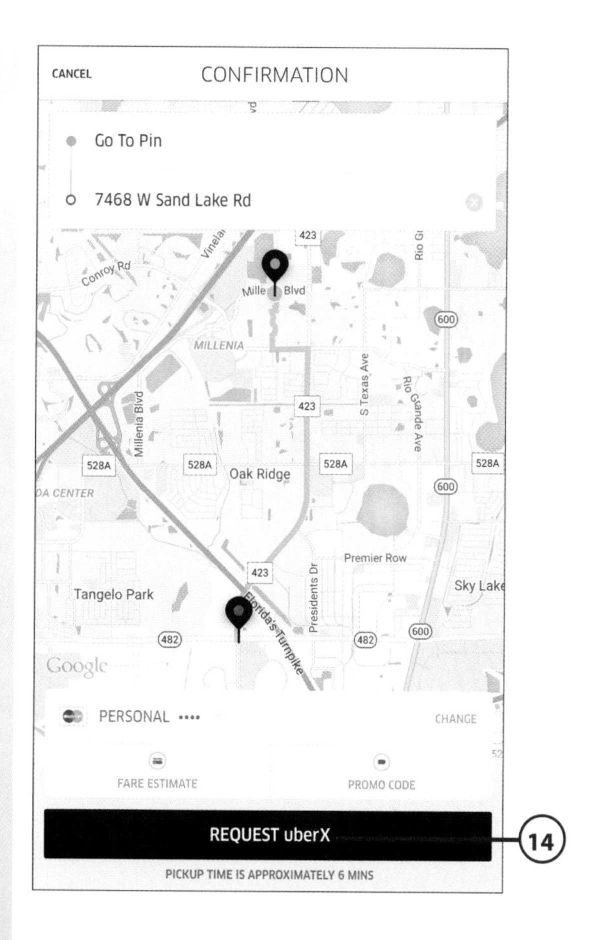

15. Wait for your ride. There is no action to take to pay the driver after you arrive at your destination. The payment is automatically deducted from your online payment method. A screen signifying that you have booked a ride appears. Just tap OK.
16. To cancel a ride, swipe the blue part of the screen upward to view more options. Notice that your driver's information appears at the bottom of the screen.
17. Tap Cancel Trip. Uber will then ask you why you cancelled the trip. Simply tap one of the response options.

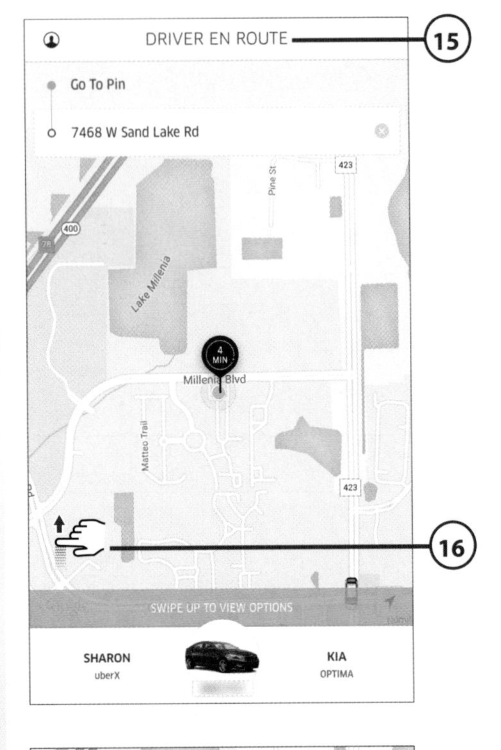

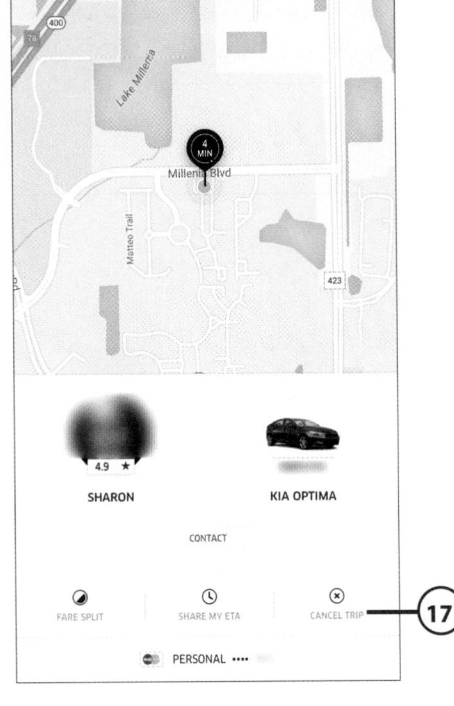

Cancellation Policy

A cancellation fee might be applied if you cancel 5 minutes or more after scheduling a pickup. If you are not at the pickup location, or if the driver cannot get in touch with you, a cancellation fee is still applied.

Finding Patient Support Communities

Having your own support network of people affected by the same health conditions as you can be a great a source of comfort and strength. Websites like Ben's Friends, CrowdMed, and PatientsLikeMe are dedicated to connecting patients with similar health conditions with one another to improve quality of life by learning from others. You can compare life experiences and treatment symptoms, and make new friends who can relate to your particular situation. CrowdMed offers an alternative solution for finding answers to an unsolved medical condition you might be struggling with by using medical experts from around the world to help solve the world's most difficult medical cases. Take a closer look at the following options to see whether one or each of them can be of help to you.

Exploring Communities for People with Rare Diseases at Ben's Friends

Bensfriends.org is an "incubator" for new communities for all diseases that don't currently have dedicated communities. How Ben's Friends works is that a member creates a group for a rare disease; when that group becomes larger, a dedicated community is created. There are a number of communities for rare disease conditions listed on bensfriends.org. If you have a rare disease, take a look at the site and see whether you can find your condition. Many people are waiting to meet you and share in a wealth of knowledge on how to live a more fulfilling life.

Ben's Friends makes it easy for you to browse conditions to find the right community for you. As of this writing, there are 30+ communities and counting. If you don't see your condition, you can follow a process to start your own group.

1. With your computer browser, go to bensfriends.org.
2. Click Our Story to learn more about the mission of bensfriends.org and about the history of the website.
3. Click Our Communities at the top of the screen, and then select Community List to see whether one fits you.
4. Scroll down to the bottom of the screen, and if you don't see your condition, click @info@bensfriends.org to learn how to create a group.

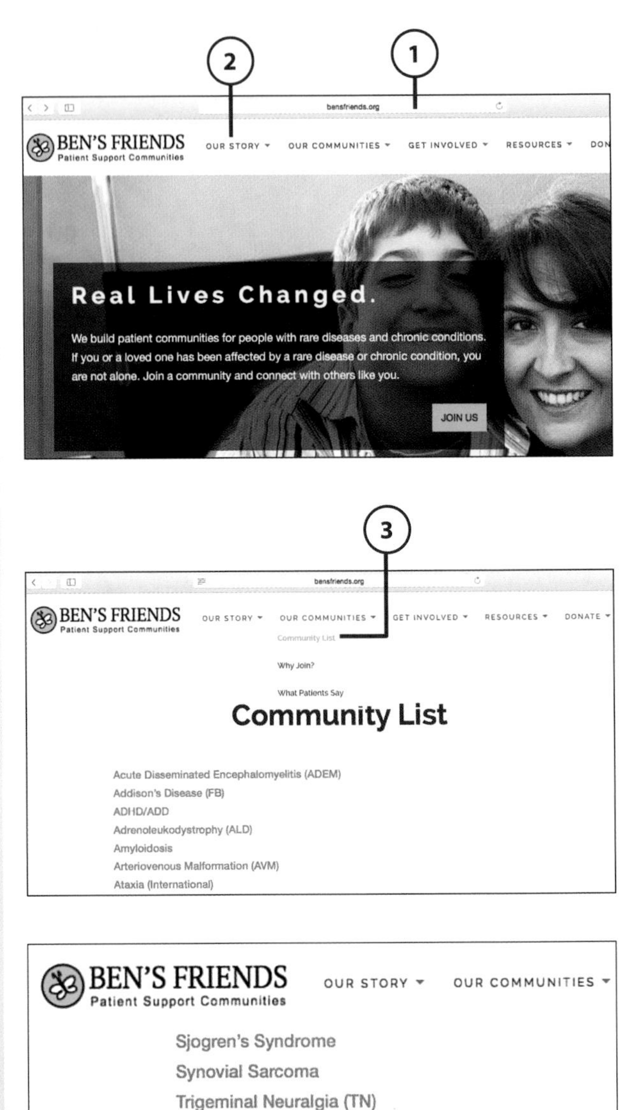

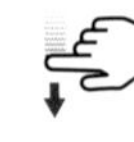

Join a Community

Tens of thousands of lives are being changed every month at Ben's Friends. If you, a family member, or a friend is living with a rare condition, you are not alone, and can join a safe and supportive patient community. Ben's Friends also has an app for your iPhone. The following examples are shown on the bensfriends.org website.

1. Click on a condition under Communities.
2. Click the Member link.
3. Fill out the information, and then click Sign Up.

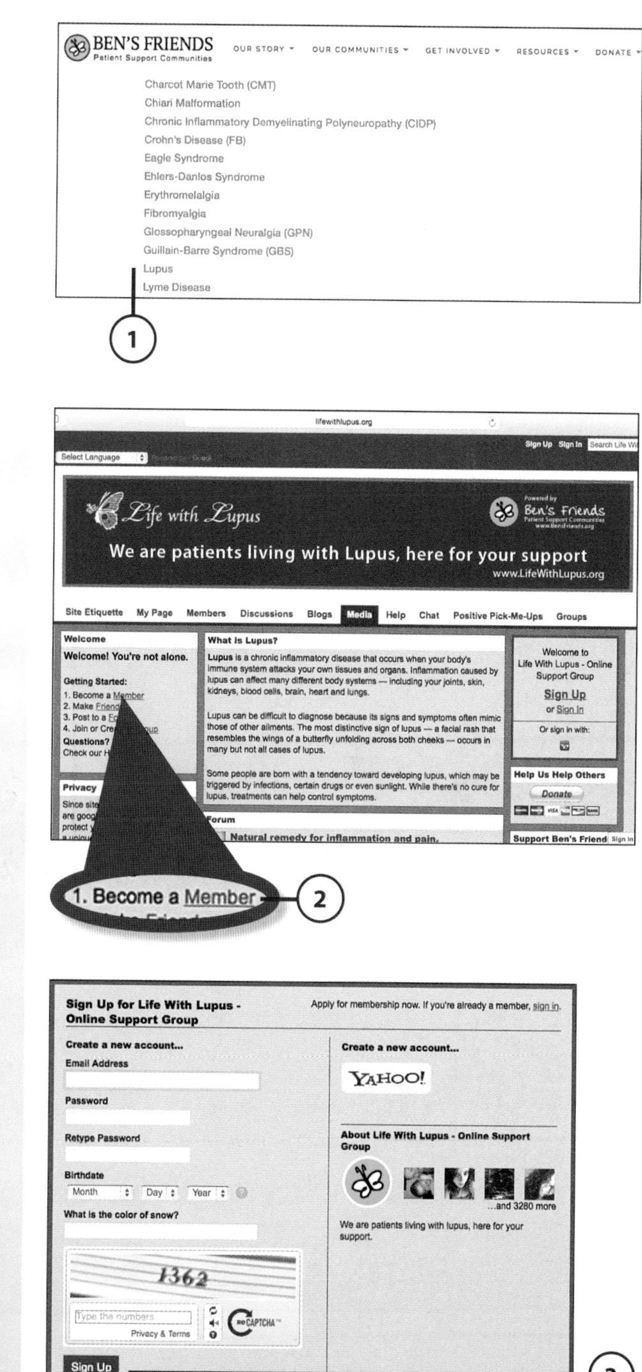

Benefiting from the Wisdom of the Experts at CrowdMed

If you are struggling with an unsolved medical condition, CrowdMed might be able to help you. CrowdMed uses an online network of medical detectives including retired physicians, scientists, nurses, physician assistants, and regular people who enjoy investigating medical mysteries to solve difficult cases. You can remain anonymous while trying to find the answers you need from CrowdMed.

After you register at crowdmed.com, getting started is quite easy. First you complete an online patient questionnaire and upload your medical information. CrowdMed then collects and filters diagnostic and solution suggestions from their medical detectives. At the end of the process, you get your detailed results containing CrowdMed's best medical suggestions, and then you can discuss those results with your doctor. CrowdMed is a paid service, but if your report proves inaccurate, you are refunded the money.

Vet this service thoroughly, and understand that CrowdMed is a tool that only offers suggestions. Only your doctor can make a definitive diagnosis and prescribe the appropriate treatment.

Submit Your Case

In the submission stage, you are asked to enter the following information: Case Info, Patient Info, Illness Info, Whole Body, Patient History, Prior Treatment, and Additional Info. crowdmed.com carefully walks you through each step after you get going.

1. With your browser, go to crowdmed.com.
2. Click Submit a Case.

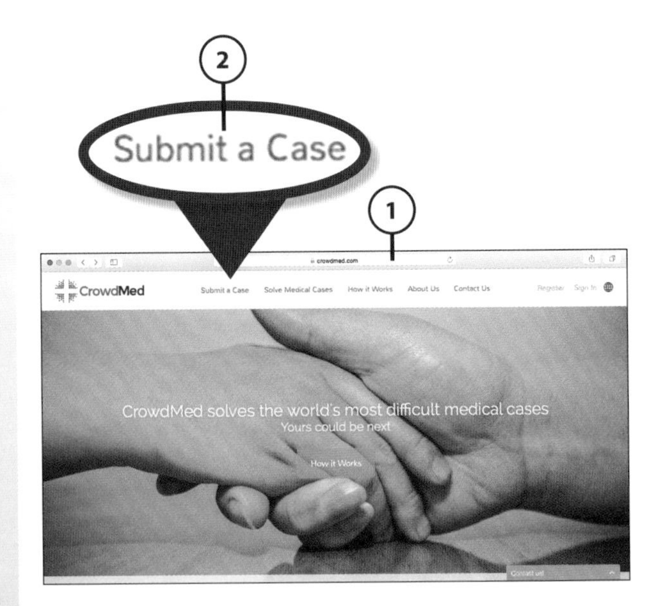

3. Click Submit a Case, again.
4. Sign up as a patient, and then click Sign Up.
5. Click to designate how you found CrowdMed, enter your phone number, and then click Submit.

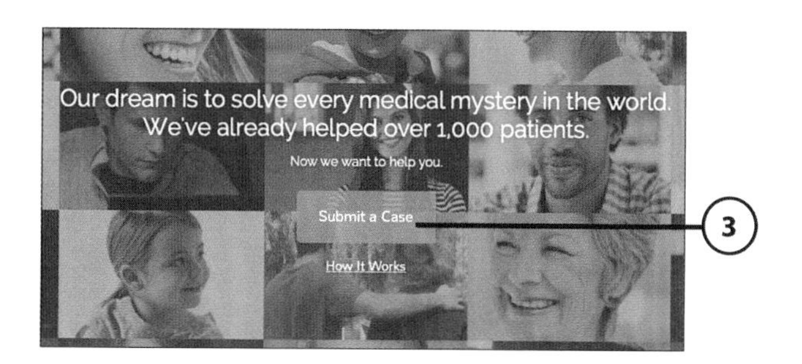

Our dream is to solve every medical mystery in the world.
We've already helped over 1,000 patients.
Now we want to help you.
Submit a Case
How It Works
3

Want to solve a case? Register as a Medical Detective.

Username:*

Connor

Email:*

Confirm Email:*

Password:*

Sign Up

*required

4

How did you find us?

- Friend, family, or colleague
- Search engine
- Newspaper, magazine, or website
- TV or radio segment
- Medical practitioner
- Partner organization
- Social media
- Advertisement
- Job posting
- Other

What is your phone number?

Submit

*required

5

6. Review the Patient Agreement information, and then click I Accept.
7. Follow the prompts to submit your medical case. CrowdMed then sends you an email enabling you to confirm your email address to gain access to its site. Follow the instructions in the email.

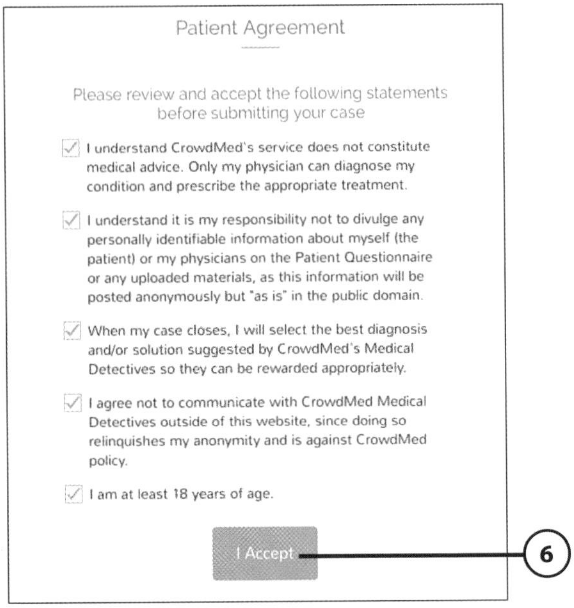

Patient Agreement

Please review and accept the following statements before submitting your case

- I understand CrowdMed's service does not constitute medical advice. Only my physician can diagnose my condition and prescribe the appropriate treatment.
- I understand it is my responsibility not to divulge any personally identifiable information about myself (the patient) or my physicians on the Patient Questionnaire or any uploaded materials, as this information will be posted anonymously but "as is" in the public domain.
- When my case closes, I will select the best diagnosis and/or solution suggested by CrowdMed's Medical Detectives so they can be rewarded appropriately.
- I agree not to communicate with CrowdMed Medical Detectives outside of this website, since doing so relinquishes my anonymity and is against CrowdMed policy.
- I am at least 18 years of age.

I Accept (6)

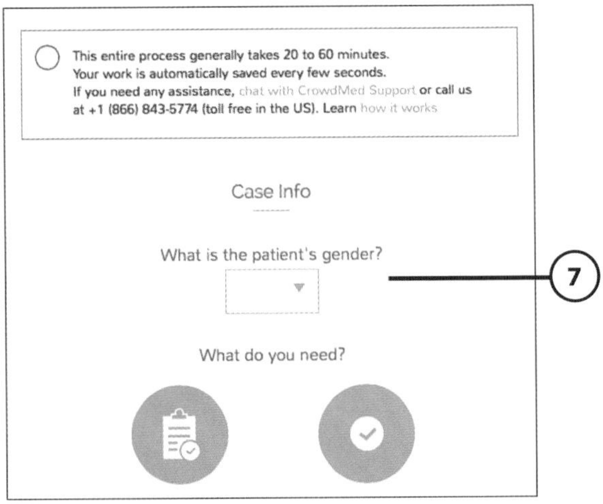

This entire process generally takes 20 to 60 minutes.
Your work is automatically saved every few seconds.
If you need any assistance, chat with CrowdMed Support or call us at +1 (866) 843-5774 (toll free in the US). Learn how it works

Case Info

What is the patient's gender? (7)

What do you need?

>>>Go Further

MANAGING YOUR CASE

You can decide how long you want your case to remain online. You can use the entire CrowdMed community to contribute to your case, or limit participation to only the top case solvers in their network.

Live Better Together with the PatientsLikeMe Online Community

The PatientsLikeMe online patient network provides a comforting, safe, and supportive environment by connecting patients who have similar health conditions. This network empowers individuals to improve the quality of their lives by providing an opportunity to learn from others and compare treatments, symptoms, and experiences. You are also given tools to track your own health over time, so you can see the larger picture of your health and contribute to research that can advance medicine for everyone. One of the most helpful parts of the site is the forum, where people go to tell what's happening in their lives. You'll find groups discussing a wide span of topics allowing you to give as well as receive support, and make new friends. Share what's working best for you and learn what's not working for others so you can better manage your condition.

Patientslikeme.com is also packed with many inspirational testimonials and news stories that keep you informed on patient surveys and how PatientsLikeMe is making a difference in the world.

As of this writing, PatientsLikeMe also has an app for your iPhone that makes a convenient companion to keep track of your symptoms and condition while on the go.

Join PatientsLikeMe

A community is out there waiting to help you. Visit patientslikeme.com to see if it's the right network for you. If it is, joining is quite easy. The following example is shown on the patientslikeme.com website.

1. Go to patientslikeme.com.
2. Click to view an introductory video and learn more about the PatientsLikeMe network.
3. Click Join now.

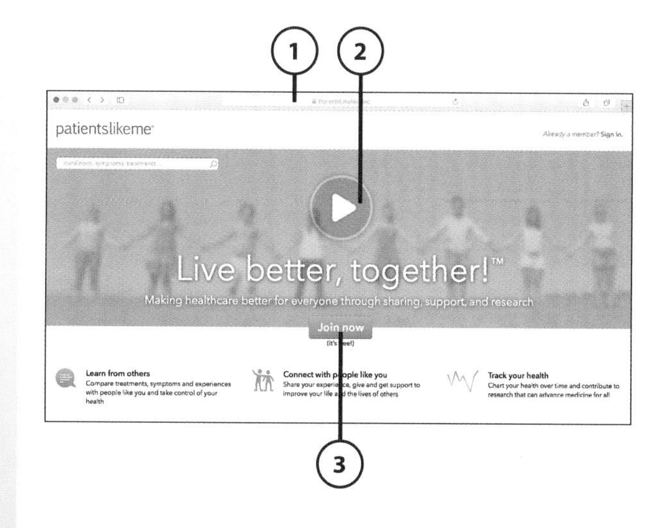

4. Fill in your account information, and then click Continue.
5. Fill in some basic information about yourself, and then click Continue.
6. Introduce yourself to the community, and then choose to Join the Conversation, Add to Your Health History, or Meet People Like You. PatientsLikeMe sends you an email that introduces you to what you can do on their website. The email also includes information about setting up your profile and provides a link to your profile so you can keep track of everything related to your health.

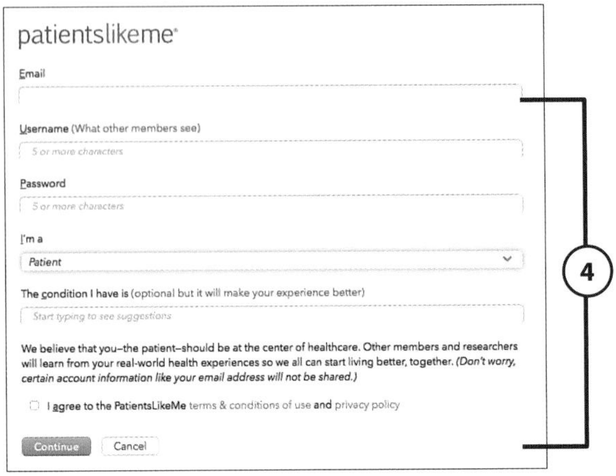

patientslikeme

Email

Username (What other members see)

5 or more characters

Password

5 or more characters

I'm a

Patient

The condition I have is (optional but it will make your experience better)

Start typing to see suggestions

We believe that you–the patient–should be at the center of healthcare. Other members and researchers will learn from your real-world health experiences so we all can start living better, together. *(Don't worry, certain account information like your email address will not be shared.)*

I agree to the PatientsLikeMe terms & conditions of use and privacy policy

Continue Cancel

4

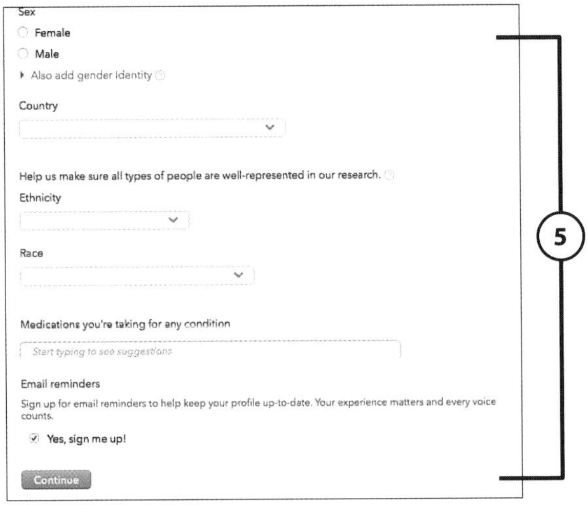

Sex

Female

Male

Also add gender identity

Country

Help us make sure all types of people are well-represented in our research.

Ethnicity

Race

Medications you're taking for any condition

Start typing to see suggestions

Email reminders

Sign up for email reminders to help keep your profile up-to-date. Your experience matters and every voice counts.

Yes, sign me up!

Continue

5

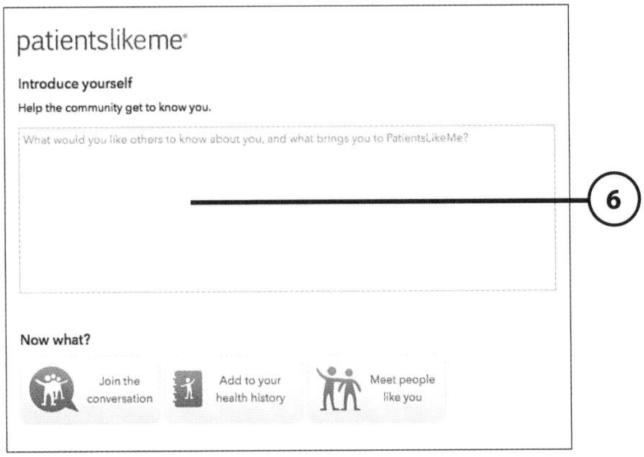

patientslikeme

Introduce yourself

Help the community get to know you.

What would you like others to know about you, and what brings you to PatientsLikeMe?

6

Now what?

Join the conversation

Add to your health history

Meet people like you

Focusing on Active Living with HealthyAging.Net

HealthyAging.net is a magazine-style website that encourages a passion for life through tips, techniques, and resources for living a healthier lifestyle. If you have the desire to live an active lifestyle and find your next great adventure, Healthy Aging might be the right source for you.

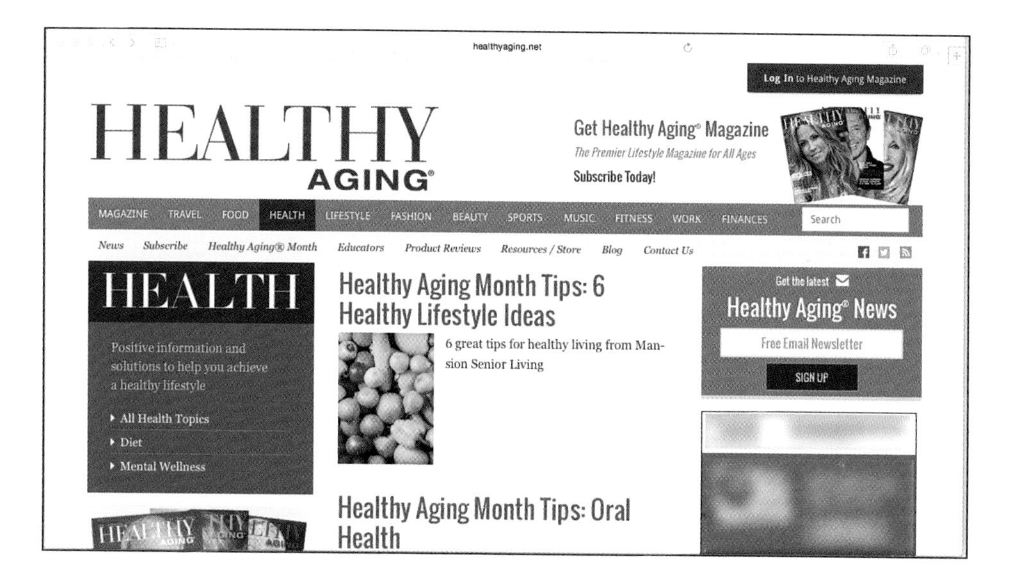

This site is constantly updated with a bounty of articles on enriching your lifestyle, travel, and food. Healthy Aging uses its online platform to promote improved physical, mental, social, and financial health. This means everything from surfing and skiing to taking on a new career. Healthy Aging is about redefining "retirement" and discovering what you can do next.

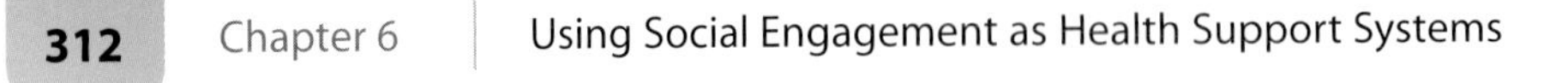

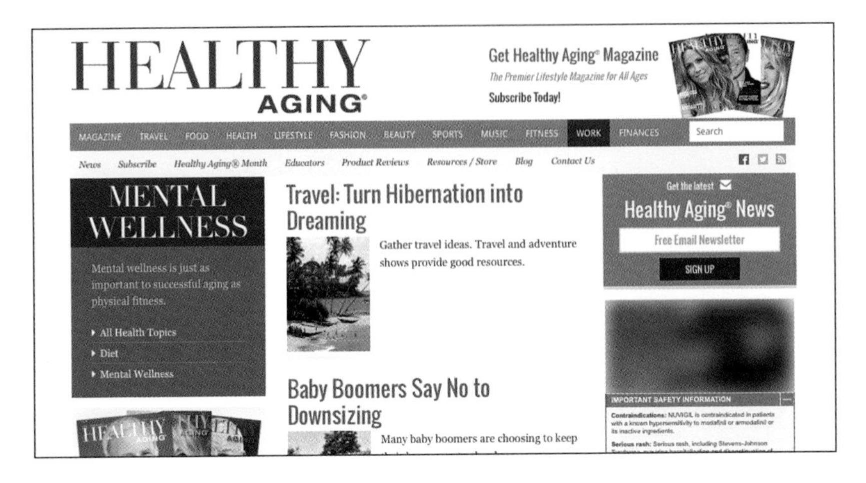

If you're looking for a vibrant resource that broadens the awareness of the positive aspects of aging, give Healthy Aging some serious consideration. You can also choose to subscribe to an email newsletter from Healthy Aging or the Healthy Aging Magazine in digital format. Simply go to healthyaging.net and click Subscribe Today! toward the top right of the page.

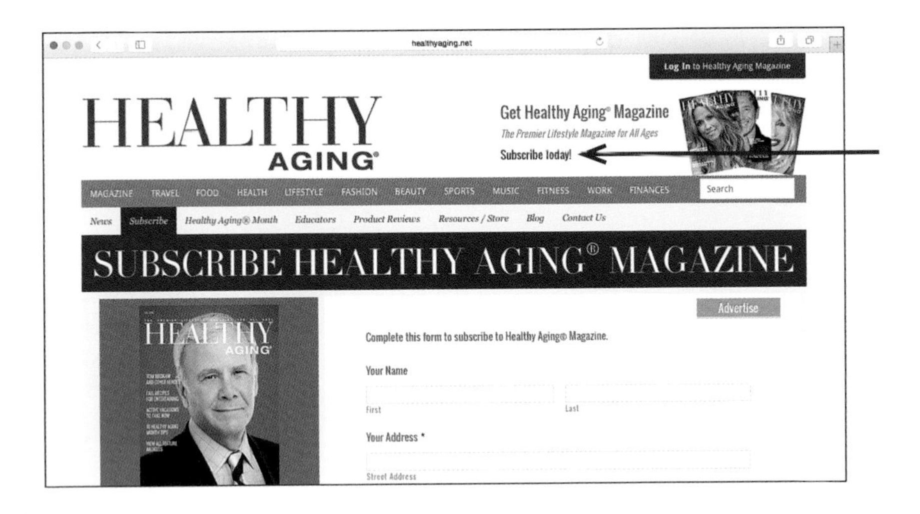

>>>Go Further

REDISCOVER WHAT MATTERS TO YOU WITH LIFE REIMAGINED

The lifereimagined.aarp.org website offers a system that takes a holistic approach to help you rediscover what matters to you. The system provided by this website helps you find your purpose; and when you know your purpose, the choices you make in life come straight from the heart of who you are.

If you are looking for a resource that can help you live the life you have always dreamed of, this website can help you determine your path forward. Think of Life Reimagined as a personalized guidance system with tools and programs that deliver inspiration, activities, and connections. Here's how it works.

Choose a program, which may focus on career, relationships, a new path for life in general, or many other areas. Sign up for one that's right for you. Follow the steps. Life Reimagined makes it easy by helping you take small steps forward by bringing you new ideas from experts and bestselling authors. Last, but definitely not least, keep going.

Life Reimagined helps you to connect with people like you so you can work with someone who has been there before. This system provides a real-world approach to change and lets you start from where you are in your life. Visit lifereimagined.aarp.org to see if what they offer can help you make positive change in your life. You can try Life Reimagined for free, and then they offer subscription services.

Combating Social Isolation Through Digital Inclusion

Over the past decade, advancements in smartphones, tablets, social media, and apps have made it much easier to stay in touch with family and friends. Facebook, Skype, Google Hangouts, and Instagram make it easy for you to stay in contact. If you want to learn more about these particular options, consider the book *My Social Media for Seniors*. Some manufacturers have sought to make social interactions even easier by creating devices that are optimized specifically for you to connect and share with family and friends. These devices and app interfaces are clutter-free and streamlined so you don't have to go looking for what you need. They are also ready to use out of the box, like the grandPad tablet. These tablets let you capture and view family photos and videos, use text messages and email, and participate with those around you in many other ways. They have their down and upsides.

The Oscar Junior and Oscar Senior apps make it convenient for you to provide or receive assistance when using a tablet. You or a family member can install the Oscar Junior app on a phone and remotely manage a loved one's tablet that has Oscar Senior installed. This is a great way to provide or receive assistance with a tablet, if needed.

If you are looking for a more complete system for independent living, the grandCARE remote monitoring system also has a community and activity management component. The grandCARE system enables you to access messages, photos, videos, letters, games, and more so you can stay engaged. Take a closer at these options to see whether they might work for a loved one or you.

Staying Closer and Caring Easier with the Oscar Tablet App

The Oscar Junior and Oscar Senior apps are great if you are not experienced with computers and tablets and could use a little help from a family member or friend from time to time. As of this writing, the Oscar apps are available only for Android devices on the Play Store. The concept is quite simple and very clever. The person providing help signs up at oscarsenior.com and then installs the Oscar Junior app on his or her smartphone. The person who needs the help installs Oscar Senior on his or her own tablet (or the helper can install it for the person) and then signs in to Junior's account. The helper (Junior) is now able to see what's happening on the other person's tablet and can solve the issue remotely or provide guidance.

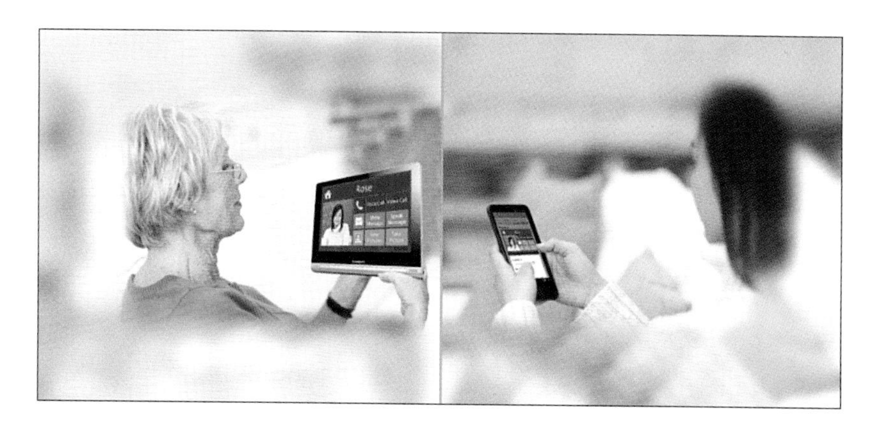

The Oscar apps are much more than remote help and control tools, though. Oscar provides a simplified interface for individuals to read news reports, e-books, or Wikipedia articles, get the weather forecast, text message, make voice and video calls, share pictures, and play games. The Oscar interface also enables you to set reminders to do important tasks like take medicine on time and remember doctor visits.

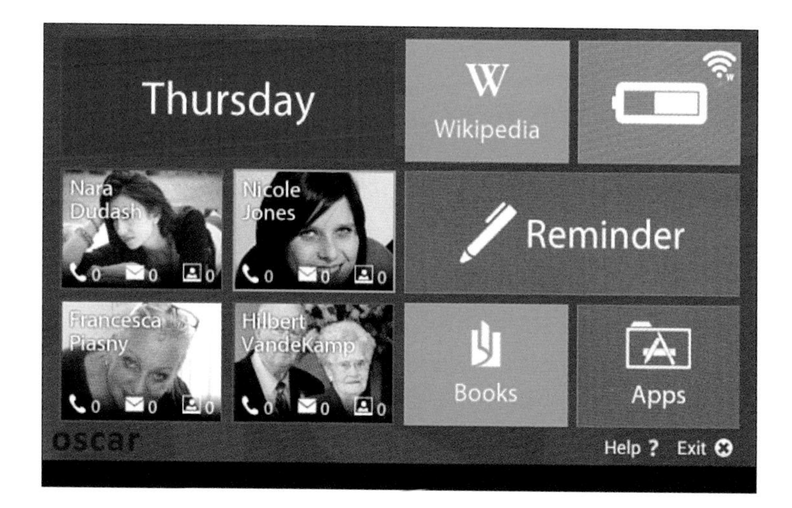

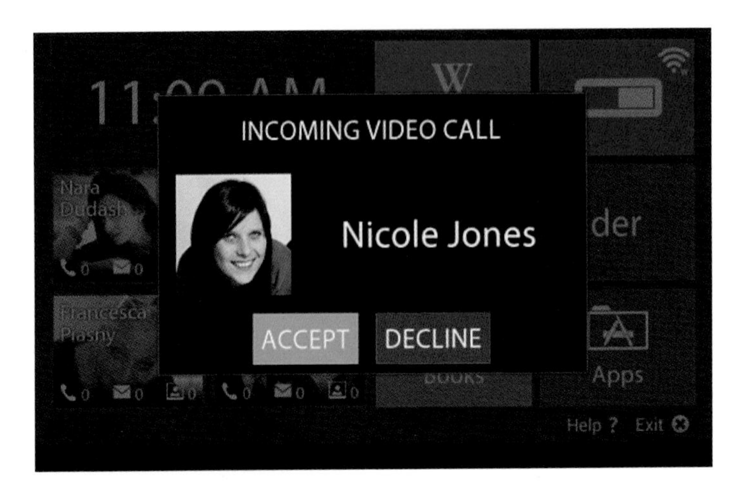

Staying Connected with Friends and Family with the grandPad Tablet

The grandPad is an easy-to-use and secure tablet that keeps you connected to family and friends. If you have taken a look at traditional tablets on the market and find that they have too many bells and whistles that you just won't use, grandPad could be the tablet for you. It's preloaded and streamlined with only the apps that you'll find yourself using the most. This tablet enables you to video chat, make phone calls, send voice messages by email, send and receive spam-free email, and view family photos and videos. You can play music and even see what the weather is like in your area and where your family and friends live before you visit.

grandPad is about making communication easy. To make voice and video calls, grandPad can be set up so all you have to do is tap a picture of the person onscreen that you want to call. You can also share photos with grandPad's free Companion App, Facebook, Instagram, and email.

Getting started with grandPad is easy. Place an order for a grandPad on grandPad.net. When you place your order, grandPad asks a few questions about your family and who would be the best point of contact to manage the device and set up contacts. This person is called the Family Admin. After your order is placed, an email is sent to your Family Admin with login credentials for grandPad Central. This will be the portal where your device is managed.

Your Family Admin sends out invitations to family and friends to install the free grandPad Companion App for Android and Apple (iOS) devices. It is through the Companion App that your invitees can interact using all the communication capabilities that grandPad has to offer. When your grandPad arrives, it is preloaded with everything you need. Just place the device in the wireless charging cradle to turn it on.

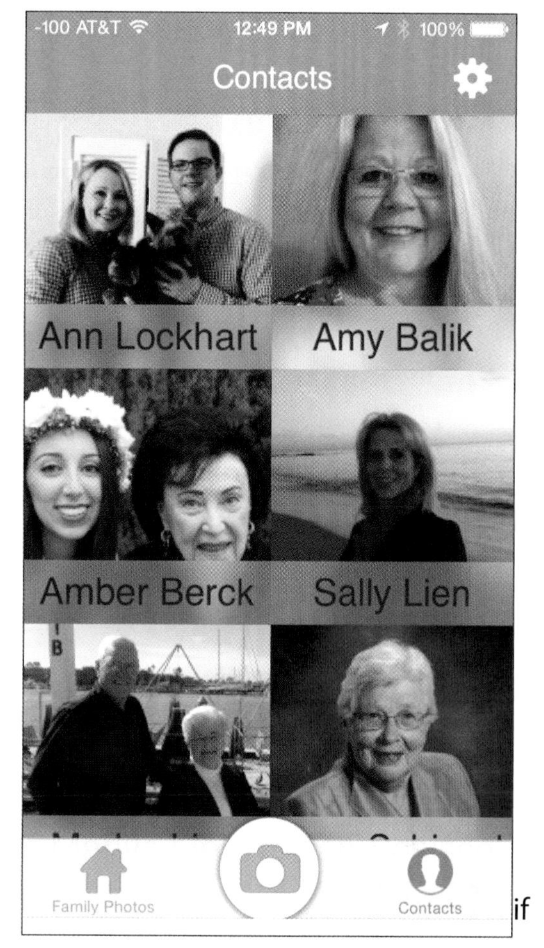

As of this writing, grandPad uses a month-to-month, no-contract membership. That membership includes a grandPad tablet, case, applications, video and phone calls, Wi-Fi connectivity, damage and theft insurance, and U.S.-based White Glove Support. The membership includes the device and all of its services. The return of your grandPad device is expected if you should cancel your membership.

Keeping in Touch with Friends and Family Using grandCARE

The grandCARE remote monitoring platform is a comprehensive service that includes telehealth, health management, activity monitoring, and social engagement. This system allows a caregiver to discreetly watch over you or a loved one and can provide alerts in case any issues arise. If you are a caregiver, or require one, grandCARE is an all-in-one subscription service that might offer the support you're looking for. This section only touches the tip of the iceberg of what grandCARE can do for you and concentrates only on its social engagement capabilities.

The grandCARE system is comprised of hardware, including health devices, and software. The system uses a touchscreen interface to keep you connected with family and friends. You can easily stay engaged in the lives of those who matter most by using video chat, photo sharing, and note and letter messaging. You can also surf the Web, read the news, and play games. grandCARE even includes a shared calendar function so that you don't forget birthdays, anniversaries, or appointments.

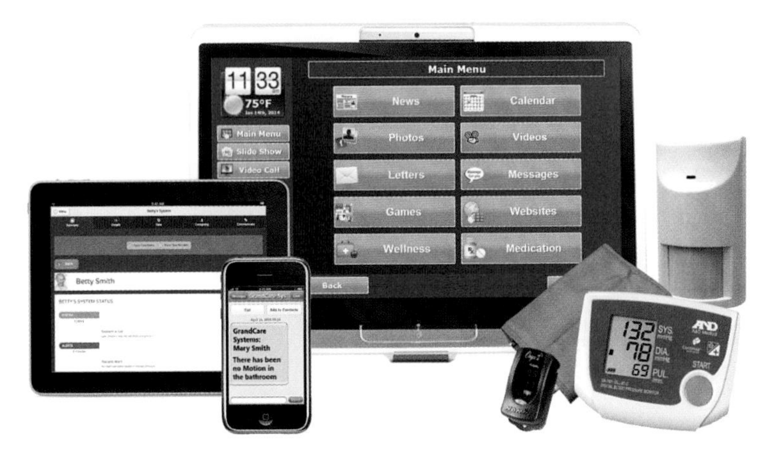

© 2005–2015 GrandCare Systems, LLC

Chapter 8, "Being Prepared for an Emergency," goes deeper into the grandCARE system as a whole and shows how in-home sensors are used to track activity online and how the system monitors vitals online. To review the grandCARE services for yourself, visit us.grandcare.com.

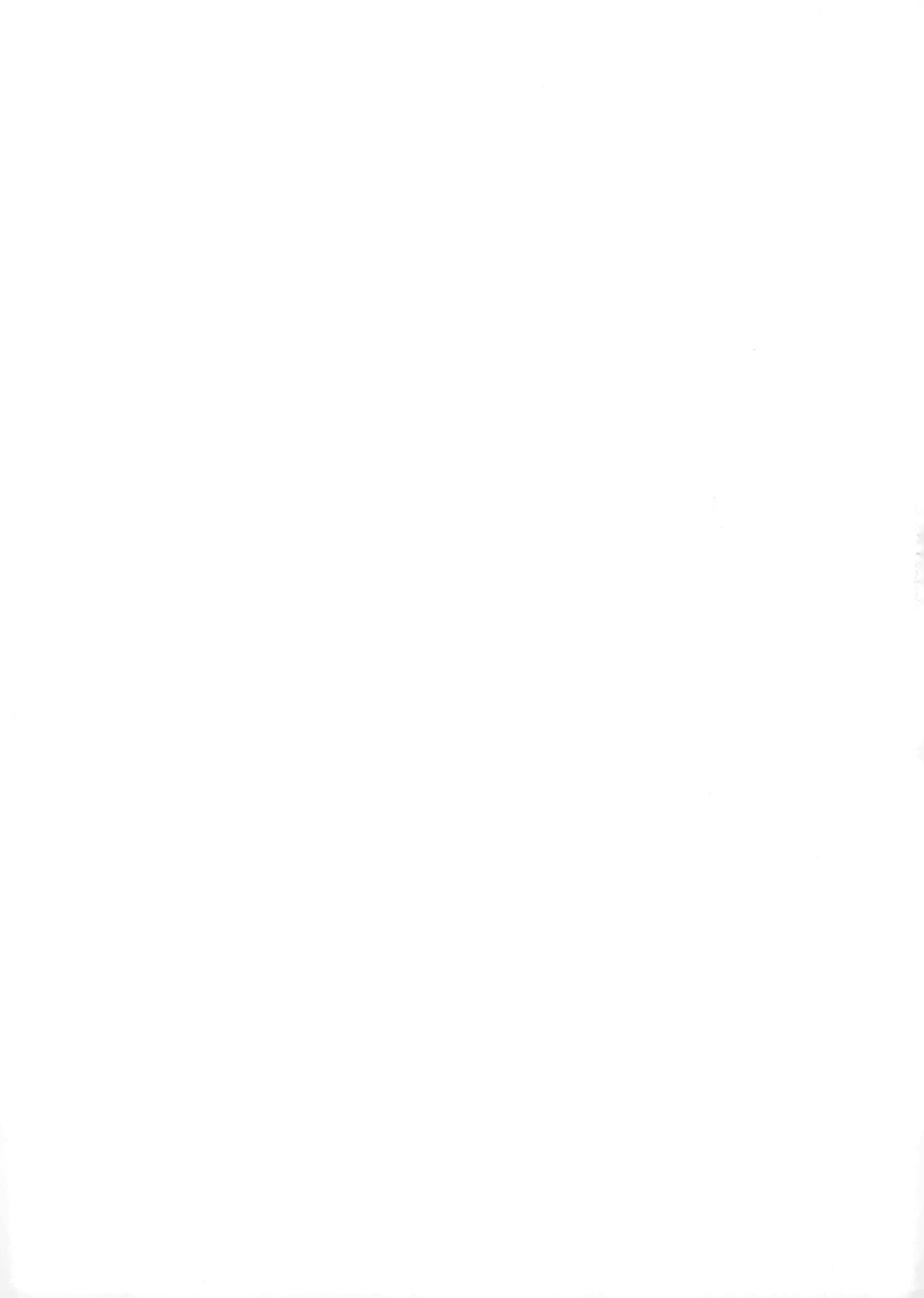

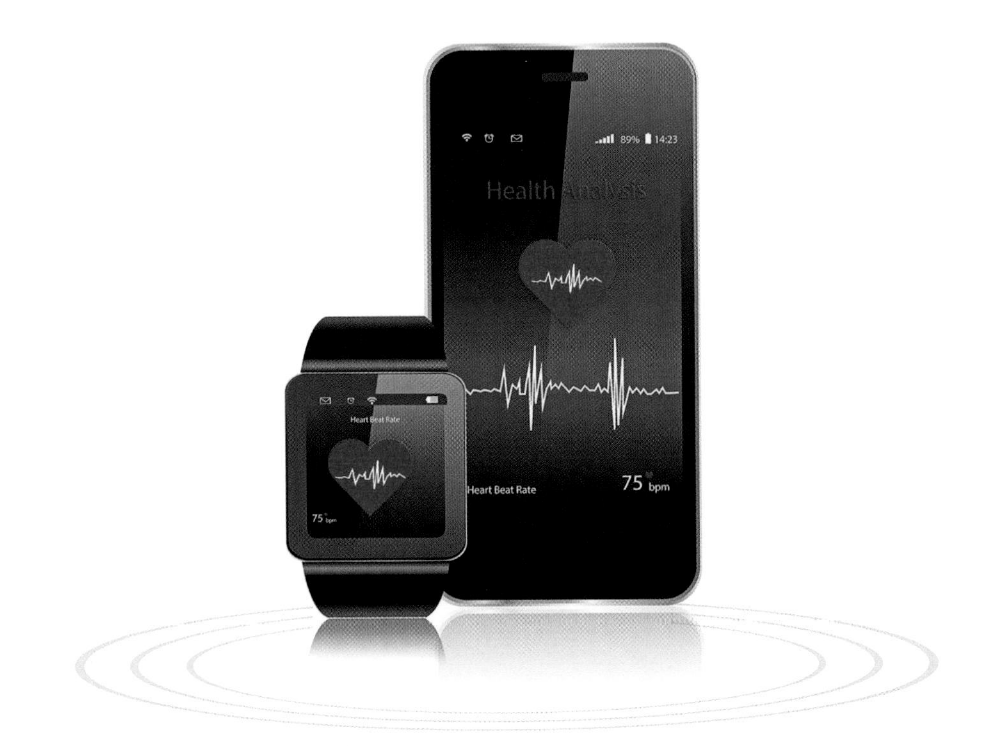

Credit: © monicaodo/Fotolia.com

Use apps, medical devices, wearables, and online resources to help manage health conditions.

In this chapter, you explore apps that can help you manage diabetes, heart-healthy technology, and resources to help control obesity. You also learn about a few resources that can help control asthma and COPD, and even assist with inner ear infections.

- → Managing Diabetes
- → Taking a Look at Heart Health Technology
- → Controlling Obesity
- → Getting Help to Control Your Asthma and COPD

Finding Solutions to Manage Specific Conditions

Mobile technology is transforming patient health management. Smartphones and tablets are being equipped as medical devices that can measure blood glucose, detect serious heart conditions, improve asthma and COPD treatments, check for inner ear infections, and even help you to get in shape. Health and fitness apps have gone mainstream. Many developers have targeted their efforts toward helping to manage some of the most widespread, adverse health conditions we face today. This new use of mobile technology as a data collection platform provides greater insight into your condition and helps you and your physician when deciding on and implementing the best course of treatment. A terrific benefit of this is that you are given more control over your lifestyle management.

Managing Diabetes

If you're living with diabetes, nothing is more effective in managing this condition than working closely with your doctor. You can use some innovative resources, under your doctor's supervision, to help you stay on top of your treatment plan. Apps such as Glucose Buddy and the Diabetes app can assist you in monitoring glucose numbers, insulin doses, carbs, and other data that can keep you on track. Devices, including the Gmate SMART and iHealth Smart Gluco-Monitoring System, make it easy to measure and track blood glucose levels. If you need more support in managing diabetes, sites like diabeticconnect.com are packed full of information. Continue reading and see whether one of these resources, or a combination of them, can help you. Keep in mind that many of the resources covered in this chapter are not medical devices. Always consult your doctor on resources you might choose. Ask your doctor whether she has any recommendations or whether a resource is truly effective.

Monitoring Your Glucose Using Apps

Frequent monitoring of your blood glucose levels is used to guide your therapy, such as insulin injections and dietary changes. If you and your doctor agree that self-monitoring is an option for you, a number of apps can assist you in tracking and sharing your blood glucose results. Some of the following apps enable you to sync your information to a website and across multiple devices. Keep in mind that this particular section is about monitoring your treatment and not the actual acquiring of blood samples. If you don't have a device that takes samples, you have a chance to review a few devices a little later in this chapter. First, let's take a look at options for tracking and sharing blood glucose measurements.

Differences in App Interfaces

An app's interface can look completely different depending on whether you download the app for Android devices or Apple (iOS) devices. The features can also be different. Throughout this chapter and this book, some apps are shown on devices that might be different from your own. When possible, the various app examples alternate between iPhone and Android devices.

Glucose Buddy App

The Glucose Buddy app lets you manually log glucose numbers, insulin injections, carbohydrate consumption, and activities. A paid version, Glucose Buddy Pro, is available as well as a free version, Glucose Buddy. The difference between the two is that the paid version enables you to track blood pressure and weight. You can review all the information you logged by signing in to your account on glucosebuddy.com. This app can also send you reminders for when it's time to log. Consider trying the free version to see how you like it before purchasing the Pro version. As of this writing, a free Glucose Buddy app is available for Android and a paid and free version are available for Apple (iOS) 4.0 or higher devices. This app can be downloaded from the Google Play Store and the App Store. To take full advantage of what this app has to offer, you must sign up for an account at glucosebuddy.com.

Sign up for an account on the website, download the app, and then use the following steps. These steps show the free Glucose Buddy app on an iPhone.

1. Open the Glucose Buddy app, read the app introduction and safety information, and then tap OK.

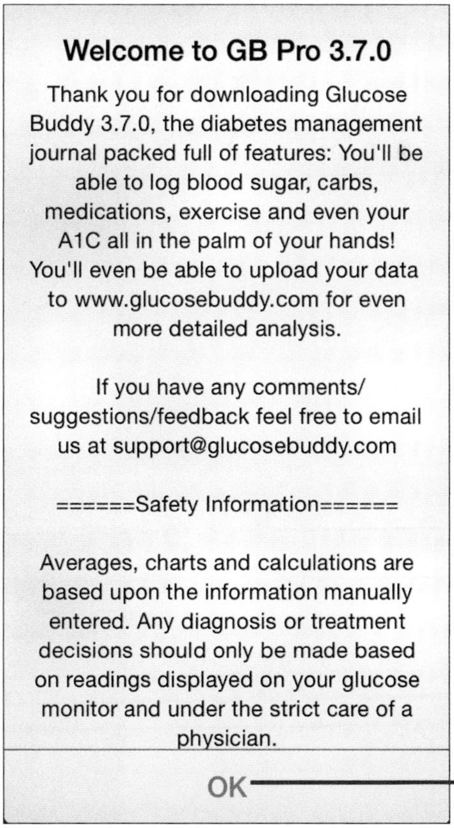

Welcome to GB Pro 3.7.0

Thank you for downloading Glucose Buddy 3.7.0, the diabetes management journal packed full of features: You'll be able to log blood sugar, carbs, medications, exercise and even your A1C all in the palm of your hands! You'll even be able to upload your data to www.glucosebuddy.com for even more detailed analysis.

If you have any comments/ suggestions/feedback feel free to email us at support@glucosebuddy.com

======Safety Information======

Averages, charts and calculations are based upon the information manually entered. Any diagnosis or treatment decisions should only be made based on readings displayed on your glucose monitor and under the strict care of a physician.

OK

1

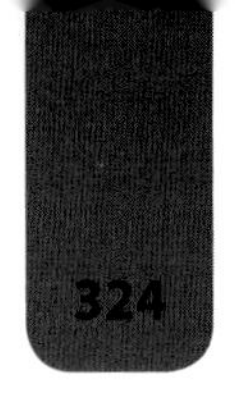

2. Tap Settings.
3. Tap Account Info, and then sign in using your credentials.
4. After you return to the main Glucose Buddy screen, tap My Info to enter information including date of birth, height, weight, and the type of medical devices you use. For example, add which type of device you use to acquire blood samples.
5. Tap Logs to review a history of the log entries you have made.

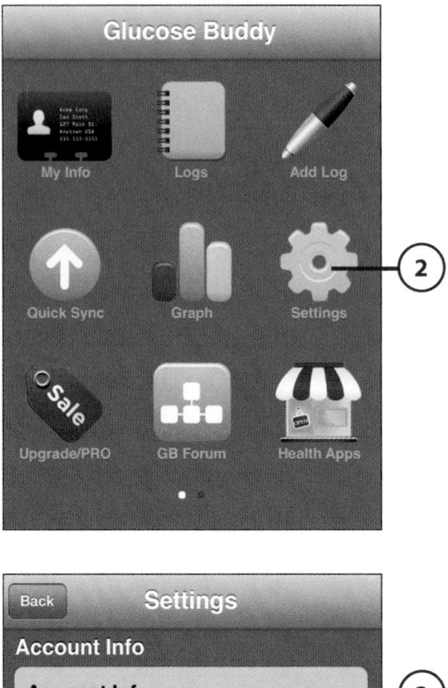

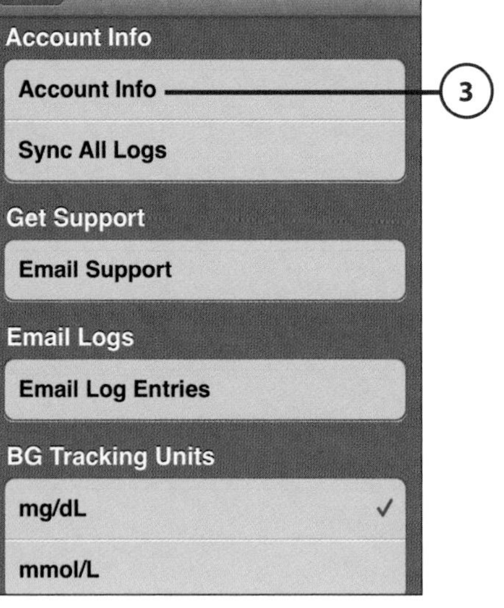

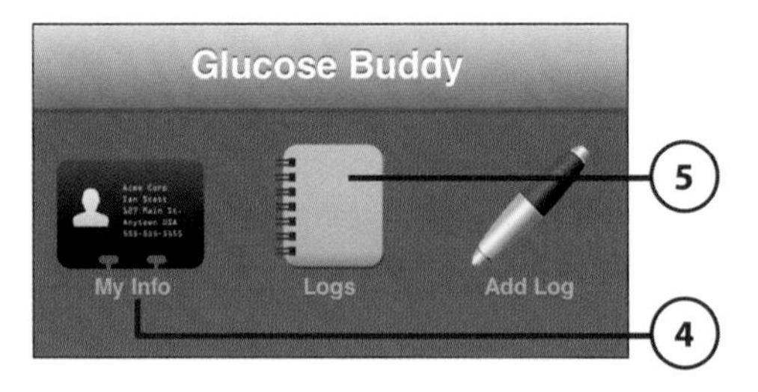

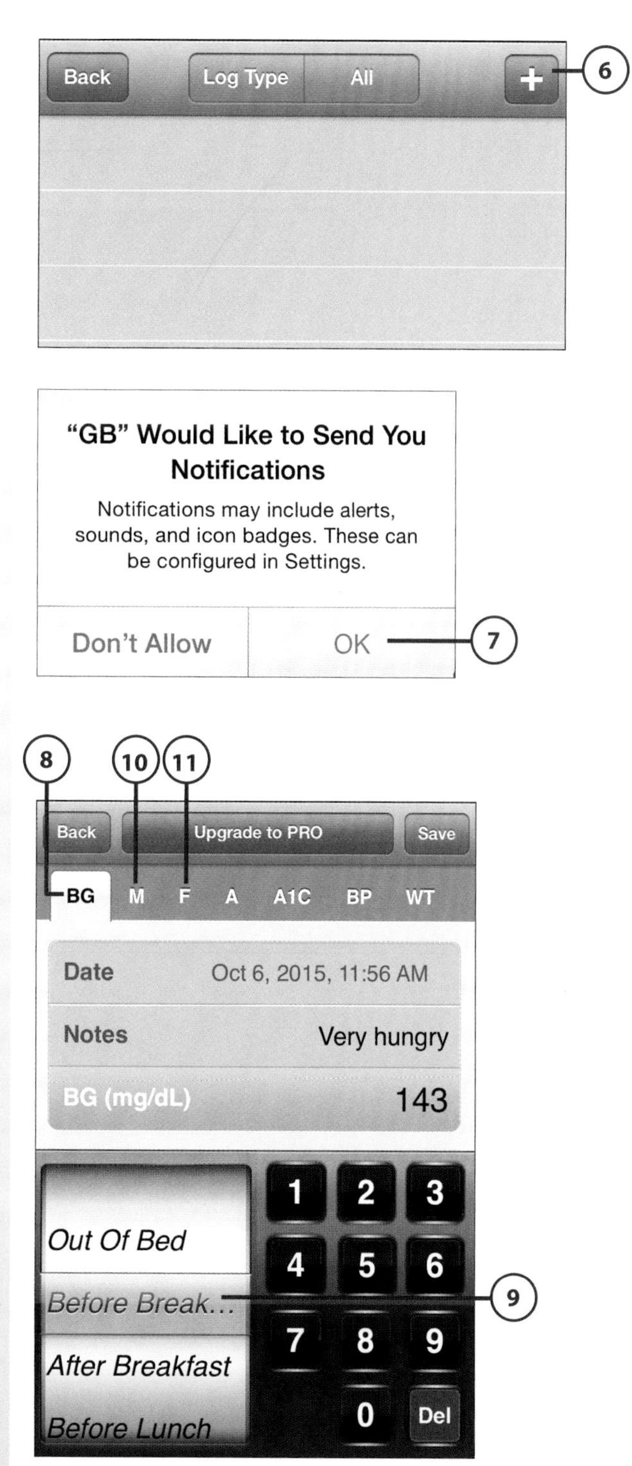

6. Tap Add Log (the plus sign) to enter a new log entry. A message box appears asking whether it's okay for your Glucose Buddy to send you alerts.
7. Tap OK.
8. After you test your blood sugar, tap BG to access the screen for entering the date, notes, blood glucose level, and when you conducted the test relative to when you ate; your activity; and other variables that might affect your test.

Types of Notes to Make

The more detailed the notes, the more helpful the log information will be to gauge how you and your doctor are managing your diabetes. For example, a note could be "Blood sugar is elevated because of a high-carb lunch."

9. Use your finger to move the scroll wheel to indicate when the test occurred in correlation to your daily meals, activity, and other variables that might affect your test.

10. Tap M to log your insulin dosages.
11. Tap F to log the foods (carbs) you eat throughout the day.

(12) Tap A to log activities including running, walking, or cleaning the house.

(13) Tap A1C to log your A1C test results.

A1C Estimator

The glucosebuddy.com website offers an A1C estimator that is not available in the Pro or free versions of the Glucose Buddy apps.

---

(14) Tap BP to record your blood pressure. This feature is only available in the Pro version of the app.

(15) Tap WT to track your body weight. This feature is only available in the Pro version of the app.

(16) Tap Save to save a log.

(17) Tap the Back button to return to the previous screen.

(18) Tap Quick Sync to sync the entries on your phone to glucosebuddy.com.

(19) Tap Graph to review a visual representation of your blood glucose levels over time.

(20) Tap Settings to edit the overall settings of the Glucose Buddy app. You can also create a Glucose Buddy account under this option.

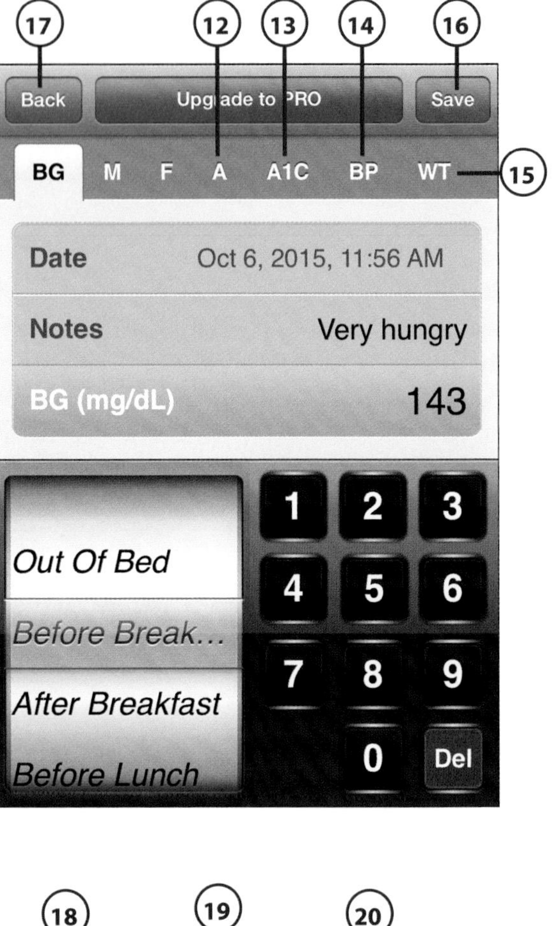

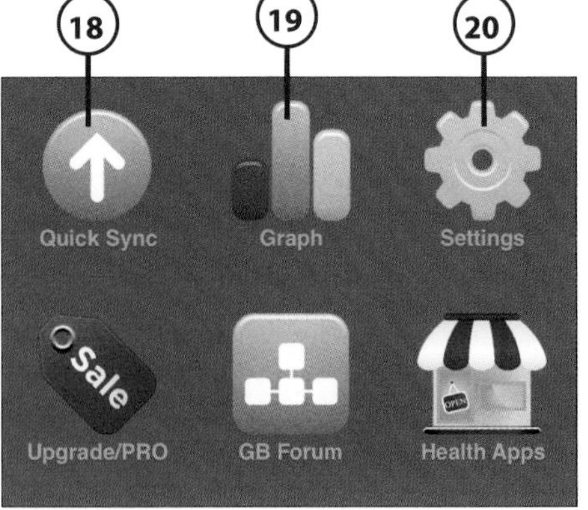

21. Because this is the free version, tap Upgrade/PRO to upgrade to the Pro version.
22. Tap GB Forum to participate in forum discussions with other people living with diabetes.
23. Tap Health Apps to view other health apps created by the developers of Glucose Buddy.

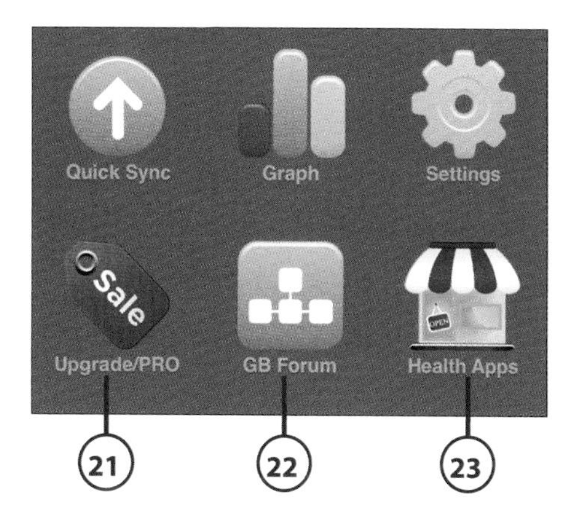

OnTrack Diabetes App

The OnTrack Diabetes app is another option for tracking blood glucose, hemoglobin A1C, food, weight, and other values. You can generate detailed graphs and reports to share with your doctor and set reminders to keep you on track. As of this writing, the OnTrack Diabetes app is only available for Android devices.

Download the app from the Google Play Store, and then follow these steps to help manage your diabetes.

1. Open the OnTrack Diabetes app, enter your email address, read the End User License Agreement, and then tap to place a check mark.
2. Tap Submit.

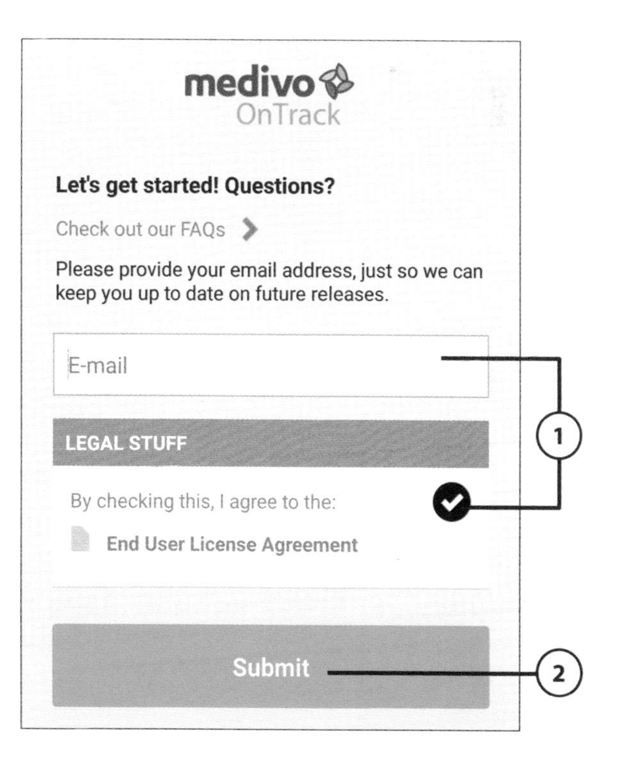

3. Tap in each field to customize the default units, and then tap Next.
4. Tap in each field and enter your low and high glucose range, and then tap Next. Consult your doctor on what your range should be. You can change these ranges at any time in the Settings and decide whether to highlight any values that fall outside of that range.

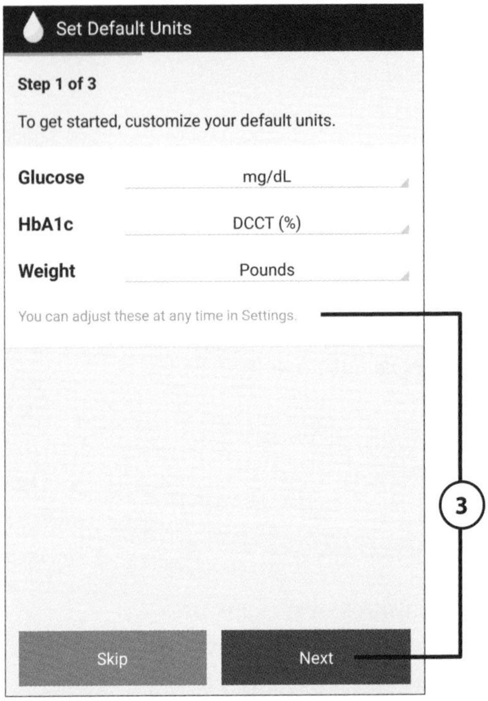

Set Default Units
Step 1 of 3
To get started, customize your default units.
Glucose mg/dL
HbA1c DCCT (%)
Weight Pounds
You can adjust these at any time in Settings.
Skip Next
3

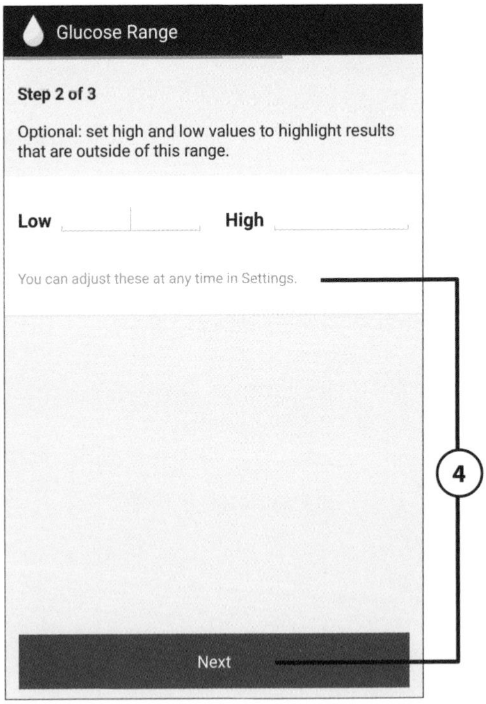

Glucose Range
Step 2 of 3
Optional: set high and low values to highlight results that are outside of this range.
Low High
You can adjust these at any time in Settings.
Next
4

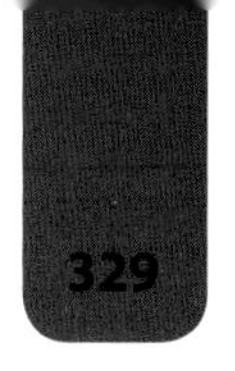

5. Tap in the field to decide whether you want the app to add a single entry, like Glucose, by default, or multiple entries at once, like Glucose, Carbs, and Medication, and then tap Finish. Multi-Add by Default was chosen for this example. You can also change this later in the Settings. The home screen opens.
6. Tap the Add button to add an entry. The Add screen opens.

Add one or many

Step 3 of 3

When you tap the Add button, you can add a single entry (like Glucose) by default, or you can add multiple entries at a time (like Glucose, Carbs, and Medication) by default.

Your current setting:

Multi-Add by Default

You can adjust these at any time in Settings.

Finish

5

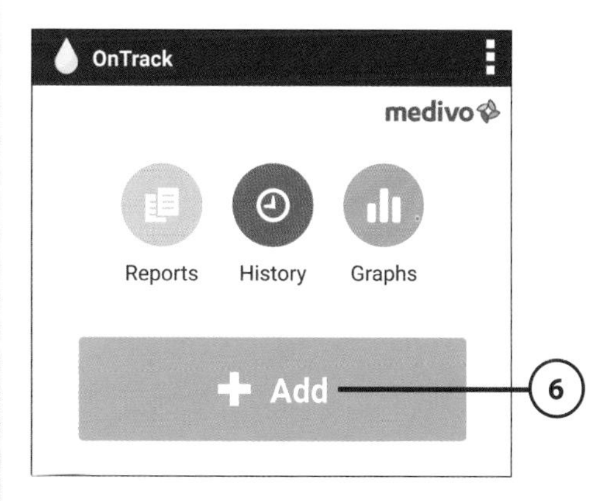

7. Tap the items you want to track, and then tap OK. You can add more items later if you decide you want to track other items.
8. Tap Reminder to add a reminder. For example, you can set a reminder to test two hours after eating.
9. Tap the gray box with dots in the first field to add more categories including Lunch, Dinner, and Snack.
10. Tap the Medication field to change the type of medication you use; in this example, from Humalin to Humalog.
11. Tap the gray box with dots in the Medication section to add another medication.
12. Tap Add Another to add another item to track, such as Blood Pressure and Hb1ac.
13. After you complete the entire entry, tap Save. The home screen reappears.

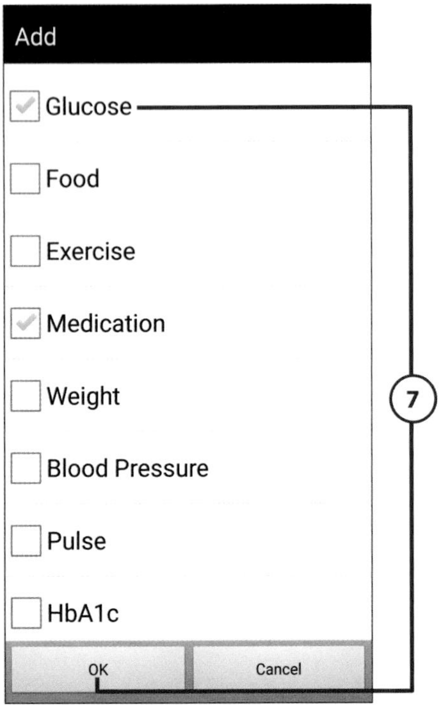

Add
Glucose
Food
Exercise
Medication
Weight
Blood Pressure
Pulse
HbA1c
OK Cancel
(7)

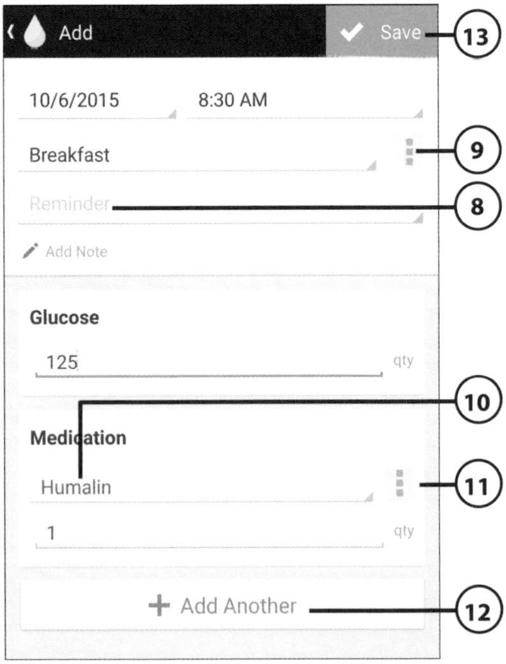

Add
Save (13)
10/6/2015 8:30 AM
Breakfast (9)
Reminder (8)
Add Note
Glucose
125 qty
Medication (10)
Humalin (11)
1 qty
+ Add Another (12)

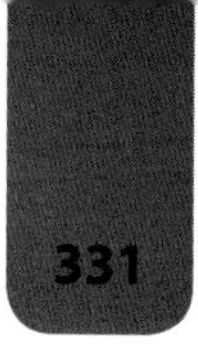

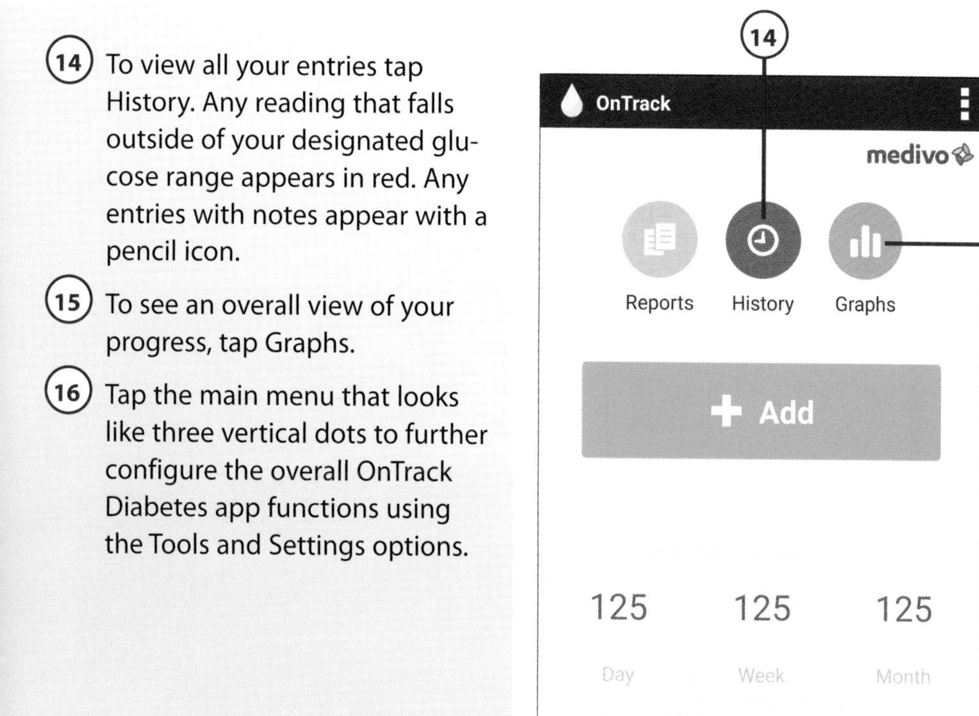

(14) To view all your entries tap History. Any reading that falls outside of your designated glucose range appears in red. Any entries with notes appear with a pencil icon.

(15) To see an overall view of your progress, tap Graphs.

(16) Tap the main menu that looks like three vertical dots to further configure the overall OnTrack Diabetes app functions using the Tools and Settings options.

Glooko App Diabetes Management System

Glooko is more than an app; it is a unified diabetes management system. The annual subscription service includes a MeterSync device—available online at shop.glooko.com or through health providers—that downloads glucose, insulin, and carb data directly to your Android or Apple (iOS) phone. Glooko makes it easy to track carbs by including nutrition data from more than 700 restaurants and 250 supermarkets. Logging food, insulin, exercise, and comments is easy, and all data entered into the Glooko app is accessible online. You can share your data by PDF or with participating health care providers using the ProConnect feature, so they can monitor trends and make adjustments to your treatment when needed. You can sync your data using more than 40 meters, pumps, and CGMs. Before you sign up to become a Glooko member, visit glooko.com/compatibility to make sure your medical device is supported. Download the app at the Google Play Store and the App Store.

Take a closer look at the Glooko management system at glooko.com to decide whether a subscription might be right for you. If you like what Glooko has to offer, it's easy to get started. The following steps show the app on the iPhone.

1. Go to shop.glooko.com, and then tap Create an Account.
2. Choose a Glooko subscription.
3. Download the app.
4. Sync your compatible device to the app using the MeterSync device.

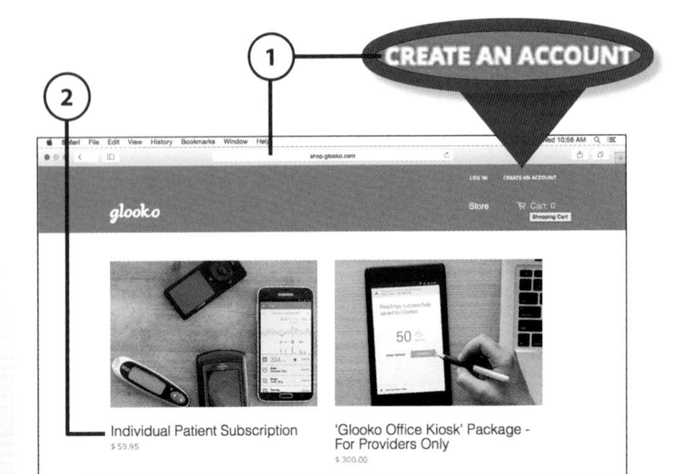

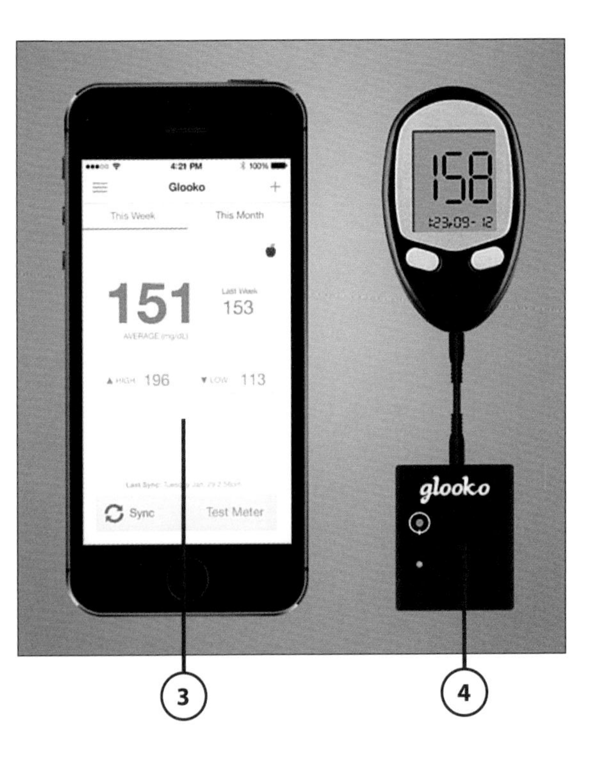

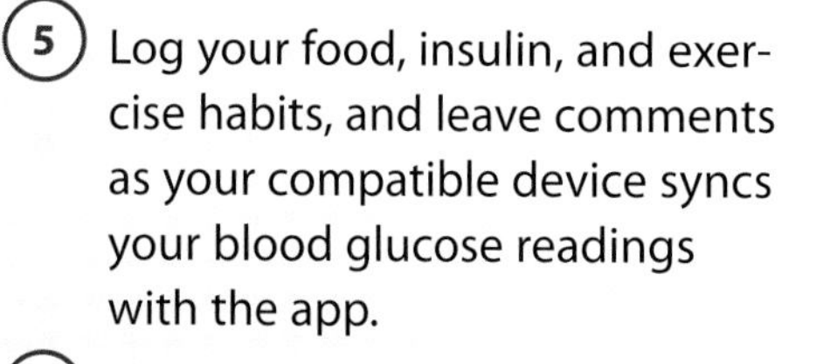

5. Log your food, insulin, and exercise habits, and leave comments as your compatible device syncs your blood glucose readings with the app.
6. View graphs to see the correlation between your glucose, insulin, and carb data.

Integration with Fitness Trackers

When you log your exercise, Glooko automatically integrates data from Fitbit, Jawbone UP, and Strava.

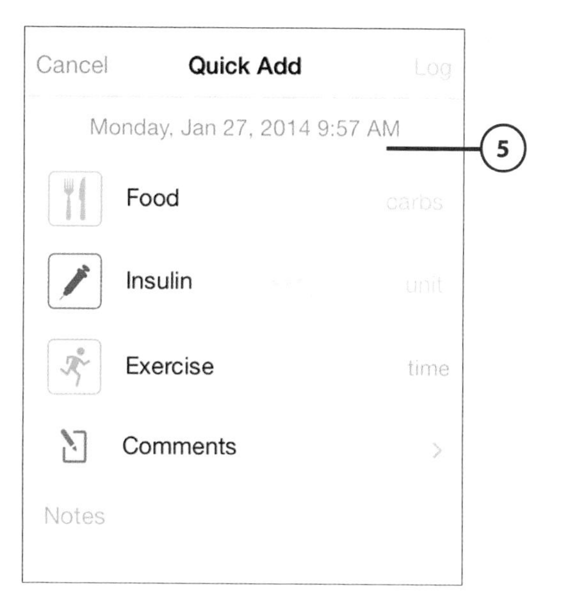

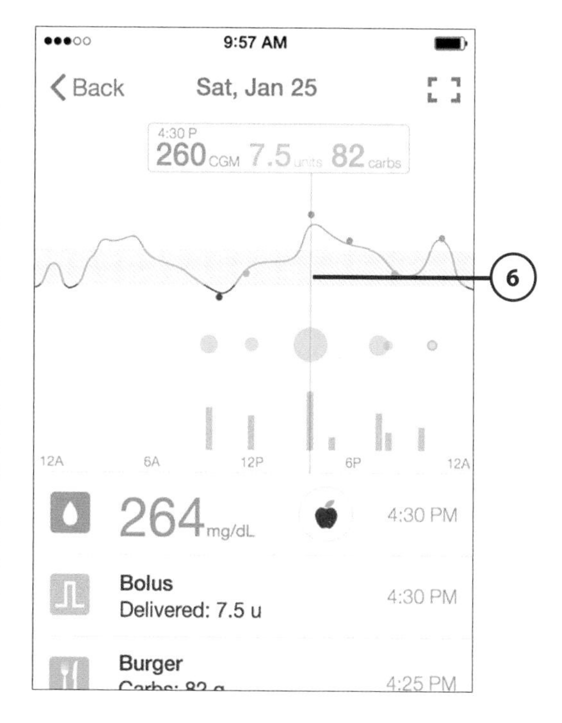

7. Share your logbook with your doctor to help improve your treatment.

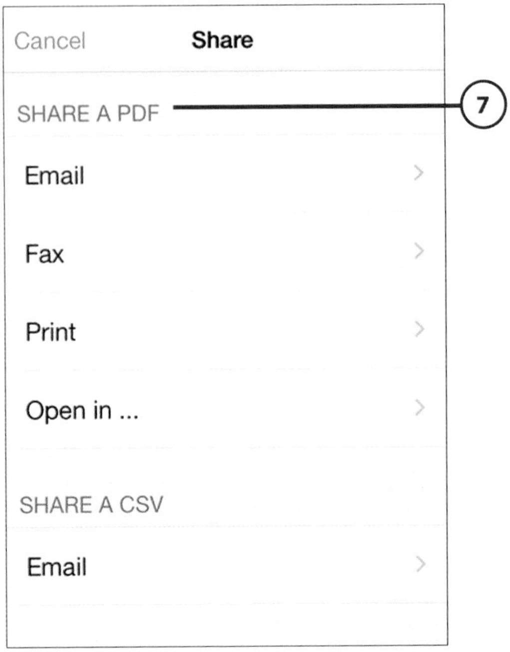

Cancel Share

SHARE A PDF (7)

Email

Fax

Print

Open in ...

SHARE A CSV

Email

Diabetes App

Diabetes App by BHI Technologies, Inc. offers a convenient resource to log and monitor your glucose levels, insulin injections, and medications taken, and to manage your activities. It also tracks how much water you drink, monitors weight and BMI changes, and helps budget your daily carb allowance. Glucose, carb intake, water consumption, and weight data are placed conveniently on a calendar. If you're looking for an app that tracks factors that influence your blood sugar level and want to share data with your doctor, Diabetes App might be another solid choice for you. The app comes in two versions: Diabetes App Lite, which is free, and Diabetes App, which is a paid app. The full version, Diabetes App, lets you create an unlimited number of logs, gives access to charts, allows you to email your data, and offers blood pressure logging. The full version is also ad free. Try out the Lite version first to see whether you like the methodology of how Diabetes App logs information compared to similar apps. As of this writing, Diabetes App is only available for the iPhone and iPad.

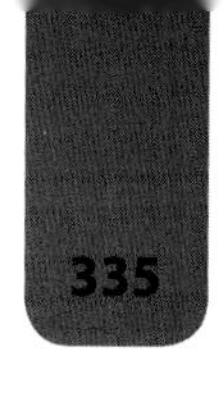

Download and then browse the app to see whether it's helpful to you. The following steps show the Lite version of the app.

1. After you open Diabetes App Lite for the first time, tap OK to let the app send you notifications.
2. Tap Overview to view all of your log information in a calendar layout. You can tap a day in the calendar to view that day's log.

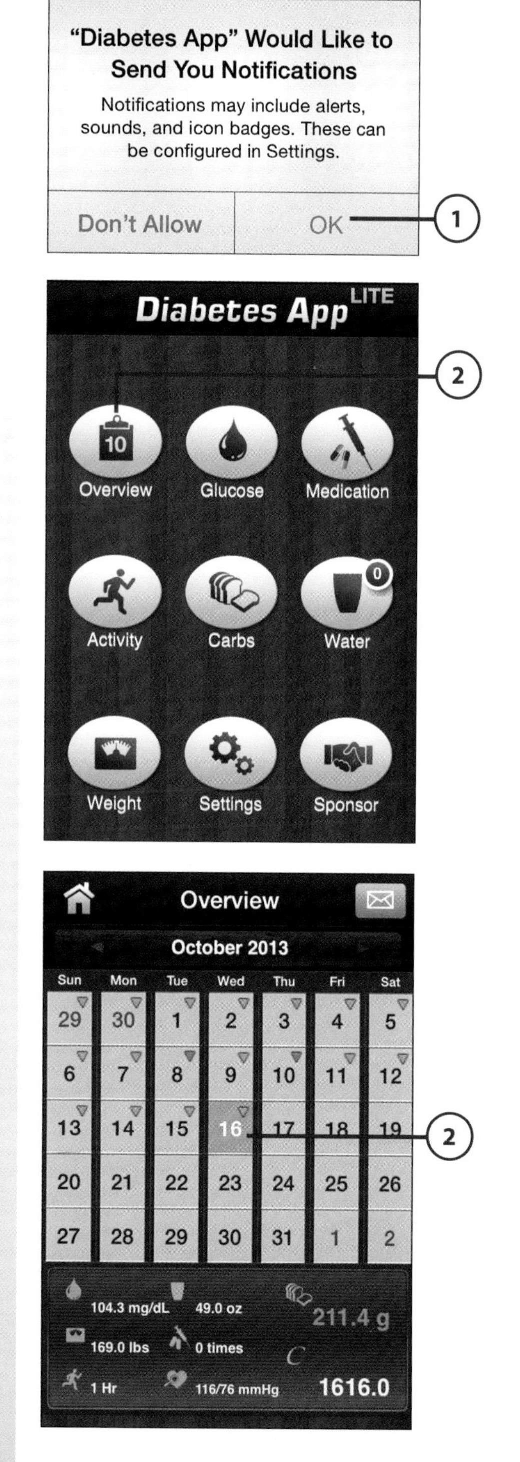

3. Tap Glucose to log glucose test results. A log of previous test results appears.

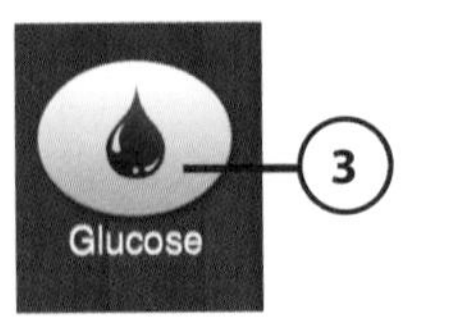

4. Tap the plus sign to add a glucose test result and time. You can tap the Home icon to return to the home screen.

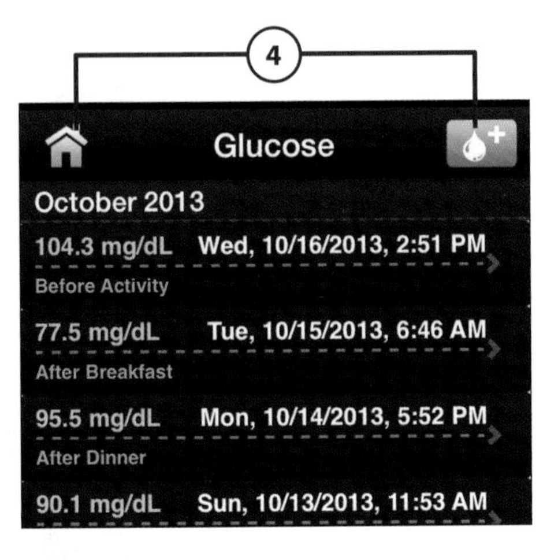

5. Tap Medication to log an insulin dose.

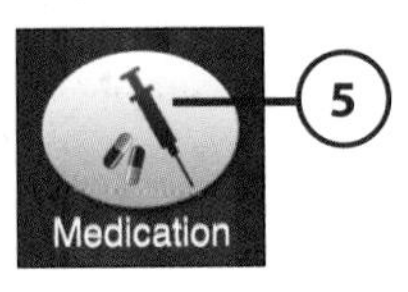

6. Tap the plus sign to add an insulin dose and time. You can tap the Home icon to return to the home screen.

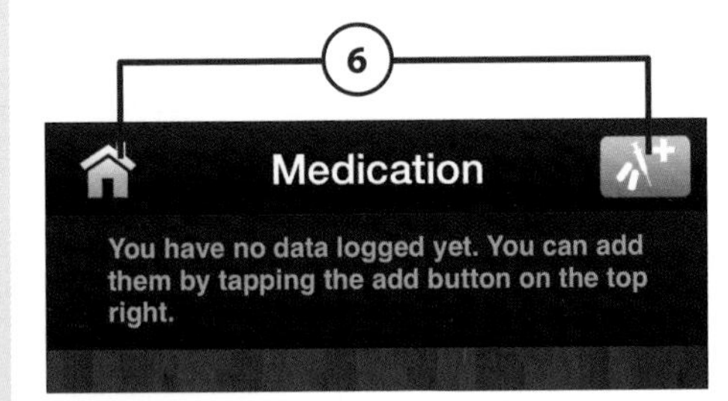

7. Tap Activity to log an exercise.

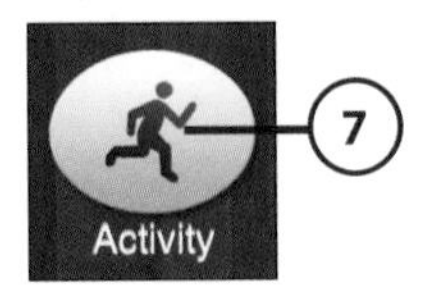

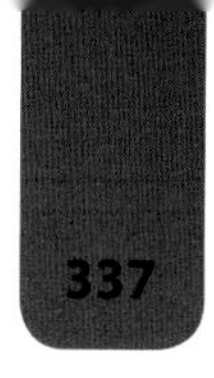

8. Tap the plus sign to add an activity including exercise level and duration. You can tap the Home icon to return to the home screen.
9. Tap Carbs to enter the nutritional value of food for meals and snacks.
10. Tap the plus sign to choose from a list of common foods from the built-in food database.
11. Tap Consumed or Remaining to view the day's tabulation of nutritional information. You can tap Back to return to the previous screen, and then tap the Home icon to return to the home screen.

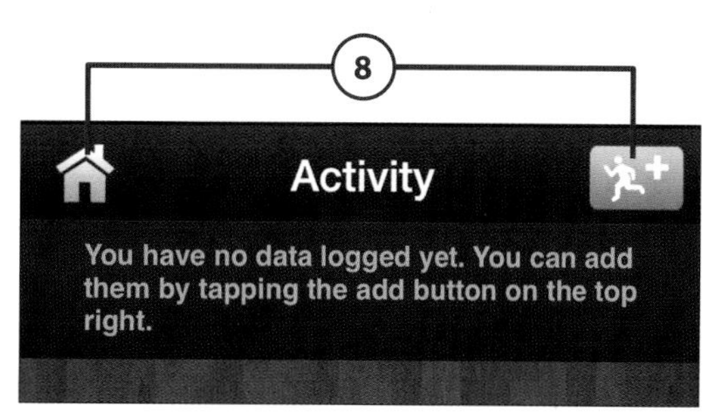

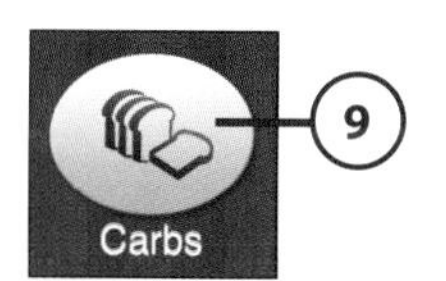

Today
Consumed 211.4 g
Remaining 63.6 g
Calories 1616.0
Fiber 7.2
Sugar 14.4
Protein 68.7
Breakfast 14.5 g
Milk sheep, fluid 13.1 g
Egg duck, whole, fresh, raw 1.4 g
10
11

Food Database

Diabetes App has an extensive food database that makes it easier for you to add carb information into your log. The database has more than 200,000 foods, including restaurant and branded food. You can save favorite foods for faster access. You can even create recipes with combinations of foods and monitor other nutritional information including calories, protein, fiber, sugar, cholesterol, and sodium. You can access this database offline, meaning it doesn't require you to have an Internet connection.

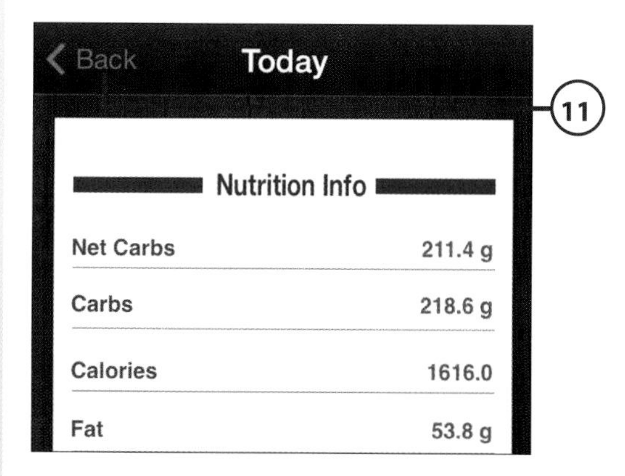

12. Tap Water to log your water intake. The zero on the water button indicates that I have not consumed any glasses of water today.

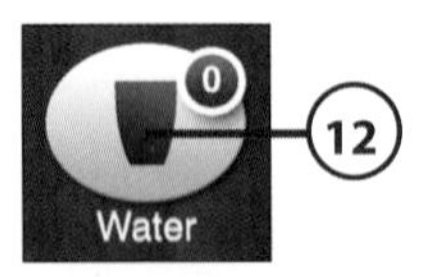

13. Tap on a glass of water to log how much water you have consumed. The glass fills with water once tapped. You can tap the Home icon to return to the home screen.

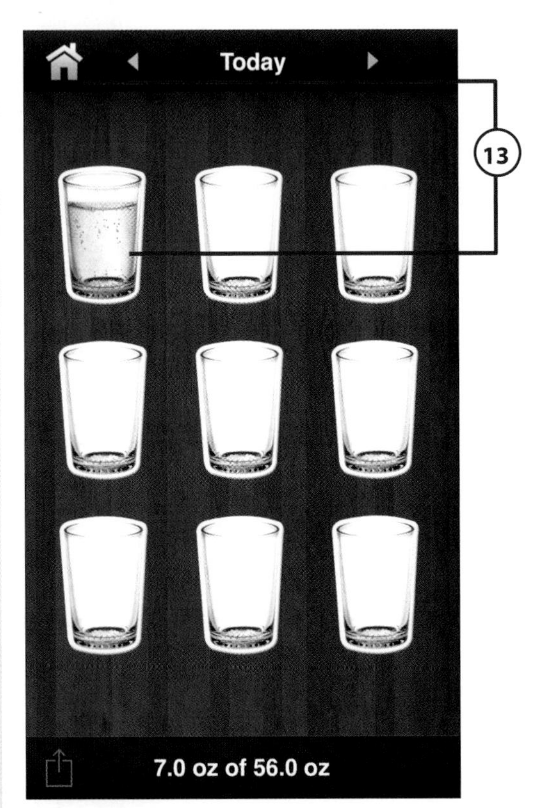

14. Tap Weight to enter your weight and calculate your Body Mass Index (BMI). A note opens telling you what information to provide to calculate your BMI.

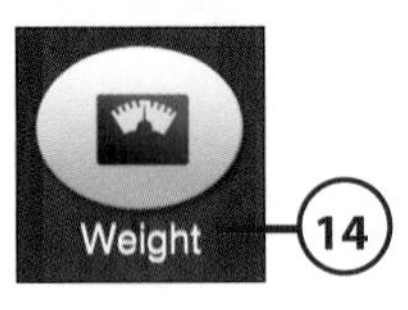

15. Tap OK in the note.

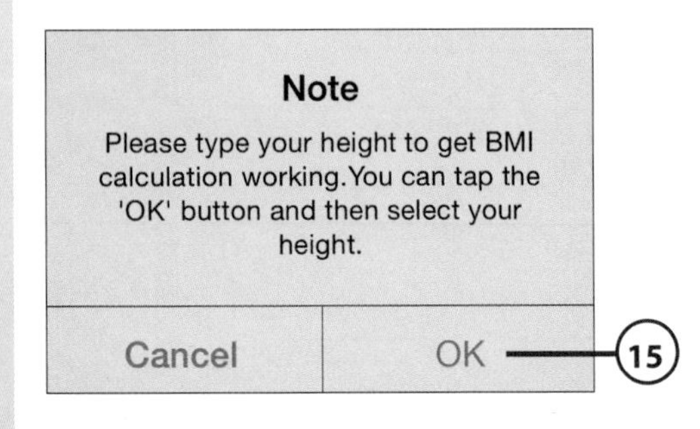

(16) Set your correct height, and then tap Save.

(17) Tap the plus sign to enter your weight and add any notes. You can tap the Home icon to return to the home screen.

(18) Tap Settings to adjust the overall settings for Diabetes App. You can tap the Home icon to return to the home screen.

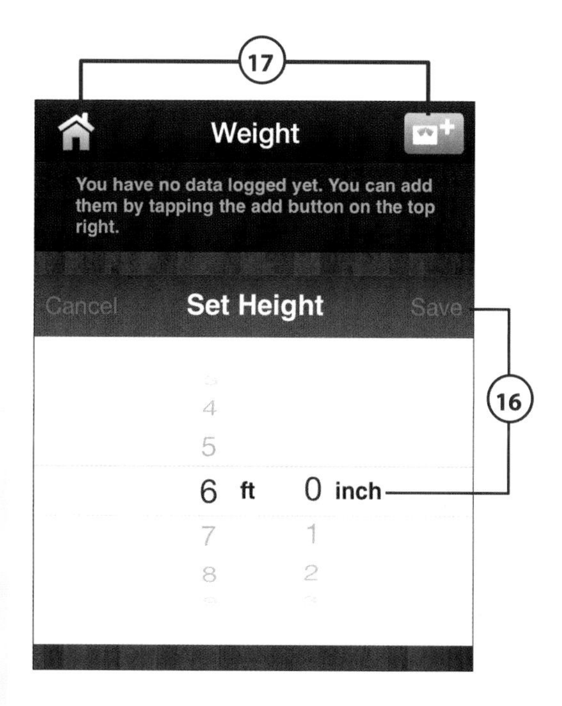

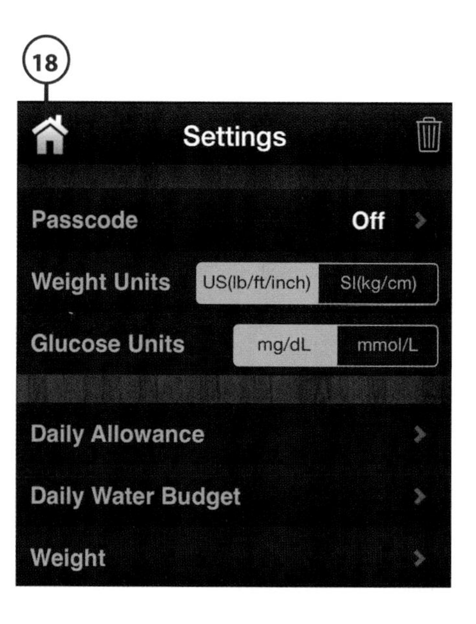

(19) Tap Sponsor to upgrade to the full version, Diabetes App.

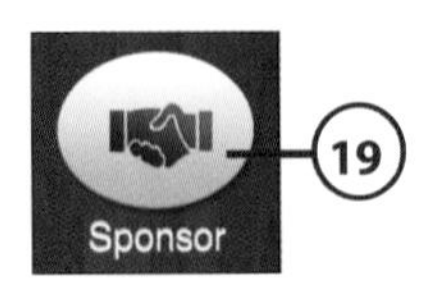

Gmate SMART

The Gmate SMART blood glucose-monitoring meter is roughly the size of a quarter and plugs in to the headphone jack of your iPhone, iPad, or iPod touch. It is used with a Gmate SMART app. As soon as you test your blood glucose, your level will show onscreen in the app. You can then email test results with notes you've made to your doctor and view past test results by date. Your data also uploads to Gmate servers and can be accessed by a nurse or caregiver. Gmate SMART also generates charts of average blood glucose test results within 1, 7, 14, 30, and 60-day periods. As of this writing, the Gmate SMART app is only available for the iPhone but will soon be available for Android in the Google Play Store. You can buy the Gmate SMART at beststrips.com. Visit gmate.com to learn more about the entire line of Gmate products including Gmate VOICE and Gmate PRO. You can also purchase the Gmate Smart on Amazon.com.

Using the Gmate SMART app is quite easy. The following steps show the app on an iPhone.

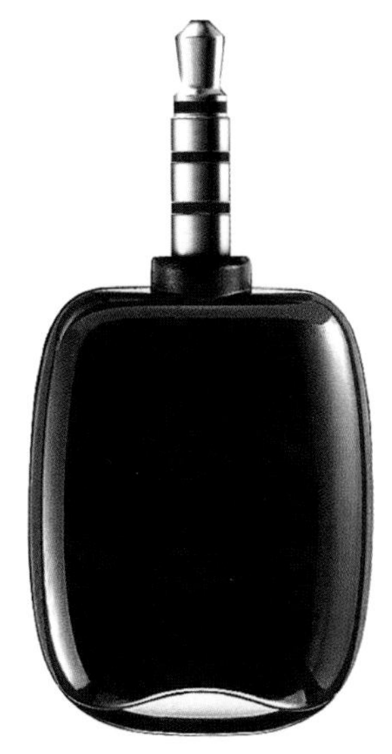

Gmate SMART Blood Glucose Monitoring System

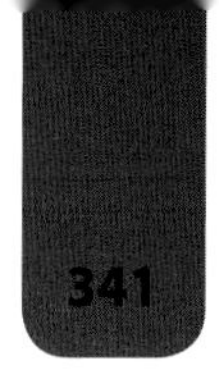

1. Download the Gmate SMART app from the App Store, and then open it on your phone.
2. Insert the Gmate SMART device into the headphone jack of your iPhone, iPad, or iPod touch. A volume control box appears onscreen. Gmate asks whether it's okay to access your iPhone's microphone. Tap OK.
3. The Gmate SMART requires the volume to be at its maximum so that the meter has enough power.
4. Set the volume to its maximum setting. The test strip port at the bottom of the device should light up when the meter is ready to use. Insert Strip appears on the screen.
5. Insert a Gmate test strip, with the electrode facing up, into the test strip port.

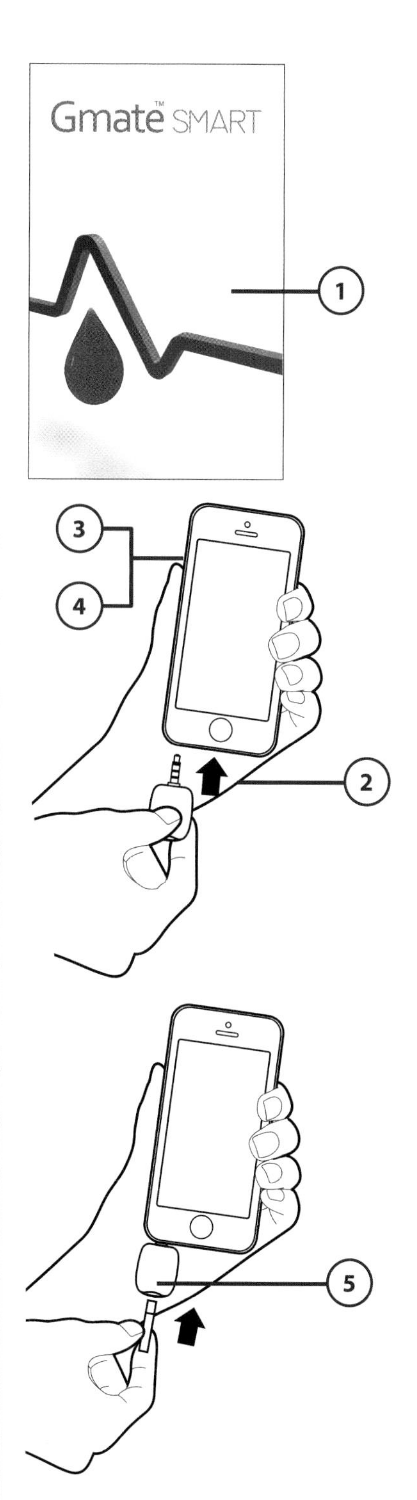

6. Apply blood to the test strip by using the lancing device. It takes five seconds for your test results to display.
7. Your test results display with times and dates when each test was completed.

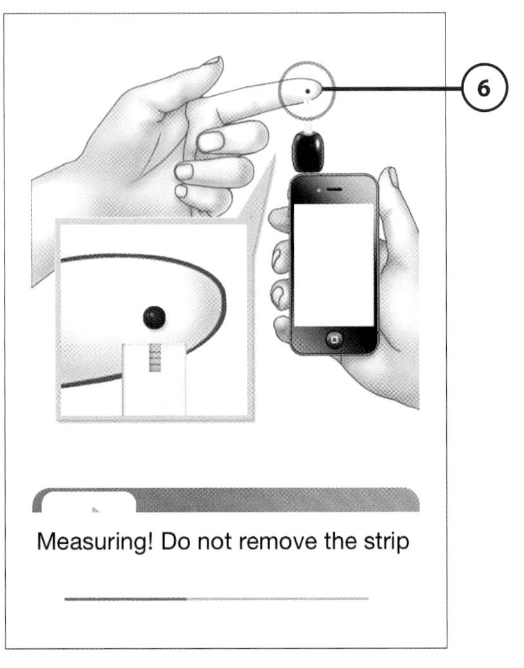

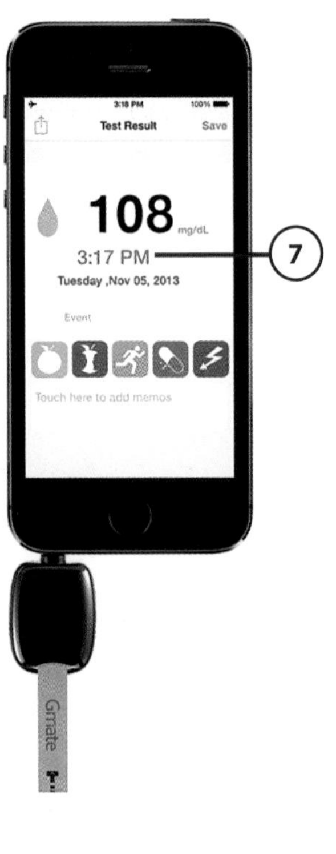

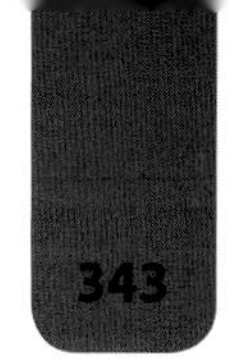

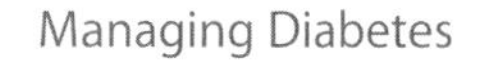

8. Tap a result to edit or add notes.
9. Rotate your device to the landscape position to view your average test results as a graph. You can email your results as a PDF file or CSV file (comma separated values file, in which your data is essentially saved in a table-structured format) to your doctor or caregiver.

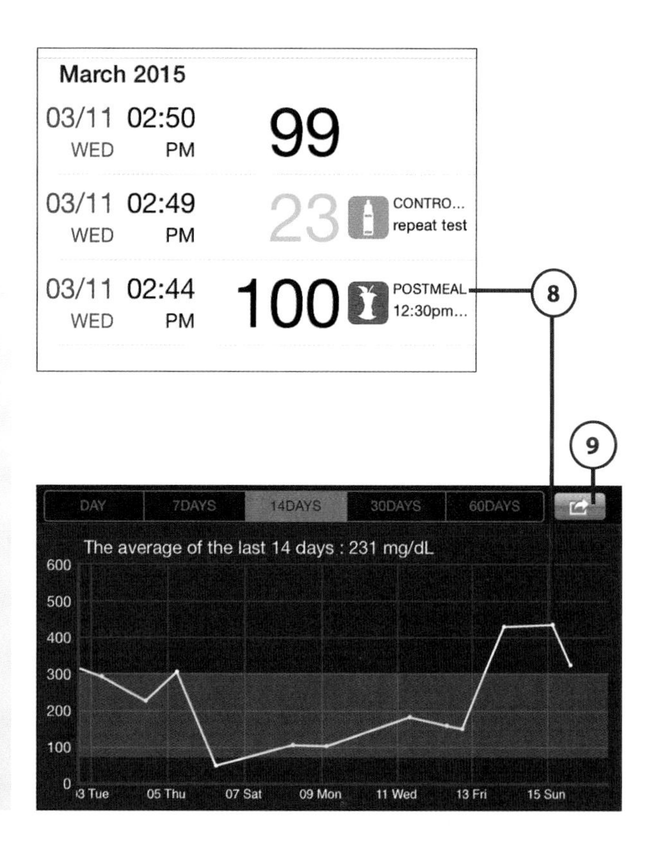

Go Wireless with the iHealth Smart Gluco-Monitoring System

The wireless iHealth Smart Gluco-Monitoring System enables you to manage your diabetes by connecting to your smartphone or tablet using Bluetooth and automatically recording your glucose readings. The device also tracks the quantity and expiration date of your test strips after a quick scan of the vial's QR code. You can view your reading on the device itself. You can record pre- and post-meal levels and medications using the iHealth Gluco-Smart app, including if you have been fasting or taking insulin. This app automatically keeps a history of your data and enables you to share it with your doctor or caregiver. You can purchase this monitoring system at ihealthlabs.com. You can use this system with both Android and Apple devices. Go to the iHealth website and see whether this monitoring system is right for you. Visit the Google Play Store and the App Store to download the app.

Follow these steps to do the initial setup for the iHealth Smart Gluco-Monitoring System on an iPhone.

1. On your computer, go to ihealthlabs.com, and click Sign In to create an iHealth Cloud account for secure data storage.
2. On your iPhone, download the iHealth Gluco-Smart app from the App Store by tapping Get. Don't open it just yet.
3. Connect the meter to your device by enabling Bluetooth on your mobile device by going into the Settings.
4. Hold down the "memory" button on the meter for three seconds, and then select the name of the device on your phone's Devices list. The meter should now appear in your Bluetooth Device list.

iHealth Gluco-Smart 4+
iHealth Lab Inc. >
iHealth
GET
Offers Apple Watch App
2

Settings Bluetooth
Bluetooth
Now discoverable as "Connor Watson's iPhone".
MY DEVICES
Anker Bluetooth Keyboard Not Connected
Bluetooth 3.0 Keyboard Not Connected
3

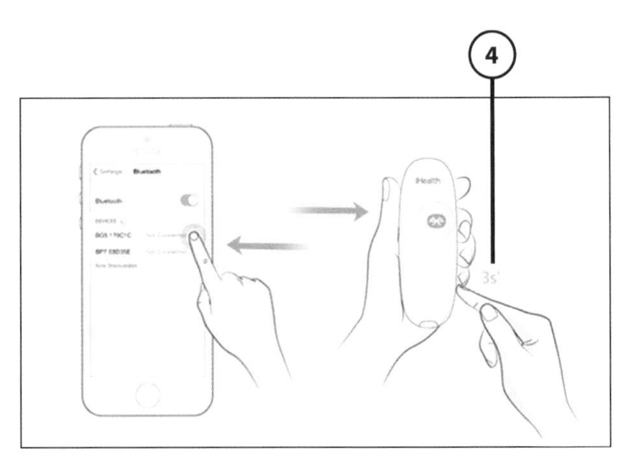

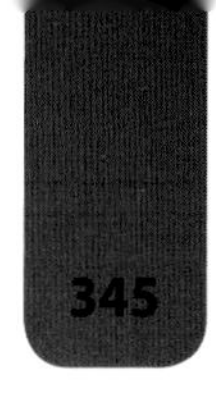

5. Open the app to connect to the device.
6. Scan the QR code on the iHealth test trip vial to calibrate the test strip with the meter. A QR code is a machine-readable code similar to a barcode on a product box. A QR code consists of black and white squares (not shown).
7. Insert a test strip into the device (not shown).
8. Apply the blood sample. Remove the test strip after you hear an alert from the device.
9. Read the test results.

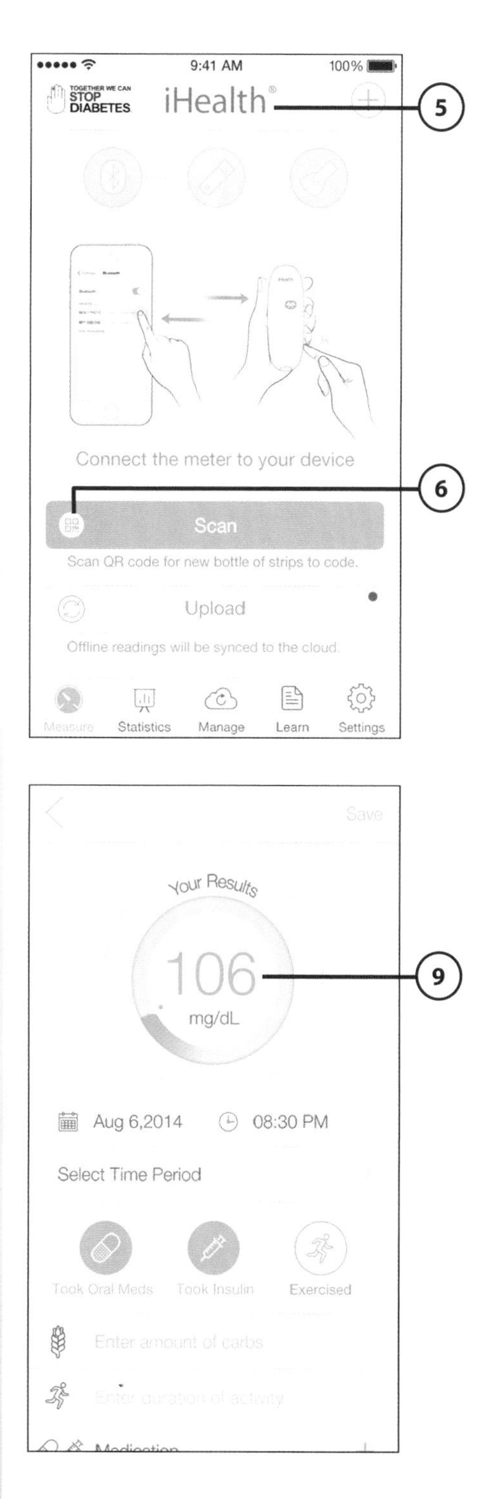

(10) Tap History to review your log history.

(11) Tap Summary to review statistics and trends.

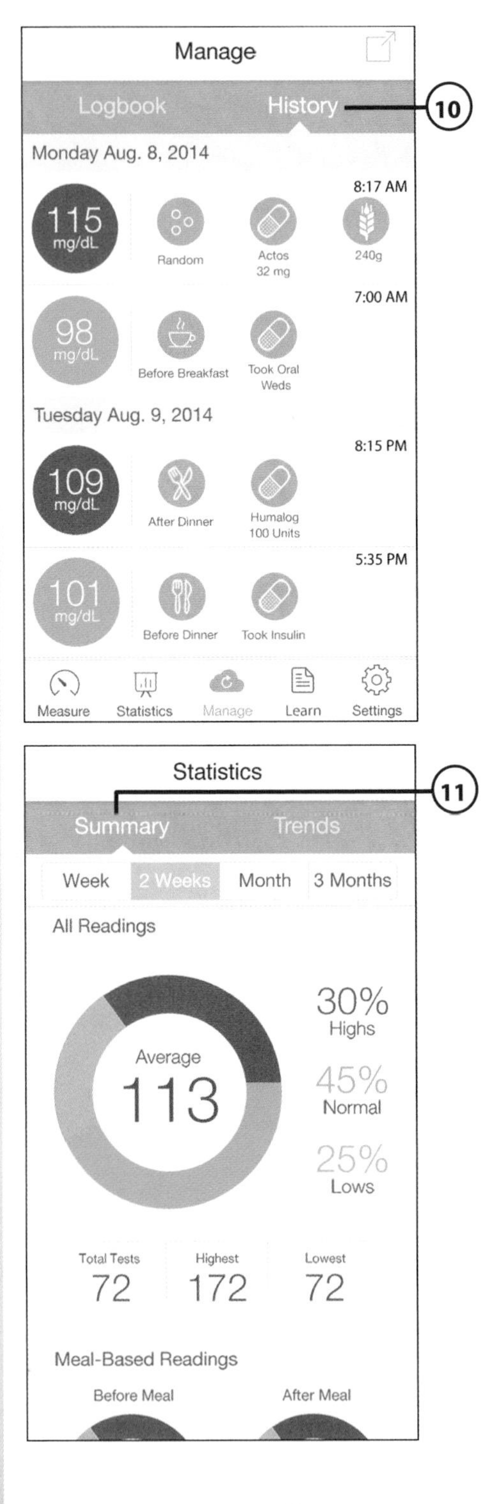

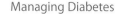

Gauge Glucose Levels Visually with the Meal Memory App

The Meal Memory app from Databetes offers a new approach to nutrition tracking and understanding how your meals affect your blood sugar. Meal Memory is food focused and the concept is very simple. Take a picture of every meal and pair them with pre- and post-blood sugars to get a clear idea of how specific meals impact your blood sugar. The design is simple, highly visual, and doesn't require an inordinate amount of manual log entry time compared to similar apps. Using it is simple, too. Take a picture of the meal you eat. Conduct a pre-meal glucose test. Wait two hours and then conduct a post-meal testing of your glucose level. The app adds color-coded dots to indicate in-range (black) and out-of-range (blue indicating high or red indicating low) blood glucose values for before the meal and for two hours after the meal. The dots are laid over the pictures that comprise your meal history so you can see the blood sugar impact of meals. When you eat the same meal again, you can take the necessary precautions in meal preparation. Depending on which devices you use, there is almost no data entry involved other than taking pictures of your food.

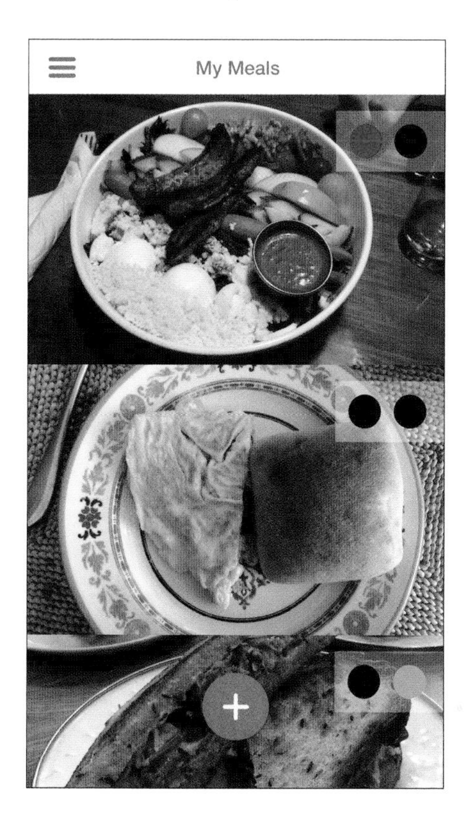

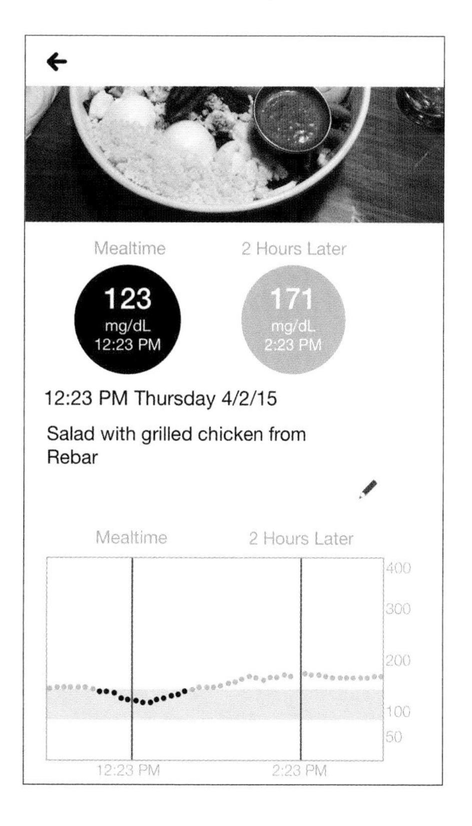

Meal Memory is available for both Android and Apple phones, but as of this writing, it is currently optimized for the iPhone and the Dexacom Share receiver. The Meal Memory app works in tandem with Apple's Health app, which pulls information from the Dexacom Share2 iPhone app. When you take a test with your Dexacom CGM (Continuous Glucose Monitoring) device, all you have do is take the picture of the food, and then come back later to view which color-coded dots it received. If you are using an Android device or a different blood glucose meter, you need to manually enter your blood glucose values before and two hours after each meal. You can set the Meal Memory app to send you a reminder two hours after you have taken a picture of the meal you are about to eat, so you don't forget.

If you have been searching for a less numbers-focused approach and less manual log entry, give the Meal Memory app some serious consideration.

Connect with Diabeticconnect.com

Diabeticconnect.com is a large community of diabetes patients where you can connect with other diabetics. You can get involved in discussion forums to ask questions, make comments, discuss treatments, and learn from others. If there is an important topic that you haven't seen posted, start a conversation of your own. By supplying a support network and a place to share experiences, Diabetic Connect can help you improve your life with diabetes.

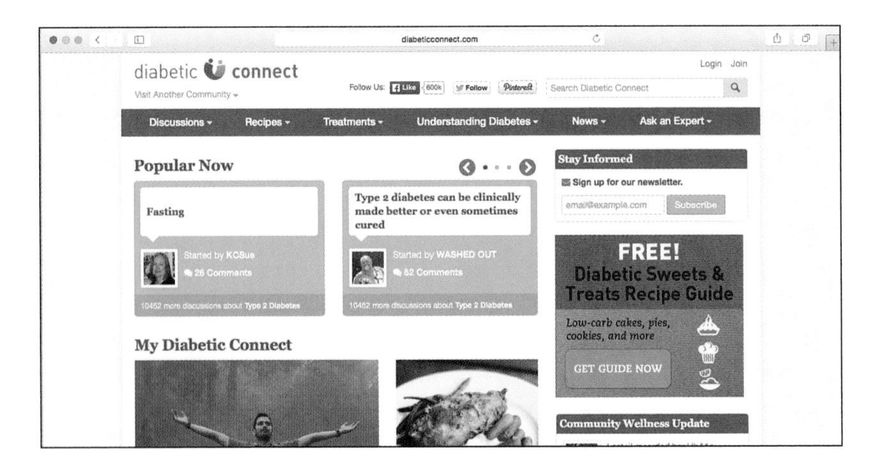

Diabeticconnect.com is a large community of diabetes patients where you can share experiences, find recipes, and get expert advice.

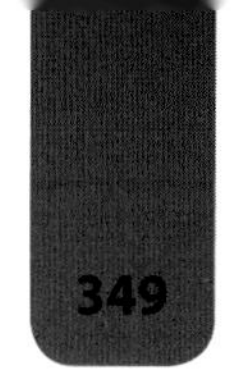

Diabeticconnect.com is much more than just a discussion forum. You will find many helpful articles on living well, treatment and care, and diet and exercise, including plenty of recipes. You find featured news stories in relation to Type 1 and 2 diabetes, diabetic diet, weight loss, diabetes research, and diabetic treatments. An Ask an Expert section offers a place where you can get answers to your most pressing questions.

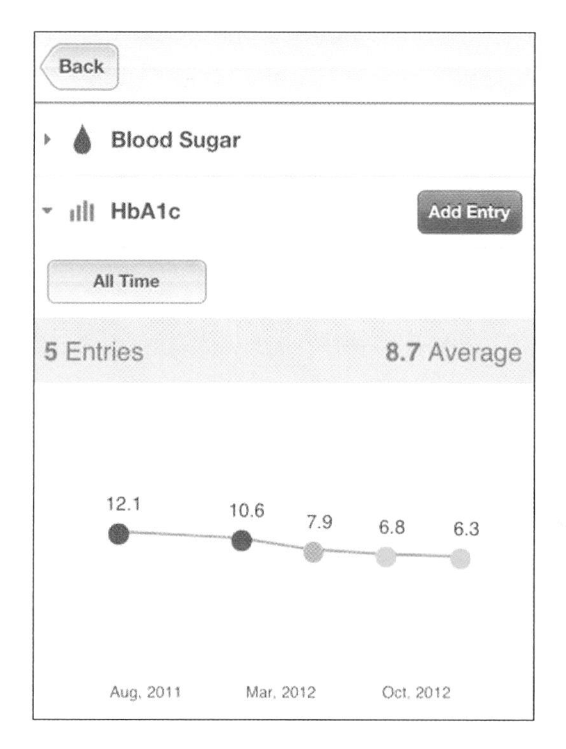

Diabeticconnect.com also offers an app with a logbook to help you track your blood glucose.

As of this writing, this site even has an app for the iPhone, but not for Android. Along with offering you the ability to participate in discussions while on the go, the app also features a logbook so you can track your blood glucose for better diabetes control.

Visit diabeticconnect.com to see what you think of the site and join the community.

Other Communities Accessible from Diabeticconnect.com

Diabeticconnect is also a portal to other support communities. If you look at the top of the screen, just under the logo, you can click a "Visit Another Community" drop-down menu to visit other support communities including arthritis, breast cancer, Crohn's disease, depression, and much more.

Taking a Look at Heart Health Technology

Many of the medical devices that were once accessible only during doctor visits are now being made for use in the home, including heart health devices. These consumer devices include heart rate monitors, ambulatory blood pressure monitors, apps that can track your heart rate over time, and electrocardiogram devices that can detect a serious heart condition. None of these devices are meant to replace your doctor, but they can provide helpful information that you can share with your doctor. While exploring consumer heart health devices and apps, keep in mind that results may vary. Not all products are up to par, so vet everything. See what others have to say about a product and above all else, ask your doctor for suggestions on devices that can help keep your ticker in shape.

This section introduces you to options for keeping an eye on hypertension and blood pressure. You get some suggestions on wearable heart rate monitors, and explore heart health apps for your smartphone. This is just a starting point for you to begin your own search and give some of these truly innovative devices a try.

Keeping an Eye on Your Hypertension and Blood Pressure

Access to blood pressure monitors outside of the doctor's office has been around for a while. For years you've been able to walk into a Walgreens or CVS and test your own blood pressure. Now you can easily keep an eye on your hypertension or blood pressure from home. Take a look at some of the more traditional devices, or progress to the more technologically savvy cuffs that make the data available in your smartphone. Whichever blood pressure monitor you choose, make sure that the one you purchase fits comfortably around the circumference

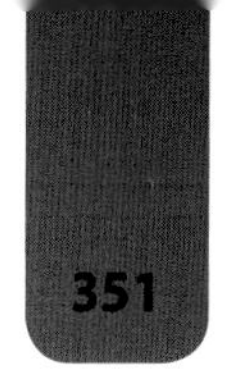

of your arm. Cuffs come in different sizes. Measurements won't be reliable if the cuff is too small or too large. Keep in mind that some monitors have cuffs that fit around your wrist.

Talk with Your Doctor

Only a doctor can diagnose if you might have hypertension and a blood pressure condition. And if you have a heart condition, such as an irregular heartbeat, this might dictate which monitoring device is right for you. This section does not provide interpretations of blood pressure readings. What it does do is introduce you to the hardware and software being used to read blood pressure.

Use a Manual Blood Pressure Cuff

Manual blood pressure monitors are the traditional blood pressure cuffs you see in your doctor's office, although automatic monitors are quickly replacing them. A manual blood pressure monitor kit usually consists of a cuff, an attached pump (bulb) that inflates the cuff, a stethoscope, and a gauge that allows you to measure blood pressure. This type of monitor requires some coordination when using the pump to inflate the cuff. Note that this type of equipment is difficult to use if you are unable to perform the hand movements or are visually or hearing impaired.

You can purchase manual blood pressure monitors on amazon.com or your local Walgreens or CVS pharmacy.

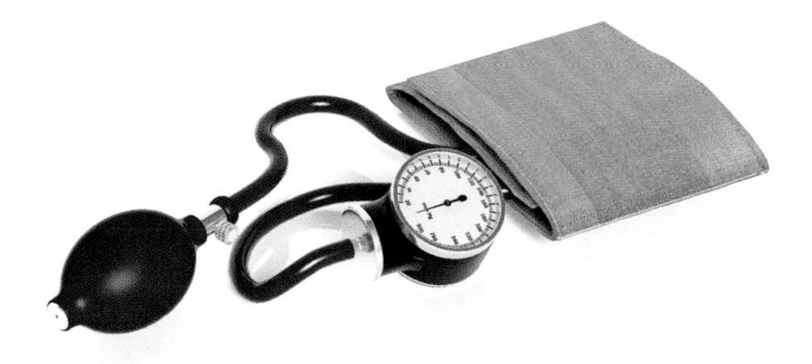

Credit: © viperagp/Fotolia.com

Manual blood pressure monitor

Use an Automatic Blood Pressure Monitor

Automatic blood pressure monitors are becoming more of the norm in doctors' offices. You've seen them before, being wheeled over to you on a five-leg stand. The nurse puts on the cuff, presses a few buttons, and then the cuff automatically begins to tighten around your arm. You can have a monitor similar to this at home, minus the stand and wheels. The Omron 7 Series and Panasonic EW3109W are both automatic, upper-arm blood pressure monitors. An automatic blood pressure monitor kit usually consists of a cuff attached to a monitor with buttons. After properly placing the cuff on your bare upper arm, you press a start button on the digital interface to inflate the cuff. The cuff slowly deflates, and a few moments later your measurement appears on the monitor.

Tracking Your Blood Pressure

Manually logging your blood pressure measurements lets you see how you are progressing over time. Some automatic wireless blood pressure monitors can upload your measurement directly to an app, or you can manually enter your measurements into a health app. We take a look at some blood pressure apps later in this chapter.

The Omron 7 Series cuff accommodates an arm up to 17 inches in circumference and can automatically average your last 3 readings taken in 10 minutes for a more accurate reading. Visit omronhealthcare.com to learn more about the device or to purchase the Omron 7 series blood pressure monitor. You can also go to Amazon.com to purchase the monitor and read customer reviews.

The Panasonic EW3109W cuff can accommodate an arm up to 15.75 inches in circumference, and the screen automatically flashes the LCD screen for hypersensitive readings. Visit shop.panasonic.com and enter a search for the EW3109W monitor to learn more and purchase the device.

Other Places to Find Automatic Blood Pressure Monitors

Check your local Best Buy, CVS, Target, Walgreens, or Walmart for these products, or talk with your local medical supply store to find more options.

>>>Go Further

AMBULATORY BLOOD PRESSURE MONITORS

An ambulatory blood pressure monitor lets you record blood pressure over a period of 24 hours by taking a reading every 15 to 30 minutes. The device is about the size of a cell phone, but thicker. It's designed to be placed on your belt, and the cuff to be worn under your shirt, where no one can see. Some units even transmit wirelessly, so you only need the cuff to be connected. You wear the device while going about your everyday activities, even while you sleep. The doctor can then analyze blood pressure variability for a more accurate estimation. Doctors use those devices to diagnose hypertension in patients and to see whether treatment for hypertension is effective. These devices are quite expensive and are usually issued by a doctor.

Use Wireless Blood Pressure Cuffs with Your Smartphone

The Wireless Blood Pressure Monitor from Withings and the QardioArm Blood Pressure Monitor provide you the convenience of recording and archiving readings to your phone wirelessly using Bluetooth. Both work with Android and Apple (iOS) devices. Each comes with an upper arm cuff and its own accompanying app that you can download from the Google Play Store and the App Store.

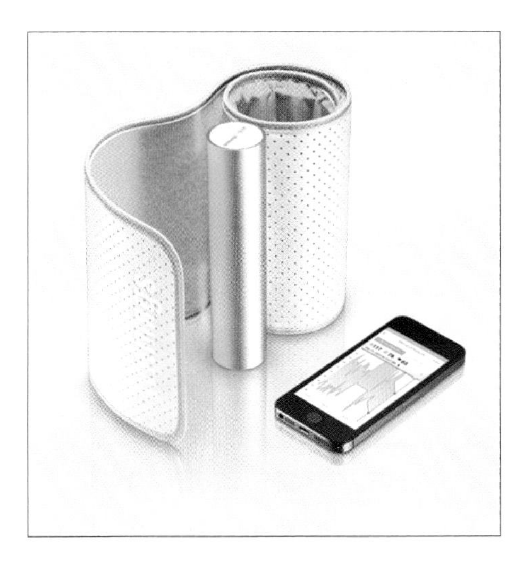

The Wireless Blood Pressure Monitor from Withings and Health Mate App

Using the Wireless Blood Pressure Monitor from Withings is as simple as downloading the Health Mate app, putting on the cuff, and then turning on the blood pressure monitor. The app automatically launches, and after some brief instructions you are ready to take a measurement. After the measurement is completed, the Health Mate app gives you color-coded feedback based on the AHA (American Heart Association) and the ESH (European Society of Hypertension) recommendations for hypertension. An archive of your past measurements and charts is built to help you monitor trends. You can share this information with your doctor straight from the app.

The cuff takes accurate measurements on arms between 9 and 17 inches. Visit www.withings.com to learn more and to purchase the monitor. You can also purchase the monitor at Best Buy stores and Amazon.com. Download the Health Mate app for Android and iPhone at the Google Play Store and the App Store.

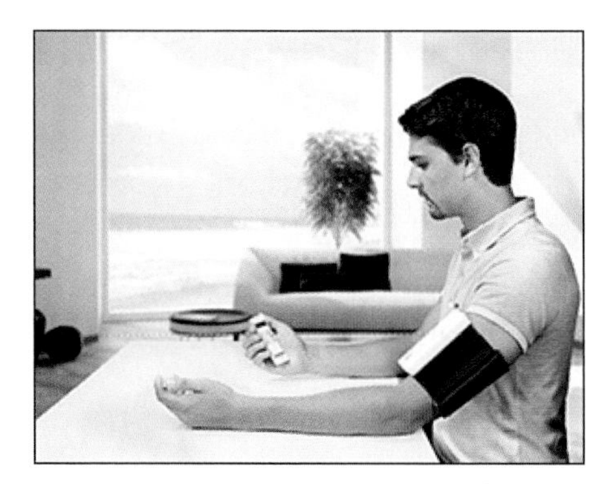

The QardioArm Blood Pressure Monitor and Qardio App

Using the QardioArm smart blood pressure monitor is easy as well. Download the Qardio app. Unroll the QardioArm, which automatically switches on the Qardio app. Slide your arm through the armband and then secure the band. Pair the QardioArm with your smartphone. Press Start on the app when you are ready to take your measurement. QardioArm tracks your measurements over time with smart charts, trends, and stats. You can share your blood pressure data with your doctor from the Qardio app.

The QardioArm cuff takes accurate measurements on arms between 8.7 and 14.6 inches. Visit Qardio.com to learn more and to purchase the device. You can also purchase the QardioArm on Amazon.com.

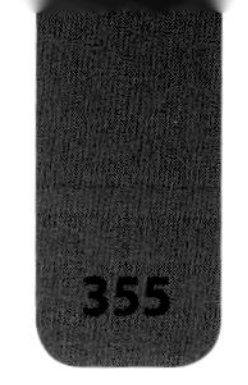

Choosing the Right Wearable Heart Monitor for You

Heart rate monitoring has gone mainstream and is a highly sought-after feature in fitness trackers, usually featured on higher-end models. It is even slowly being built directly into smartphones. You can log your heart rate before, during, and after physical activity to track your cardiovascular progress over time, and hopefully, see improvement.

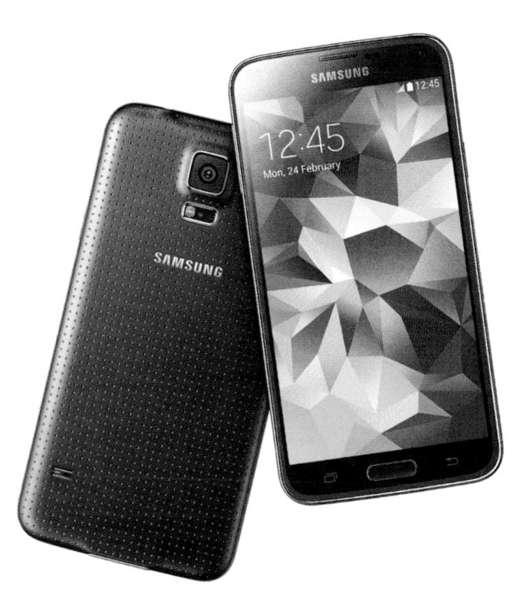

The Samsung Galaxy S5 with heart rate sensor

Heart rate monitoring options include the following:

Smartphones: Your phone doesn't technically fall under the term *wearable*, but if you already have a Samsung Galaxy S5, it might be all you need. Before making this decision, be aware of what it means to use a heart rate scanner on your phone—you have to stop what you're doing to take a reading. As of this writing, the Samsung Galaxy S5 has incorporated this technology. To find your heart rate, you place your finger on the sensor located on the back of the phone as it shines a red light through your finger to measure your heart rate in beats per minute (bpm). The results appear in the S Health app where you can log your heart rate over time and see visual representations in charts. This is a good option if you don't mind the interruption. If you're looking for a more passive monitor, an activity tracker is what you are looking for.

Fitness trackers: Fitness trackers such as the Fitbit Charge HR and the Basis Peak are continuous heart rate monitors. This means that they take measurements as you are walking, running, eating, sleeping, or doing anything else. A continuous heart monitor on your wrist also does a better job than stand-alone measurements at tracking your sleep and how many calories you burn during an activity. Fitness trackers measure your heart rate using LED lights pressed against the wrist. Monitoring your heart rate using activity trackers is good for gathering mostly non-interrupted averages of the intensity of your workouts. If you are a walker or a runner, activity trackers are great for taking a quick glance at your heart rate to see whether you're in the "cardio zone," so you can increase or lower your intensity. Many products other than the Fitbit Charge and Basis Peak are available that can serve as quality heart rate monitors.

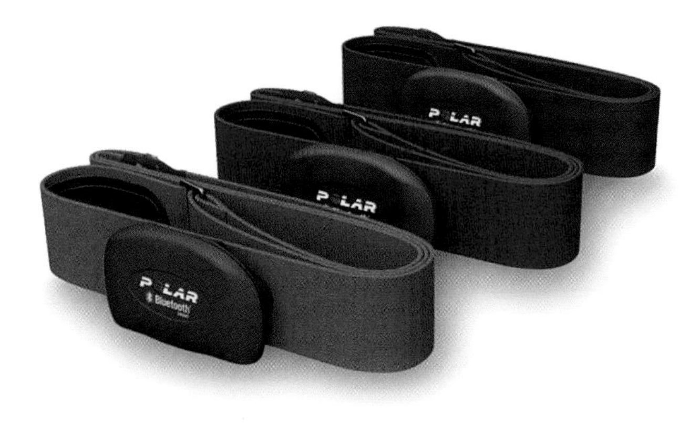

Heart rate sensor straps from Polar

Some heart rate monitors use wireless straps with built-in sensors that detect your pulse electronically, and then send that data to a watch or an app. These devices give you continuous, average, high, and low heart rate data. Polar and Garmin offer quality products in this area.

Let's take a look at some heart-rate-focused features you might find helpful in a fitness tracker.

The ability to set target zones: A fitness tracker with programmable fitness zones offers more direction in getting the most from your workout. For example, you can enter heart rate data for a series of different workouts such as endurance, aerobic, and anaerobic variations so you can tailor your workouts.

Fitness trainer capabilities: This high-end feature provides alerts for intensity levels that go above or below your chosen target zone.

A recovery heart rate mode: Fitness trackers with this feature track the time it takes your heart to recover to its normal resting rate after a workout. This is a good indicator of cardio fitness, especially if you do a lot of running or interval training.

Understand Heart Rate Target Zones

Heart rate zones are a great way to gauge your intensity and help you maintain an optimal target heart rate for a specific goal. First, you need to know your maximum heart rate. The American Heart Association calculates maximum heart rate by subtracting your age from 220. For example, if you are 55, subtract 55 from 220 to get your maximum heart rate of 165. This is the maximum amount of times your heart should beat in 1 minute while you are exercising. Now that you know your heart maximum heart rate, you can calculate personal target zones where your heart is being worked but not overexerted.

The Mayo Clinic places moderate exercise intensity between 50 to 70 percent of your maximum heart rate. Vigorous exercise intensity is 70 to 85 percent. First and foremost, gauge your intensity level by how you feel. If you feel like you're over exerting yourself, you probably need to back off. If you're not fit, the Mayo Clinic says to stay around 50 percent and then work your way up. If you are very much overweight, you might want to start even lower. Talk with your doctor and use your best judgment.

To calculate your zones, take your maximum heart rate—we'll use the 165 calculated earlier—and multiply that number by 0.7 (70 percent) to find out the lower end of the vigorous range. We get 115.5. Rounding up, that's 116. For the top end of vigorous intensity, do the same for 0.85 (85 percent). We get 140.25. In this example, the Vigorous intensity zone is somewhere between 116 and 140 beats per minute. You can do the same calculations for moderate exercise. Again, use your judgment. Age is just one factor we're using for this example. Listen to your body when you're working out.

There are specific target heart rate zones for weight loss to increase endurance and stamina, and for conditioning. The "Investigating Apps for Heart Health on Your Smartphone" section introduces a tool provided by the makers of the Instant Heart Rate app that can help you identify these zones.

Talk to Your Doctor Before Using HR Target Zones

Some medications can lower your maximum heart rate and lower your target heart rate zone. Ask your doctor if you need to lower your target zones because of medication you are using or other conditions.

Use Heart Rate Monitoring Data

You can use heart rate monitoring data to engage in activity levels that are right for you. Some high-end fitness trackers enable you to enter heart rate zones into the device and use them as workout goals. Some of these trackers can even alert you when your beats per minute are out of the specified zone. With other trackers, you might only be able to determine whether you stayed within a zone by viewing a graph of your activity measurements after you have finished. A great perk of having your heart rate data is the ability to use today's data to motivate yourself to do better tomorrow. Today you stayed mostly in your "moderate" range (50 to 65 percent). Tomorrow you can try going faster for longer.

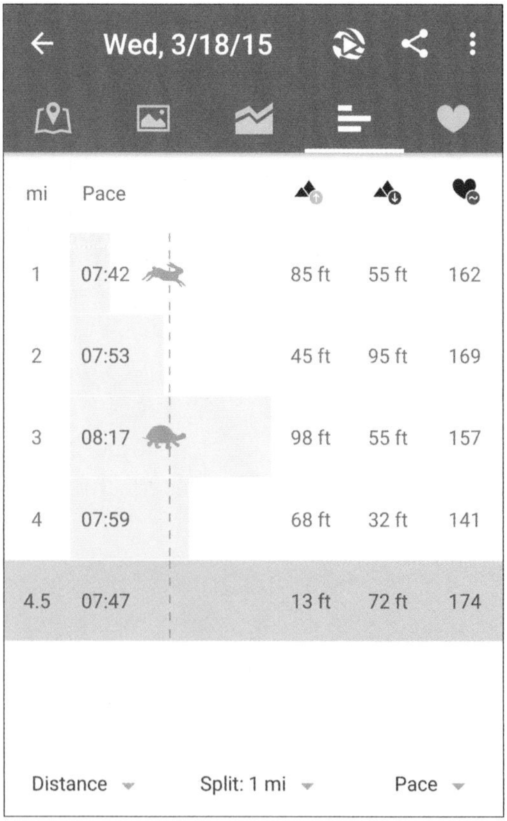

Wed, 3/18/15

mi	Pace			
1	07:42	85 ft	55 ft	162
2	07:53	45 ft	95 ft	169
3	08:17	98 ft	55 ft	157
4	07:59	68 ft	32 ft	141
4.5	07:47	13 ft	72 ft	174

Distance Split: 1 mi Pace

Consider using heart rate target zones to improve running and workout performance

If you are a runner, using heart rate data for the first time could be a breakthrough moment in your performance. There are different heart rate target zone formulas that some runners say work much better for them than the calculations mentioned in the previous section. There are even workout percent of maximum heart rate suggestions for various race distances. You can check out this information on runnersworld.com, which includes the experiences of runners who are 50+ using heart rate monitoring to push to the next level.

Investigating Apps for Heart Health on Your Smartphone

You don't need an activity tracker or a dedicated monitor to measure your pulse. Apps for Android and Apple (iOS) devices are capable of acquiring accurate readings. There are even apps, coupled with small devices, that enable you to take an electrocardiogram (ECG) at home or on the go, to let you know whether any abnormalities were detected.

Find Your Target Heart Rate with Instant Heart Rate

The Instant Heart Rate app makes it easy for you to measure your pulse and find your target heart rate, so you can optimize your workout or simply track your exertion for any activity. This app is available for Android, Apple (iOS), and Windows phone devices and comes in a free and a paid version. Download the app on the Google Play Store, the App Store, or the Windows Phone Store. Instant Heart Rate uses your smartphone's camera flash to measure your pulse. This app works best on devices that have a flash. If your device does not have a flash, make sure you use it in a well-lit room.

Let's take a look at how you can take a heart rate measurement and also find your target heart rate using Instant Heart Rate. The following steps are shown on an iPhone and in the paid version that, as of this writing, is $1.99.

What Are In-App Purchases?

When you go to download some of the apps this book covers, you might see "In-app purchases" written underneath the price (or the Get or Install option) for Apple or Android devices. In-app purchases means you have to purchase extra content and subscriptions within the app to gain access to specific features. If you tap on a feature that requires an in-app purchase, you are alerted to the fact. The in-app purchases usually are listed in the app description on the Google Play Store or the App Store.

---

1. When you open Instant Heart Rate for the first time, the app asks for permission to send you notifications; tap OK. The app then asks whether it can access your camera.
2. Tap OK. The Camera light comes on.
3. Place your finger over the camera until it completely covers the lens. Press gently. The app uses the change in color in your fingertip to detect the blood flow so it can take the measurement. Your heart rate displays.

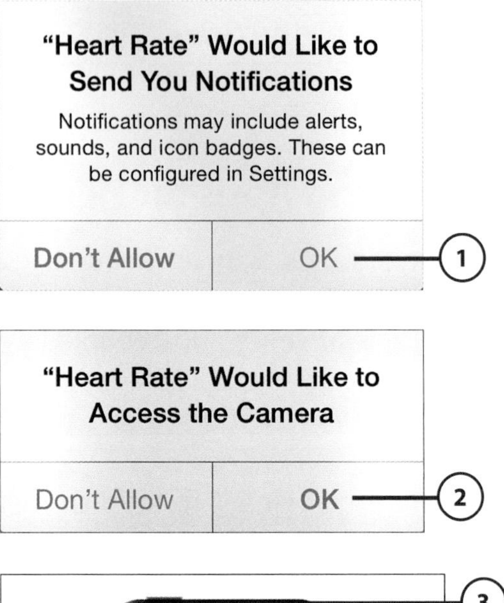

"Heart Rate" Would Like to Send You Notifications
Notifications may include alerts, sounds, and icon badges. These can be configured in Settings.
Don't Allow
OK
1
"Heart Rate" Would Like to Access the Camera
Don't Allow
OK
2

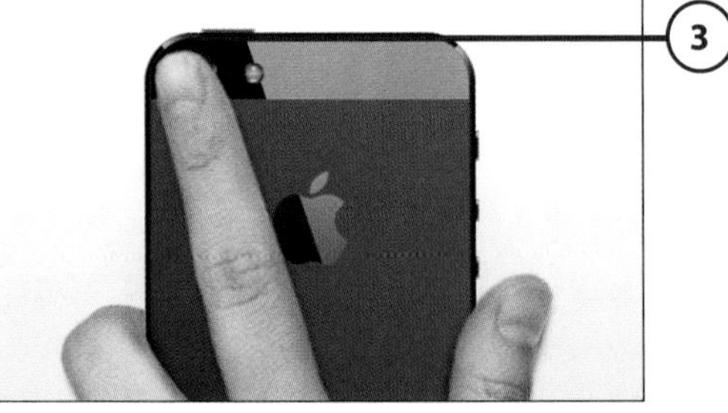

4. Tap the Settings button that looks like a gear.
5. Scroll down the page to Heart Rate Zones Calculations and tap Based On Age. Scroll wheels open, letting you enter your birth date.

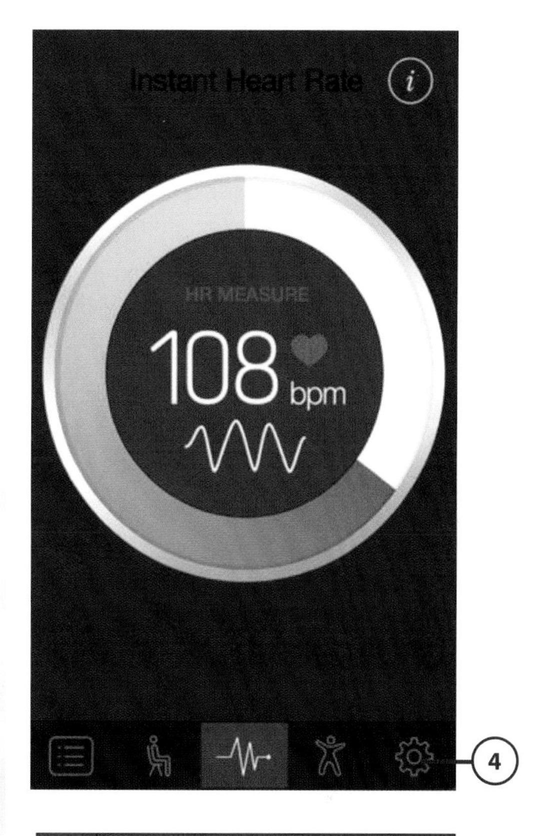

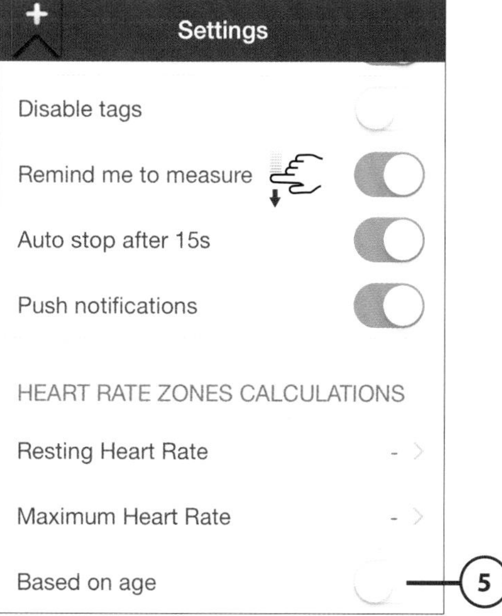

6. Swipe up and down on the scroll wheels to enter your birth date, and then tap Done.
7. Scroll the menu to select your gender, and then tap Done.
8. Scroll up to view your Heart Rate Zones Calculations. On the developer's website, you can calculate what your heart rate should be at your age for various exercises.

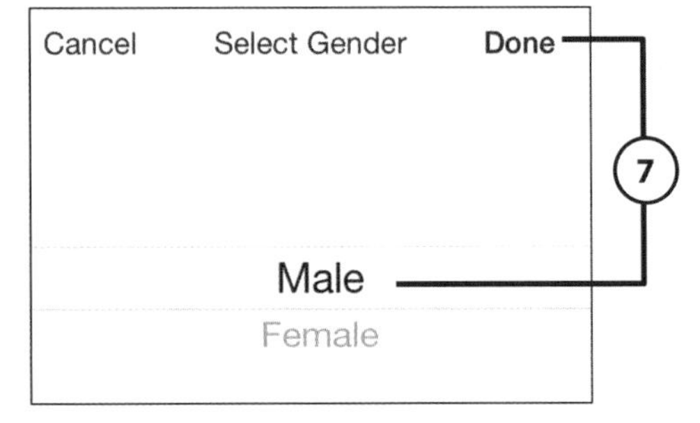

9. Go to azumio.com, scroll down the page, and then tap the Instant Heart Rate App.
10. Scroll down to the "What's In Each Beat" section.
11. Drag the slider to your appropriate age, and the numbers change for each activity. Now you have a clear map of what range you need to be in for weight loss, to increase endurance and stamina, and more.

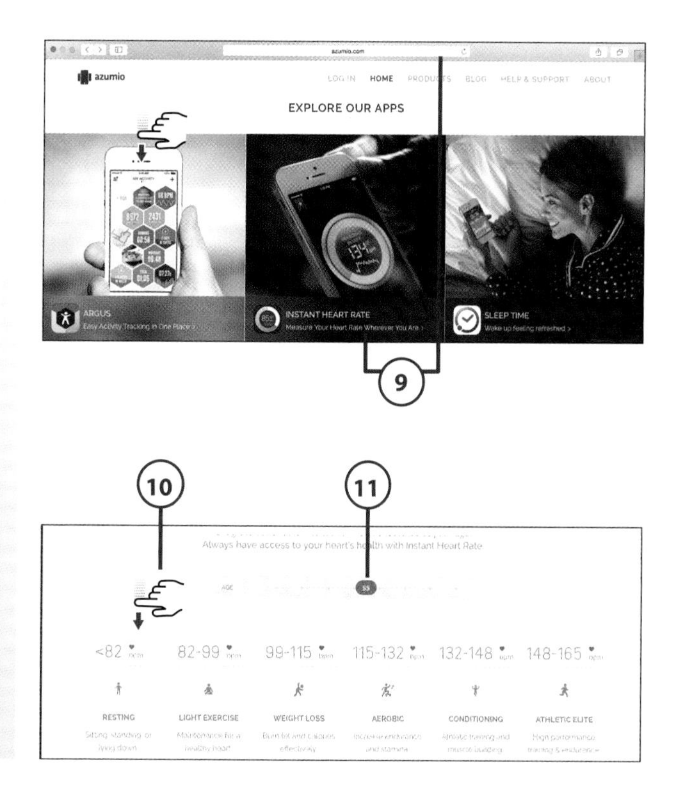

Detect a Serious Heart Condition with AliveCor ECG

The AliveCor Mobile ECG (echocardiogram) is FDA cleared and is both an app and hardware solution for detecting a serious heart condition. After an ECG reading, you can track your symptoms, activities, and diet to help you and your doctor see what might be causing heart rhythm disturbances.

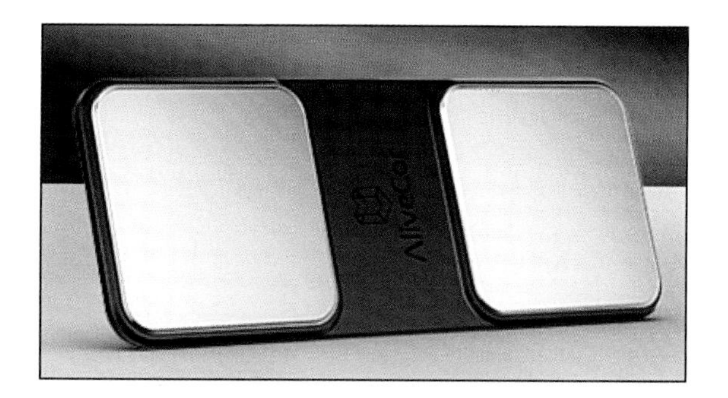

The AliveCor Mobile ECG

Each ECG shows how your heart changes from beat to beat. You can know right away if your ECG is normal or if atrial fibrillation (AF) is detected. The AliveECG app makes it easy for you to create entries between readings— just to track how you're feeling, what you've been eating, and your activities. The AliveCor ECG hardware and app are compatible with both Android and Apple devices. You can download the app at the Google Play Store and the App Store. Visit alivecor.com to learn more and purchase the mobile ECG.

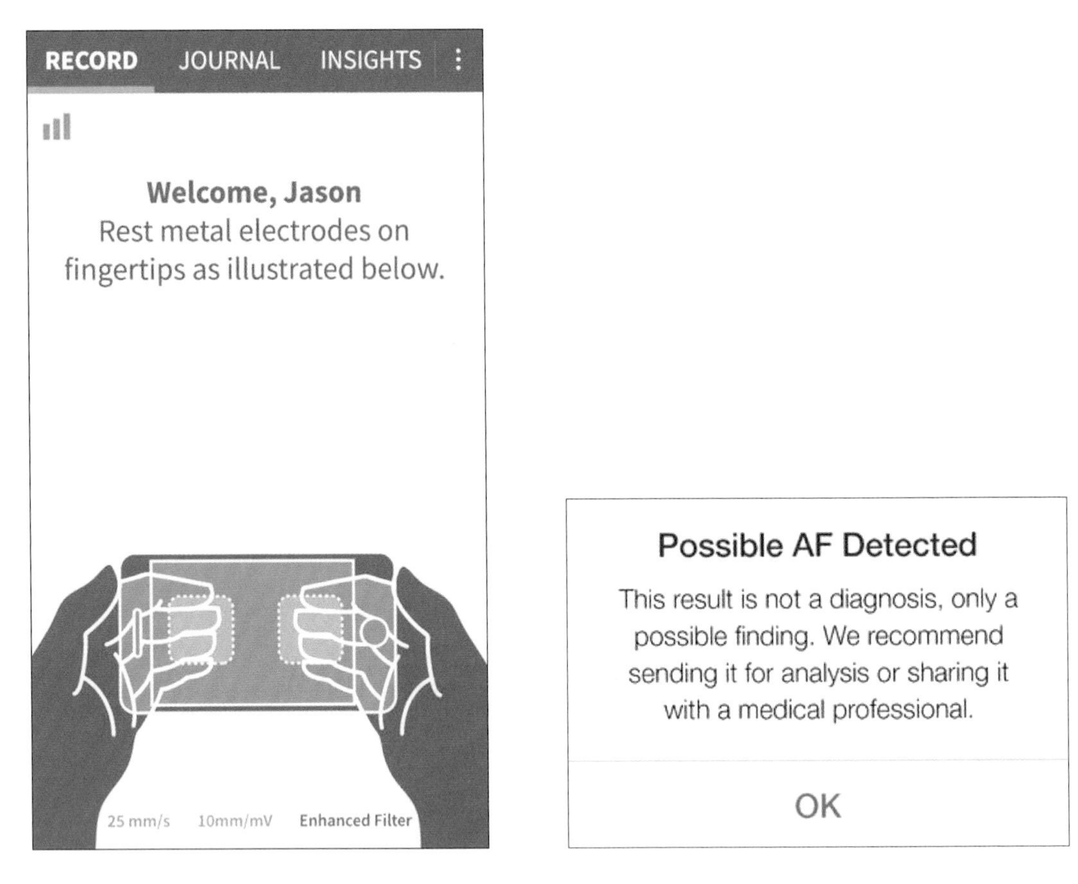

The AliveECG App **The AliveECG AF Warning**

AliveCor comes with a special case for your Android or Apple phone, where the case holds the monitor on the back of the phone. After you've launched the app, simply rest your fingers on the AliveCor heart monitor and find out in just a few seconds if possible AF is detected.

Controlling Obesity

Proper diet, physical activity, and behavioral changes can counteract many risk factors for obesity. Resources such as online-guided programs, fitness trackers, food logs, workout trackers, and virtual coaches can help you get started. Making fitness a habit is a great way to improve overall health. Be sure to consult your doctor before starting any exercise program or using any of the products in this section. Only your doctor and you can accurately assess where you need to begin in your journey to becoming the healthiest version of you that you can possibly be. This section offers one highly structured approach to taking control over obesity and some options for helping you stay the course. You will even learn about some resources that can aid you in the efforts you might have already begun on your own.

Making a Lasting Lifestyle Change at Omada Health

If you could use a support system to help achieve a healthy weight, Omada Health offers a 16-week health program that might offer the support you have been looking for. The online program is called Prevent, and it conveniently coordinates the resources that you need to embrace lasting change for a healthier you.

The Prevent program includes a full-time health coach who monitors your progress as well as gives feedback 24/7. A wireless scale is delivered right to your door, already synced to your account, and you don't even need Wi-Fi for it to work. Other special gear is delivered at key points in the process to ensure you have the tools you need for success. Participants are also placed in support groups and paired with like-minded online peer groups so that you get the encouragement and accountability you require. There will be homework; over 16 weeks you are guided through an interactive curriculum designed to tackle the physical, social, and psychological challenges of chronic conditions such as obesity. You are also engaged with interactive games that help you make connections to real-world scenarios. After your 16 weeks, you continue to receive support for as long as it is needed to help maintain a healthier lifestyle.

Visit omadahealth.com to review more information on their Prevent program and find out how to get started. You can sign up on your own for the Prevent program, but Omada Health also works with employers and health plans, so talk to your provider to see whether they cover some or all of the costs.

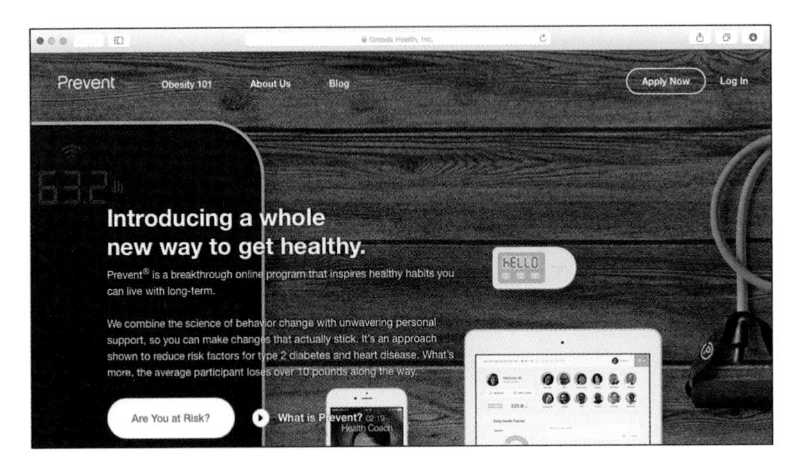

The Prevent program from Omada Health helps you find long-term solutions to obesity to prevent more serious health problems.

Keeping a Food Journal and Using Fitness and Dietary Apps

Keeping a journal of everything you eat, having daily fitness goals, and having a support network can help you reach a healthy weight. A good dietary app not only helps you document what you eat, but also provides the nutritional value of what you eat, such as how much sugar, how much protein, or how many carbs you are consuming. Knowing what you're actually putting into your body can help you make better food choices. A good dietary app also lets you enter a target body weight and calculate a daily calorie limit you can adhere to and work toward that target weight. Fortunately, some great apps are out there that can help you make healthier choices and reach your weight goals including MyFitnessPal, Fooducate, and many, many more.

Fitness apps can also help you reach a healthy weight. Many fitness apps are specialized toward people who are already physically fit. You can tell by the exercises they promote in the app description page. Make sure you do your due diligence and look for apps that match your physical capability. Features to look for in any fitness app are those that will help you get and stay motivated by presenting you with daily goals to meet, including setting goals for how many steps you take during a day. As you reach milestones, you should be able to elevate and fine-tune your exercise regimen to more challenging tasks. Another important feature to look for in a fitness app is if it can work in tandem with fitness trackers. For example, can you feed information gathered from a Fitbit or Jawbone UP straight in to the app, regarding how many steps you've taken and calories you've burned? Here are a few food/dietary apps and fitness apps to consider.

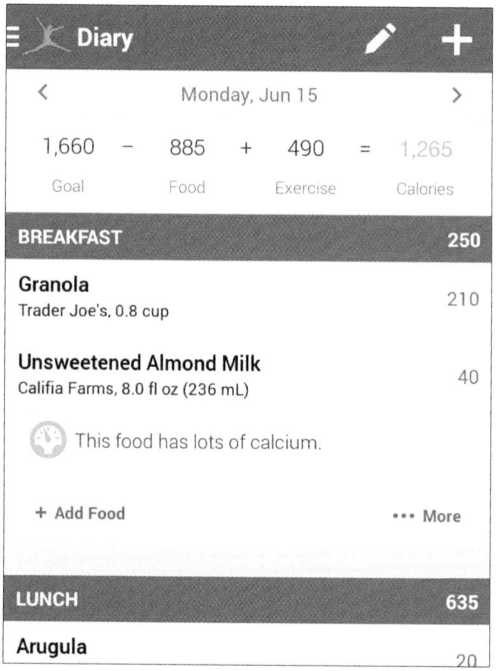

Diary
Monday, Jun 15
1,660 Goal − 885 Food + 490 Exercise = 1,265 Calories
BREAKFAST 250
Granola 210
Trader Joe's, 0.8 cup
Unsweetened Almond Milk 40
Califia Farms, 8.0 fl oz (236 mL)
This food has lots of calcium.
+ Add Food ••• More
LUNCH 635
Arugula 20

The MyFitnessPal app tracks your progress against a daily calorie goal.

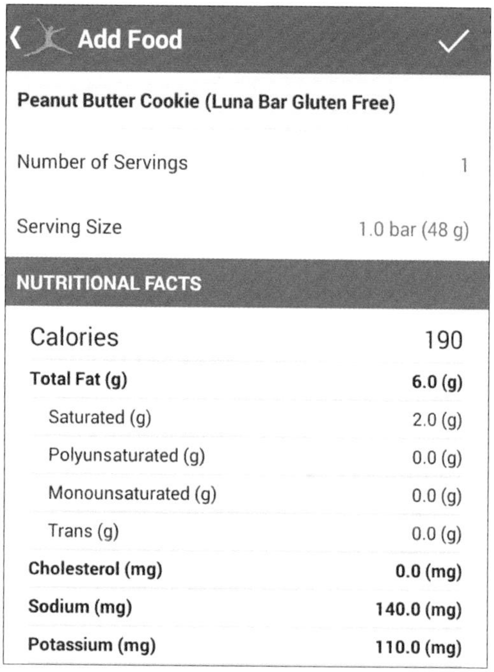

Add Food
Peanut Butter Cookie (Luna Bar Gluten Free)
Number of Servings 1
Serving Size 1.0 bar (48 g)

NUTRITIONAL FACTS	
Calories	190
Total Fat (g)	6.0 (g)
Saturated (g)	2.0 (g)
Polyunsaturated (g)	0.0 (g)
Monounsaturated (g)	0.0 (g)
Trans (g)	0.0 (g)
Cholesterol (mg)	0.0 (mg)
Sodium (mg)	140.0 (mg)
Potassium (mg)	110.0 (mg)

MyFitnessPal allows you to choose food from a database by scanning the barcode or manually entering the food.

- **MyFitnessPal** creates a personalized diet and exercise program. The app lets you set a target goal weight, asks you how active you are, and then calculates the maximum number of calories a day that you should eat. It also tells you how much weight you can expect to lose each week and gives you milestone dates for when you can expect to lose a specific number of pounds. This app has a large food database that allows you to choose your food and portion, and then automatically adds the nutritional value for that meal. If you don't

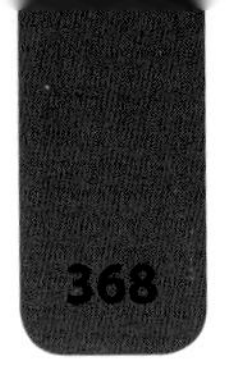

see your meal in the database, you can scan barcodes and manually enter food into the app. MyFitnessPal remembers foods that you have eaten for breakfast, lunch, and dinner so you don't have to go looking for them again. The app can also sync your information with other popular fitness apps and allows you to connect with others for support. MyFitnessPal is available for Android and Apple devices.

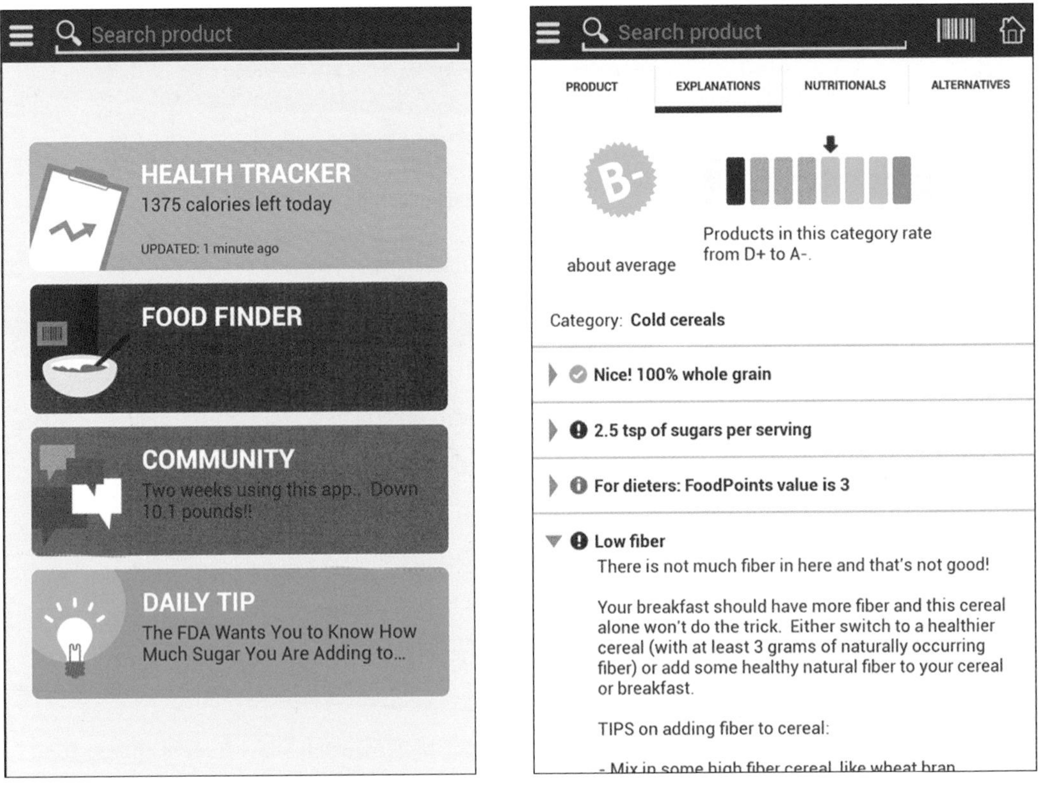

The Fooducate app helps you set a personalized diet and exercise program.

Fooducate helps you make healthier decisions about the foods you eat.

- **Fooducate** is an educational app that sets personalized goals for desired weight loss and tracks your exercise. As you journal each meal, you can easily see how many calories you have left for the day. This app helps you lose weight by providing suggestions for healthy alternatives for food that you already eat and by grading foods by nutritional value from A (Great) to D (Avoid). This app has a huge food database enabling you to view the food and

calories per serving and where the food rates on Fooducate's grading scale. Fooducate also does a good job in revealing additives and preservatives that you might be unaware of in a food that you eat. If you upgrade to Premium within the app, you can tailor your diet even further by choosing a low-carb diet, paleo diet, gluten-free diet, and more. This app also helps you stay motivated by having community features that let you share your progress with others. Fooducate is available for both Android and Apple devices.

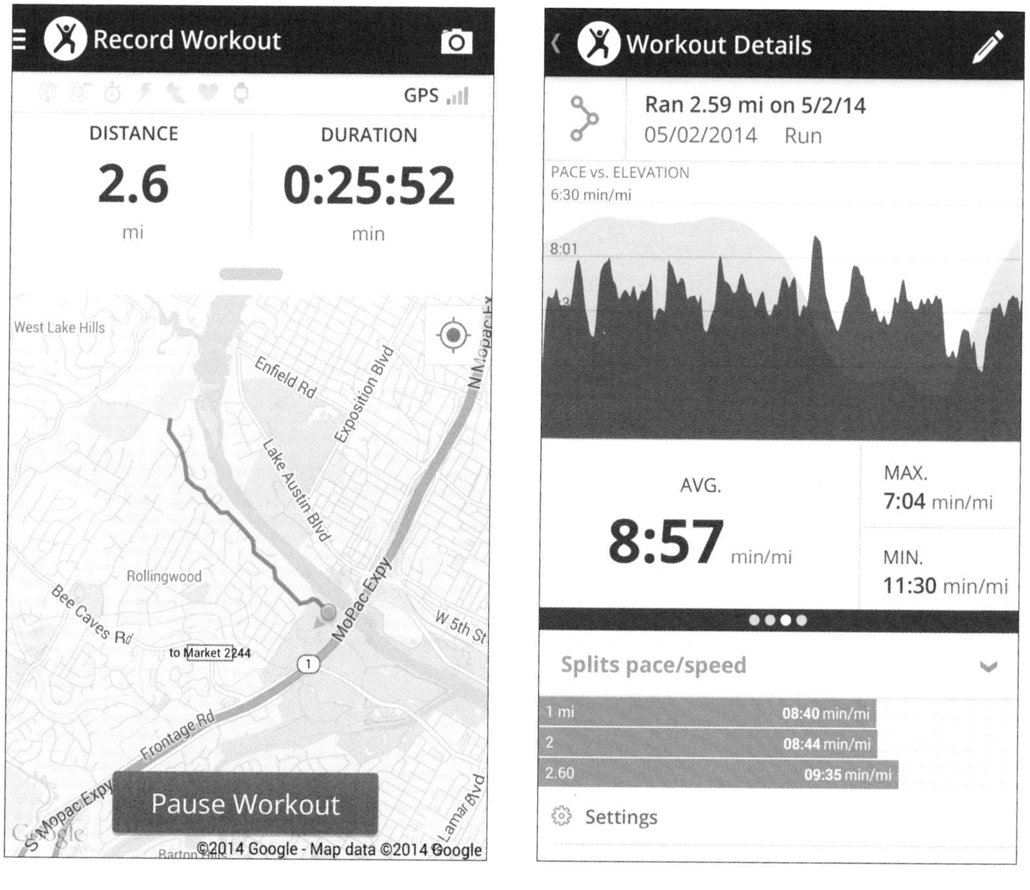

MapMyFitness allows you to track how far you have walked, run, or cycled.

MapMyFitness can share data between other fitness apps and tracking devices.

- **MapMyFitness** enables you to track distance traveled while running, cycling, and walking, and is even a calorie counter. You can also log and record work-out data from more than 600 exercises including yoga and walking. This

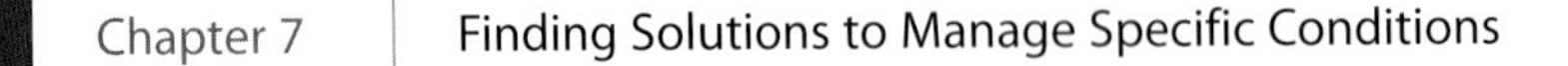

fitness app can share nutrition data with other apps, including MyFitnessPal, when you sync your accounts. It also shares data with the Google Fit app and the Apple Health app. MapMyFitness also connects with fitness tracking devices, enabling you to import data such as steps, calories burned, weight, and sleep quality. Don't underestimate the benefits of a good night's rest when it comes to weight loss. Map My Fitness is available for Android phones and the iPhone.

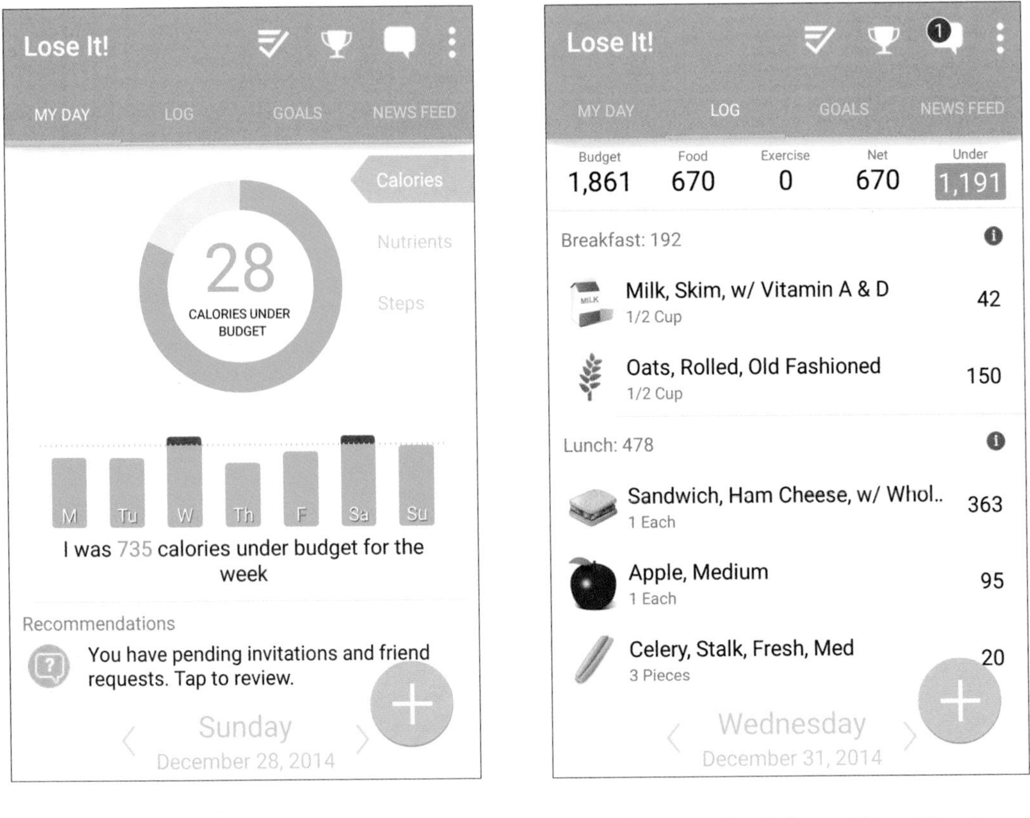

Lose It! is a comprehensive app for weight loss, exercise, and nutrition.

Set your goal weight, and Lose It! puts together your daily calorie budget.

- **Lose It!** is a great all-in-one resource for losing weight. It tracks your meals, exercise, and nutrition. Set your goal weight, and Lose It! puts together your daily calorie budget. If you upgrade to Lose It! Premium, you can track steps and exercise calories, access exercise planning, and track body fat and body

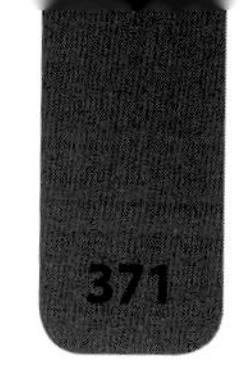

measurements such as neck, hip, and waist. You can even track your hydration and monitor your sleep. Without the Premium upgrade, Lose It! syncs with activity trackers including the Nike FuelBand, Fitbit One, and Jawbone UP. This app even works with wireless scales like the Withings Scale and Fitbit Aria. For motivation and support, Lose It! lets you connect with friends and family and connect to social apps such as Facebook and Twitter. Lose It! is available for Android and Apple devices and can be downloaded on the Google Play Store and the App Store.

Getting Help to Control Your Asthma and COPD

Anyone living with asthma and COPD knows these are serious chronic diseases that only a doctor is best prepared to help treat. The good news is that you can still live an active and healthy life with proper management of these conditions. You can incorporate some resources into your treatment, doctor permitting, that can help you stay on top of your symptoms. Personalized devices such as Propeller and Care TRX can each help you track your symptoms and help you and your doctor come up with the most effective treatment.

Using Propeller

Propeller is comprised of both a hardware and software component. It is a sensor that you attach to the top of your inhaler to wirelessly sync data with your smartphone app. It can be used on controller medication (for example, Flovent) or rescue inhalers. Any time you experience symptoms and then use your inhaler, Propeller tracks this meaningful event so you can better understand your asthma over time through logging triggers, symptoms, and medication. The sensor also logs the time and place you used your inhaler. Personalized feedback and education based on your symptoms are sent to your phone, and you can access this information at propellerhealth.com.

You can share your Propeller data with a family member and your doctor. You can also track how often a loved one is taking his inhaler and receive alerts. You can take your Propeller data with you on your next doctor's visit and review it. Ask your doctor whether this resource could benefit your treatment. You can access the Propeller mobile app on Android and the iPhone, iPad, and iPod touch devices. Visit propellerhealth.com to learn more, and download the app at the Google Play Store and the App Store.

Using CareTRx

The CareTRx Journal app lets you track and record asthma and COPD triggers, symptoms, medications, and peak flow measurements in one place. This resource is also comprised of a hardware and software component. The Care TRx sensor attaches to the top of metered dose inhalers and wirelessly transmits data by automatically pairing to your smartphone. The sensor even helps patients improve medication adherence by lighting up and sending contextual alerts when it's time to take a dose. Remote monitoring by a family member or caregiver is also an option.

The information from the CareTRx app is uploaded to the cloud and can be accessed online through the Dashboard. The Dashboard enables caregivers to track patient progress online and use direct communication and automatic flagging system for patients with higher risk factors. As of this writing, CareTRx is only compatible with Android devices, but iOS compatibility is coming soon. Visit caretrx.com to learn more.

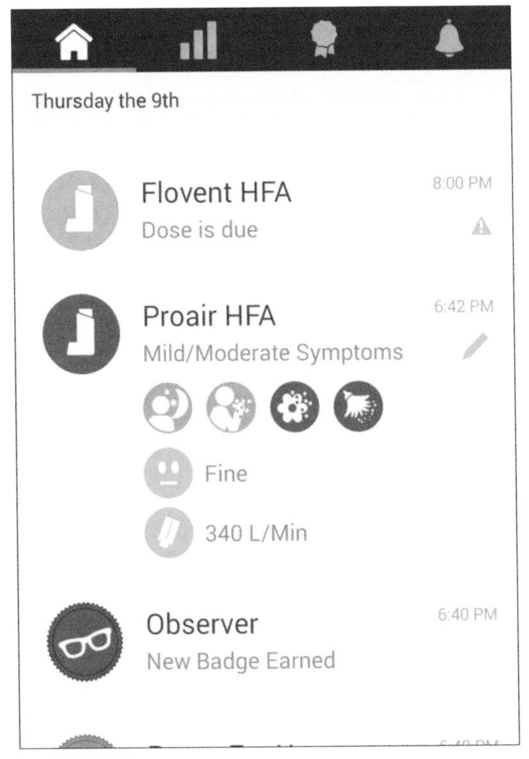

The information from the CareTRx app uploads to the cloud for easy review.

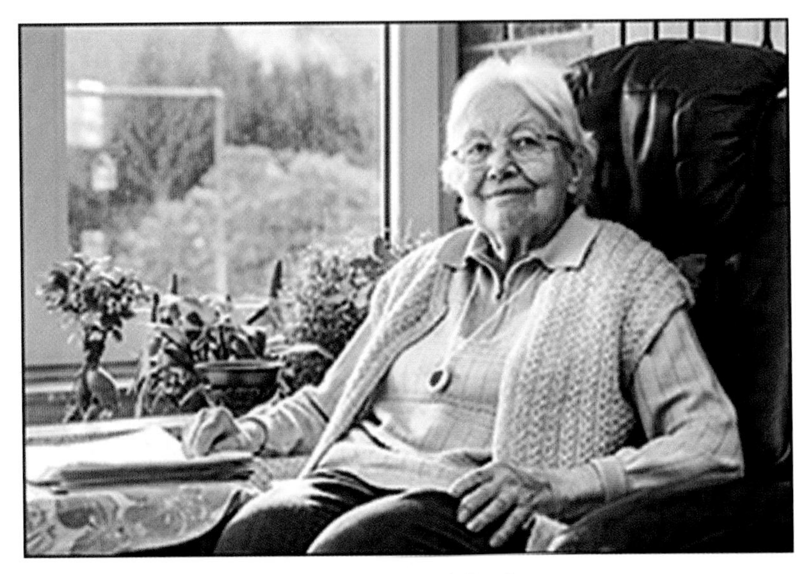

Credit: © Ingo Bartussek/Fotolia.com

Use medical IDs, location sharing, and home safety technology to be prepared for emergencies.

In this chapter, you take a closer look at emergency preparedness ranging from medical IDs to comprehensive home medical alert systems. You also get a chance to see some simple but effective resources you can use in your home to help prevent accidents.

→ Understanding the Importance of Medical IDs for Emergencies
→ Using Apps and GPS Tracking Devices as Safety Measures
→ Choosing the Right Medical Alert System
→ Turning On Lights in Your Home Remotely

Being Prepared for an Emergency

There is peace of mind in knowing that you and your loved ones are prepared in case of an emergency. Having a medical ID on your person is a simple and minimal precaution that could actually save your life. GPS (Global Positioning System) technology, placed in something as small as a pendant or watch, allows you to stay on the go, knowing that someone will be there if you need them, while keeping your family members informed of your whereabouts. Medical alert systems range from a pendant with a button you can push if you need help, to comprehensive monitoring systems with sensors that can detect if something has gone wrong.

This chapter provides insight into a wide range of tools that you can consider for yourself or a loved one. At the least, let these resources serve as a starting point for you to find the best solution for your situation.

Understanding the Importance of Medical IDs for Emergencies

The "In Case of Emergency" (ICE) practice is not a new concept. The gist is to keep personal information, including health data and emergency contacts, on you in case of a medical emergency. When first responders arrive on the scene, they use this information to identify you, gauge drug interactions based on the meds you're taking and known drug allergies, and determine whom to contact on your behalf. Your smartphone offers an enhanced version of this practice by allowing you to carry this information electronically. You can use a number of apps for this task, and depending on the type of smartphone you have, your phone might already possess the means for creating a medical ID.

It's Not All Good

Privacy and Efficacy Concerns

Smartphone medical IDs are gaining popularity; but if you use that technology, you might consider also wearing a medical ID bracelet or necklace, or even carrying a card in your wallet, just to be safe. If your phone is lost or stolen, a medical ID on the lock screen makes your medical information vulnerable. Also, a first responder or good Samaritan's first instinct might not be to check your cell phone for your medical ID. Think of your phone as a backup for emergency information. First and foremost, you want whoever is responding to the emergency to be able to find your ID. If you're walking, a first responder might search your purse or wallet. Because medical bracelets and pendants have been around for a long time, your wrist, neck, or ankles may be secondary places checked. If you're in a vehicle accident, the glove compartment could be the first place someone looks.

Create a Medical ID on Your Android Phone

Many medical ID apps, including the ICE—In Case of Emergency by Appventive and the ICE Standard app, are available that you can download for your Android phone. If you lock your phone with a security PIN or finger print scanner, read app descriptions carefully and make sure that your medical ID can be accessed from the lock screen. Many apps don't have this feature, and it does you little good if a first responder or good Samaritan can't access your information. Also, check your phone to see whether it allows you to place widgets on the lock screen. A widget is an icon or text that is a shortcut to launch an app. In this case, it will be a symbol for the ICE app that can be pressed to open the full app so all of your information can be seen. Consider a medical ID app that doesn't only send notifications to your contact(s), but also includes a hot button for your contact's phone number that can be tapped to automatically call your contact. First responders need to know for sure that your contact has been notified.

If you already use a security PIN or fingerprint scan to lock your phone, then you already know that an Emergency Call button appears at the bottom of the screen, allowing a 911 call. Let's take a look at how you can upgrade your emergency preparedness and add personal, medical, and contact information.

The following example shows how to use the ICE - In Case of Emergency app by Appventive to create a medical ID on an Android (Nexus 6) phone's lock screen. As of this writing, the app is $3.99. Download the app, and then follow these steps.

1. Open the ICE – In Case of Emergency app, read the app Getting Started information, and then tap anywhere off the screen to continue.

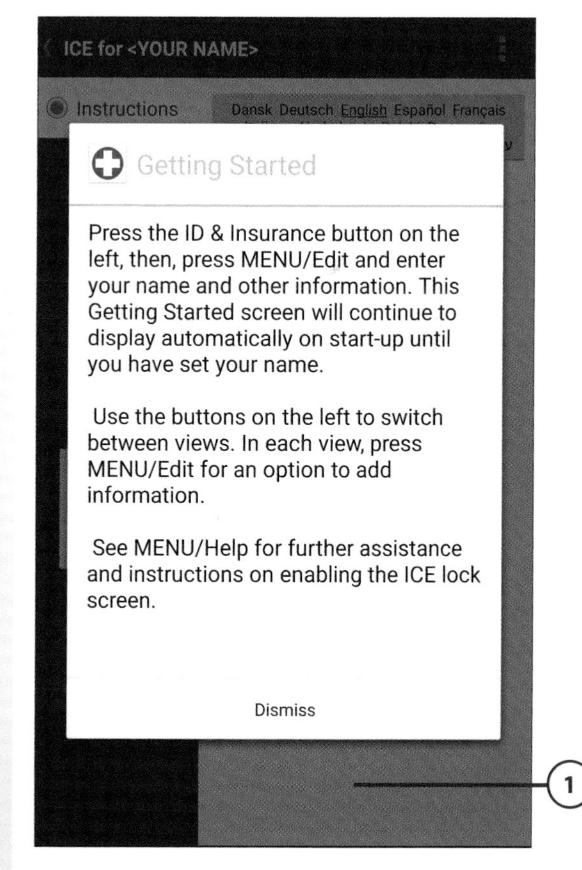

2. Tap ID & Insurance.
3. Tap the main menu in the upper-right corner that looks like three vertical dots.
4. Tap Edit to enter edit mode.
5. Tap the Edit icon that looks like a pencil on the right of the screen to enter your personal information. The Details screen opens.

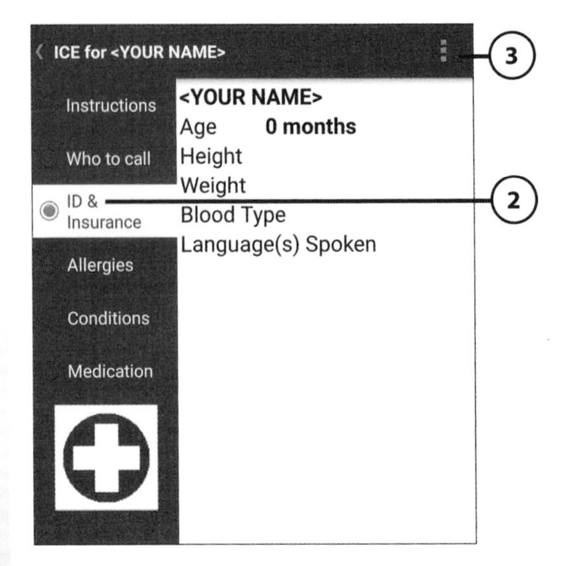

Edit
Settings
About & What's new
Send
Get Family Medical Info
Help
Backup or restore
Export profile
4

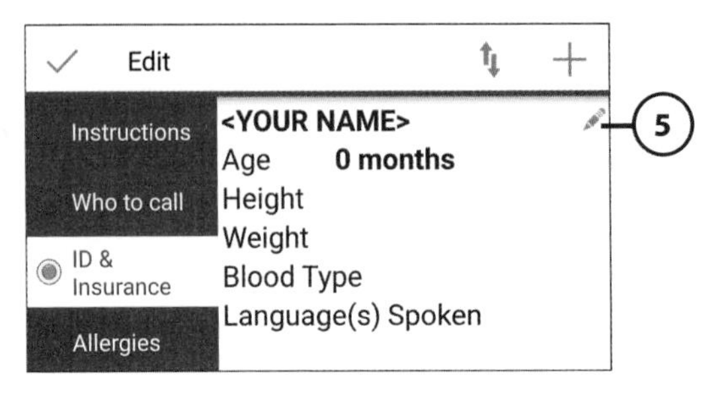

6. Enter your information.
7. Tap the profile picture just to the left of the name to add a picture of yourself.
8. Tap the back arrow to return to the Home screen.
9. Tap the Add icon (the plus sign) to add insurance information and doctor information. Tap away from the menu that appears to make these options go away and return to the home screen.
10. Tap Who to call.
11. Tap the Add button.

Details
<Connor Watson>
Date of birth Jun 21, 1957
Height 6'0"
Weight 185
Blood Type O+
Language(s) Spoken
English, Spanish

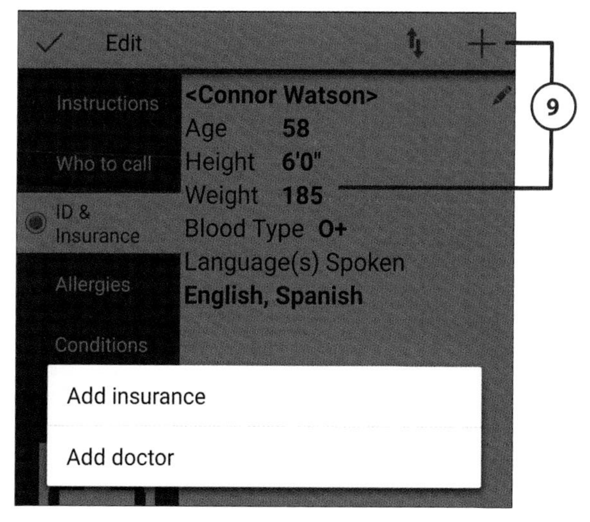

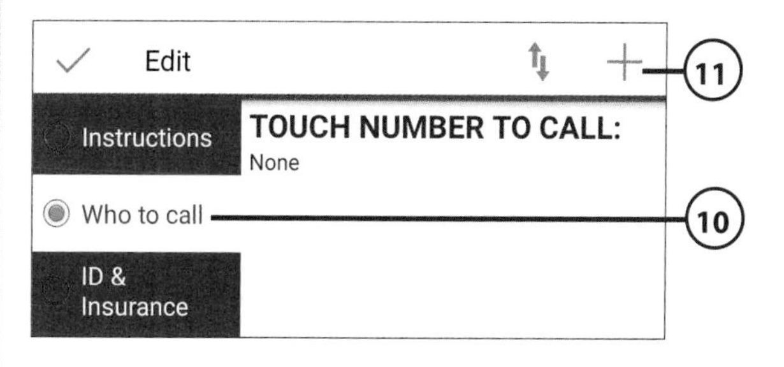

12. Enter your emergency contact's information, and then tap the back arrow.
13. Tap Allergies.
14. Tap the Add button.
15. Enter any allergies that you may have. Even if a field does not apply to you, don't leave it blank. For example, enter "No known allergies" just so that the person responding to the emergency knows you haven't simply overlooked a category.
16. Tap the back arrow.
17. Tap Conditions to enter any medical conditions you have. For any entry that you make, you can tap the pencil icon to the far right of the field to edit the current entry or tap the Add button to enter more information.

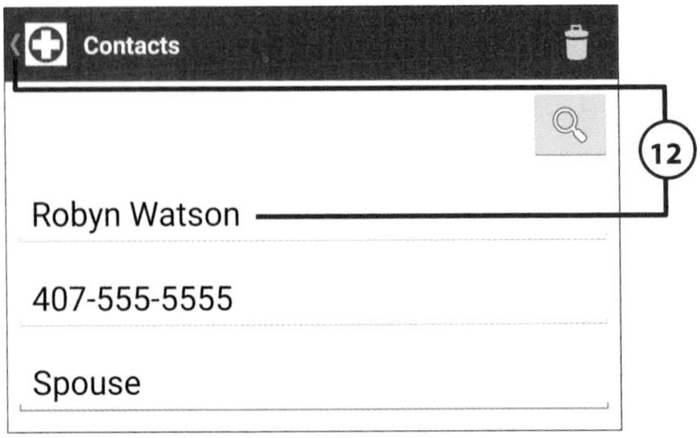

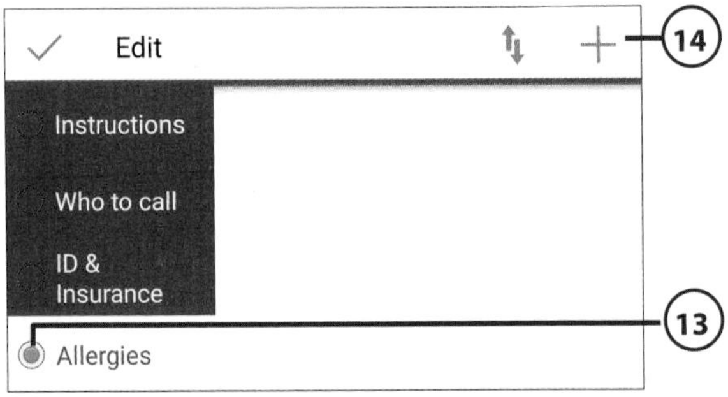

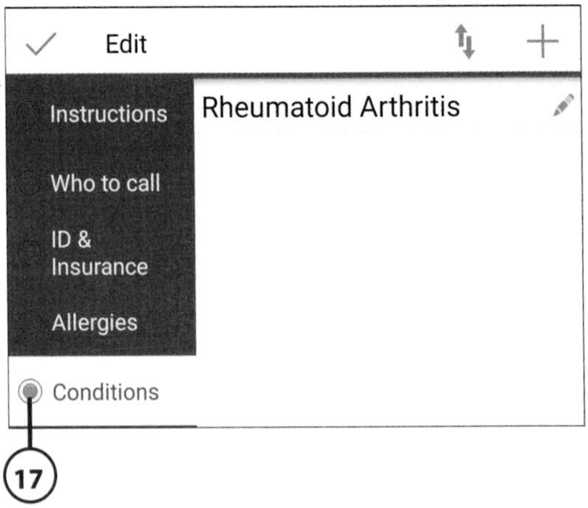

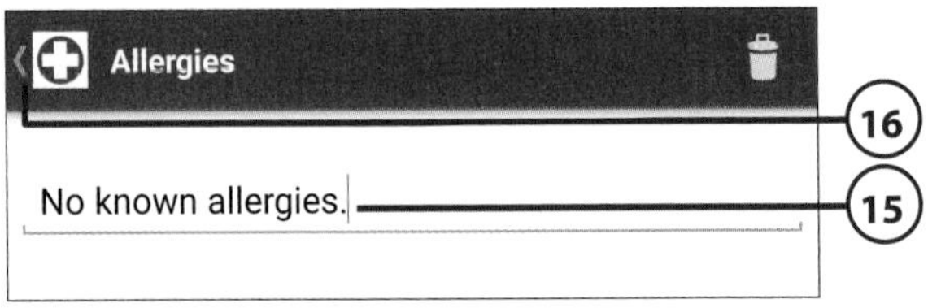

Contacts
Robyn Watson
407-555-5555
Spouse

Edit
Instructions
Who to call
ID & Insurance
Allergies

Allergies
No known allergies.

Edit
Instructions
Who to call
ID & Insurance
Allergies
Conditions
Rheumatoid Arthritis

18. Tap Medication to list your medication regimen.
19. Tap the main menu icon (three vertical dots).
20. Tap Settings.
21. Tap Show on Lock Screen to place a check mark in the box.

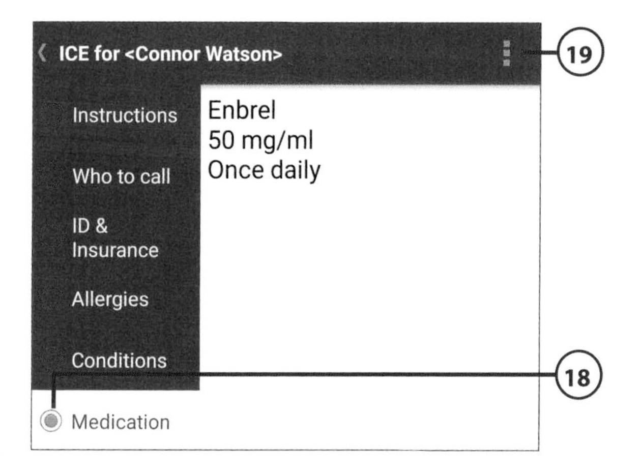

Edit

Settings — 20

About & What's new

Send

Get Family Medical Info

Help

Backup or restore

Export profile

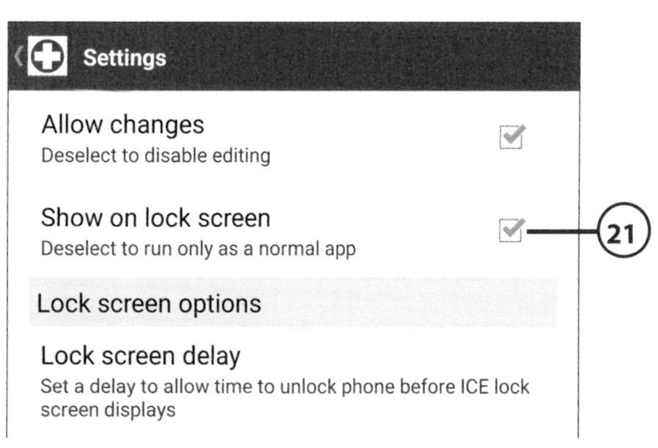

(22) Read the note that pops up, and then tap OK. Now your medical ID is ready to go.

(23) To make sure it worked, lock your phone, and then wake it, but don't fully unlock it by entering your security PIN. View your medical ID on the lock screen.

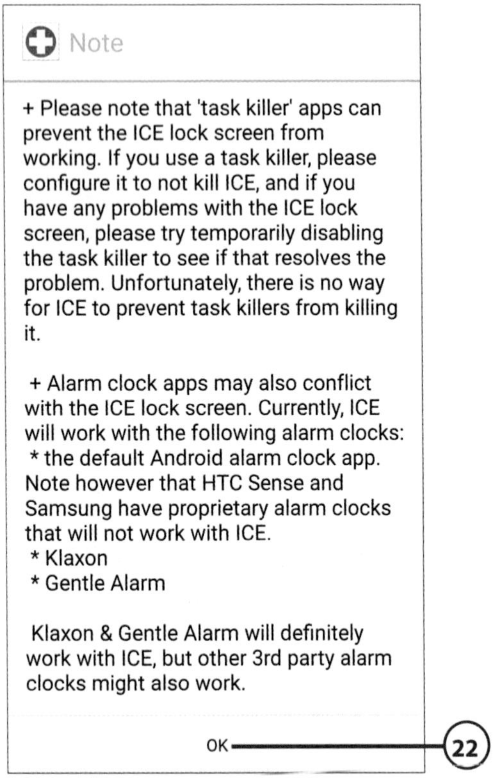

Note

+ Please note that 'task killer' apps can prevent the ICE lock screen from working. If you use a task killer, please configure it to not kill ICE, and if you have any problems with the ICE lock screen, please try temporarily disabling the task killer to see if that resolves the problem. Unfortunately, there is no way for ICE to prevent task killers from killing it.

+ Alarm clock apps may also conflict with the ICE lock screen. Currently, ICE will work with the following alarm clocks:
* the default Android alarm clock app. Note however that HTC Sense and Samsung have proprietary alarm clocks that will not work with ICE.
* Klaxon
* Gentle Alarm

Klaxon & Gentle Alarm will definitely work with ICE, but other 3rd party alarm clocks might also work.

OK (22)

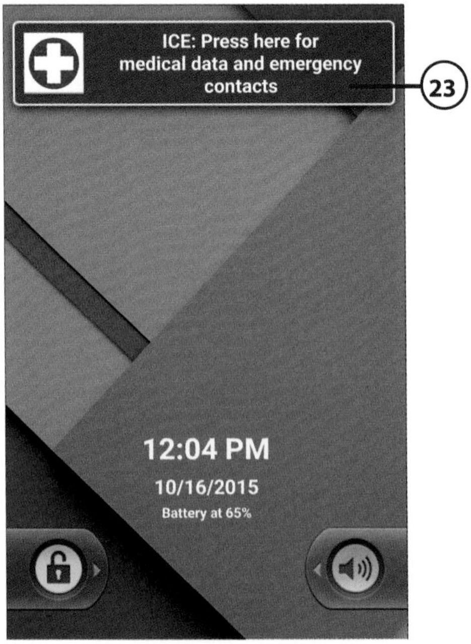

ICE: Press here for medical data and emergency contacts (23)

12:04 PM
10/16/2015
Battery at 65%

>>>Go Further

ANOTHER MEDICAL ID OPTION

If you don't lock your phone with a PIN or fingerprint scanner, the ICE Standard app is another popular option for an Android phone. This app uses color-coding to flag medical information and helps first responders determine the severity of a health condition. Red indicates an individual has severe allergies, medical devices, health conditions, or takes medications. Yellow indicates that the individual is taking medication. Green indicates the individual has no health complications.

Create a Medical ID on Your iPhone

Starting with the introduction of iOS 8, the preinstalled Apple Health app has a medical ID feature that makes your ICE information accessible from the lock screen.

If your iPhone runs iOS 8 or later, follow these instructions to create a medical ID:

1. Tap the Health app to open it.

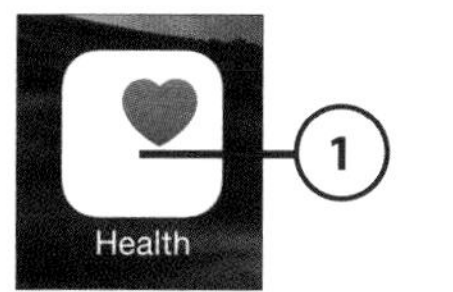

2. Tap Medical ID at the bottom of the screen.
3. Tap Create Medical ID.
4. Make sure that the Show When Locked option is set to the on position (green). This should be on by default. Just below, your name should also be entered by default.
5. Tap Add photo to add a photo of yourself to the profile. If by default there is a picture already in there from one of your social media feeds, just tap Edit to add your picture.
6. Tap Add Birthdate.

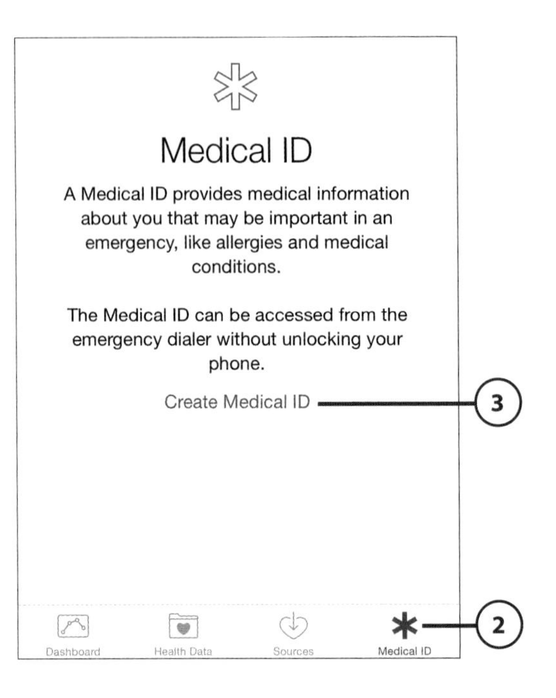

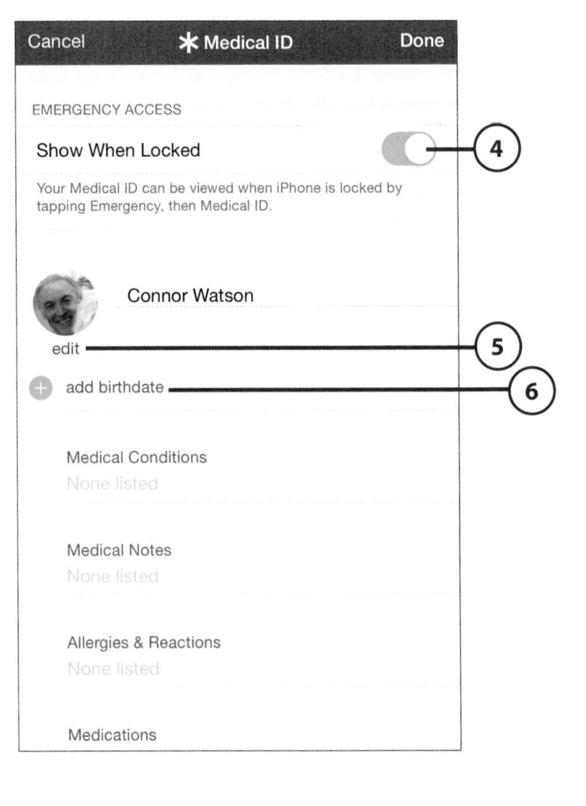

7. Use the scroll wheels to enter your birth date.
8. Tap Medical Conditions and enter any medical Conditions you might have. The scroll wheels disappear.
9. Tap Medical Notes to add any information a first responder might need to know before administering treatment.
10. Tap Allergies & Reactions to add information. Don't leave any fields blank. This ensures that responders know you did not unintentionally miss adding that information.
11. Scroll up the screen, and then tap the green plus sign next to Add an Emergency Contact. This person must already be listed in your contacts. Choose a contact from your Contacts list.
12. Tap each green Add button to enter information into the remaining fields.

Birthdate June 21, 1957
Medical Conditions (8)
None listed
Medical Notes
March 18 1954
April 19 1955
May 20 1956
June 21 1957 (7)
July 22 1958
August 23 1959
September 24 1960

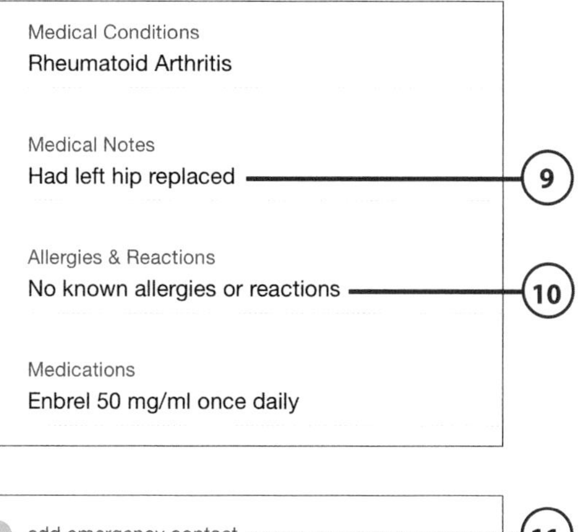

add emergency contact (11)
add blood type (12)
add organ donor
add weight
add height
This information is not included in your Health Data or shared with other apps.

13. Tap Done when you are finished. Your medical ID profile appears.
14. Tap Edit to edit any information.

AT&T 3:46 PM
Cancel
Medical ID
Done
13
Medical Notes
Had left hip replaced
Allergies & Reactions
No known allergies or reactions
Medications
Enbrel 50 mg/ml once daily
spouse Robyn Watson
add emergency contact
Blood Type O+
Organ Donor Yes
Weight 185 lb
Height 6′0″
This information is not included in your Health Data or shared with other apps.

Medical ID
Edit
14

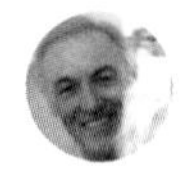

Connor Watson
June 21, 1961 (54)

15. To make sure it worked, lock your phone and then wake it, but don't fully unlock it by entering your security PIN.
16. Tap Emergency in the lower-left corner.
17. A new screen opens with Medical ID located in the lower-left corner. 911 can also be dialed from this screen by first entering the numbers and then tapping the green Phone button.

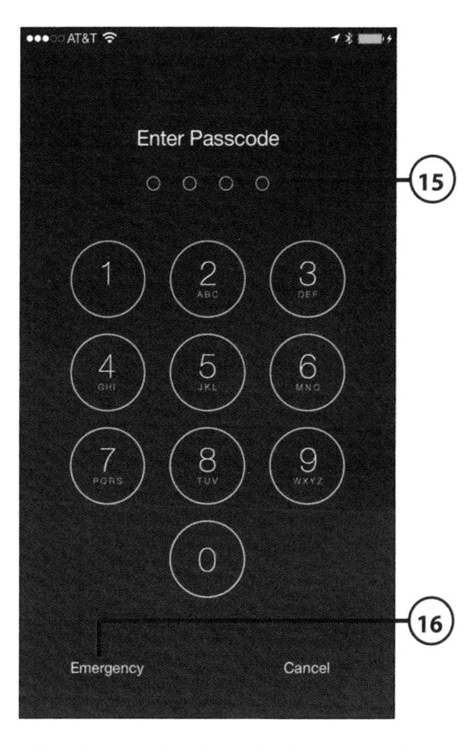

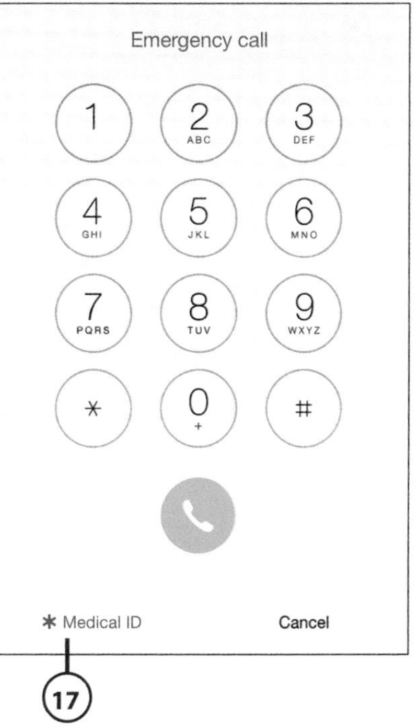

Consider the ICE Standard with Smart911 App

The ICE Standard with Smart911 app is only available for the iPhone and is for people who are looking for an app that offers a little more than just a medical ID. This app puts your emergency health information on the lock screen and, if you're registered in a Smart911-enabled community and 911 is dialed on your phone, the operators and police get your medical information automatically. Visit smart911.com to learn more about the free Smart911 public safety service and to see whether the service is available in your area. The ICE Standard with Smart911 app not only allows you to add your medical information including conditions, medications, allergies, and contact information, but if you upgrade, it also allows for automobile information.

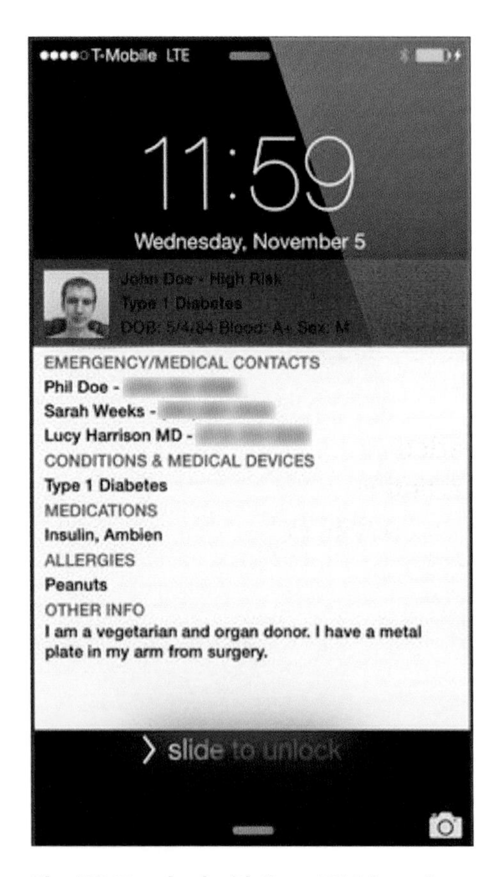

The ICE Standard with Smart911 App shows emergency medical information on your lock screen.

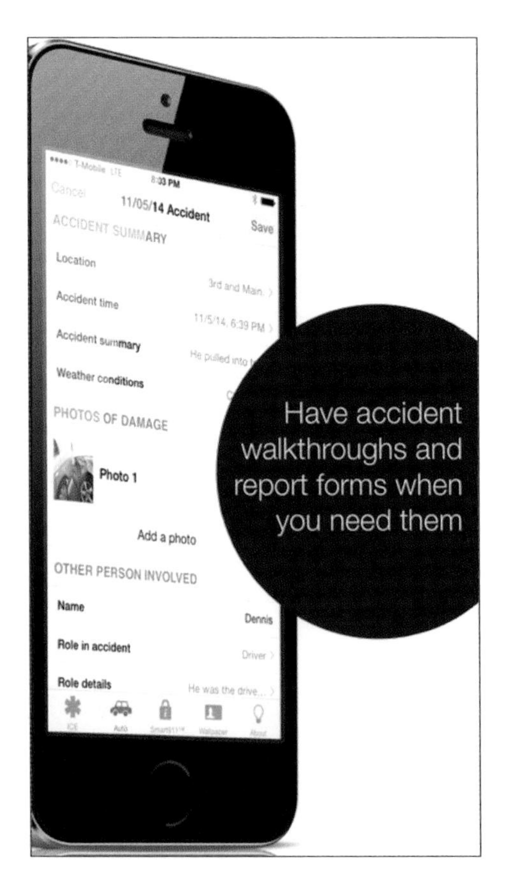

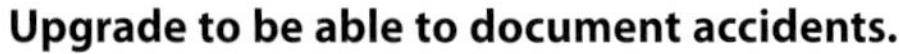
Upgrade to be able to document accidents.

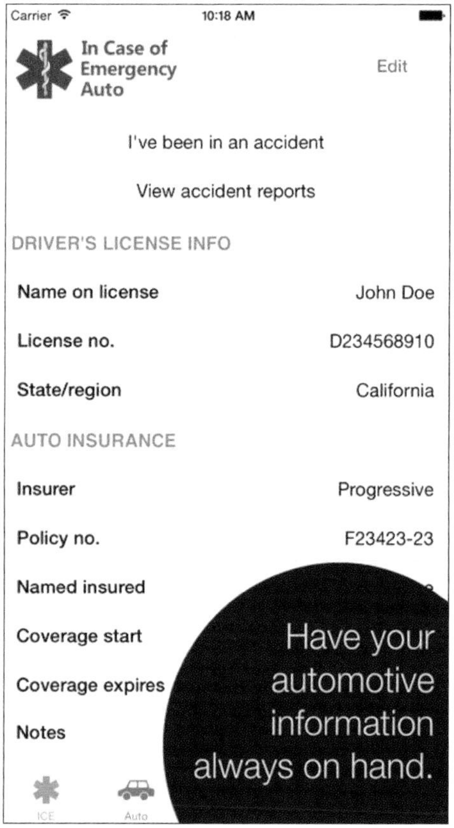

You won't have to worry about fumbling for your automotive details in an emergency.

If you are in an automobile accident, the upgraded app enables you to document accident walk-throughs, including report forms and photos of the damage. The ICE Standard with Smart911 app enables you to input all of your automotive information so that you can always have it on hand.

Register a New Phone Number

If you change your phone while using Smart911 emergency services, make sure that you unregister your old number and register the new number. If your community does not currently participate in Smart911, visit smart911.com to see how to get the process started.

Using Apps and GPS Tracking Devices as Safety Measures

A simple app can serve as a medical alert system in case of an emergency, letting you stay mobile but also quickly reach out to a trained professional who can dispatch the appropriate emergency services, or to an emergency contact. Some apps and devices use GPS, allowing you to create a safety network regardless of physical distance, so friends and family can know a loved one's location and offer help, if needed. We discuss more comprehensive medical alert systems later in this chapter, but the resources discussed in this section add an extra layer of security so that, if an emergency does occur, you have what you need to take care of the ones you love, including yourself.

Consider GreatCall 5Star Urgent Response

The 5Star Medical Alert Service app from GreatCall is a virtual medical alert system. No extra hardware is needed other than your phone. Along with being a medical alert service, 5Star is a personal safety app, ICE app, and emergency help button that you download to your Android phone or iPhone.

5Star uses your phone's GPS capability to access Certified Response Agents trained in CPR and other medical procedures. GPS information can also be passed on to emergency services. The app gives responders easy access to your medical profile as they evaluate your situation. If needed, agents can dispatch emergency services or the police, and connect you to a nurse or doctor. 5star can even conference in your family and friends.

The app requires a subscription to the 5Star service. You get a 30-day trial when you sign up in the app. Visit greatcall.com to learn more about this service and go to the Google Play Store or the App Store to download the app.

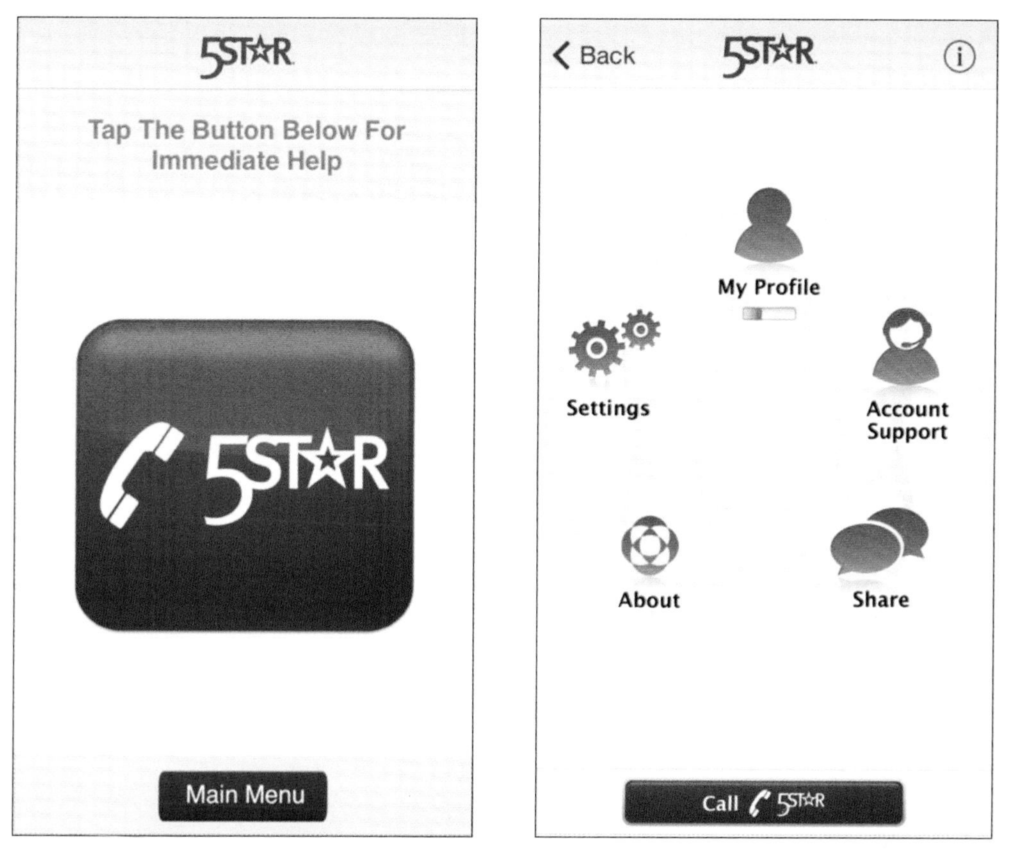

Upgrade to be able to document accidents.

Your 5Star profile includes your medical information, and allows agents to connect you to family members, doctors, nurses, or other emergency response services.

Stay Connected to the People Who Matter with the Life 360 Locator App

The Life 360 Locator app helps you stay connected and know that your family is safe, even if they are far away. This app uses GPS to let you view your family members' locations on a map and communicate with them using real-time location data. You can even receive alerts when your loved ones arrive at home, school, or work. It also eliminates the need for "Did you arrive safely?" phone calls by allowing you to "Check in." Just install the Life 360 Locator app on your phone and have your family and friends install it on their phones. After everyone has registered, each member appears as a unique icon on a map. You can create private groups for location sharing, send messages, and keep family and friends separate using the Circles feature. A Circle can be created for caregivers so that you can keep track of an individual's whereabouts and text with him or her. Your whereabouts are personal. Location sharing is up to you. If you don't want everyone to know where you are at all times, you can turn it off whenever you want. The Life 360 App is available for Android phones and the iPhone. Download the app, and then continue reading.

Create Circles for the Important People in Your Life

Create Circles and create private groups for family, friends, and caregivers for location sharing and sending messages. The individuals whom you want to add in your Circle must first be in your address book on your phone.

Download the app, and then follow these steps, which are shown on an Android phone.

 Open the Life 360 app, and then tap Get Started.

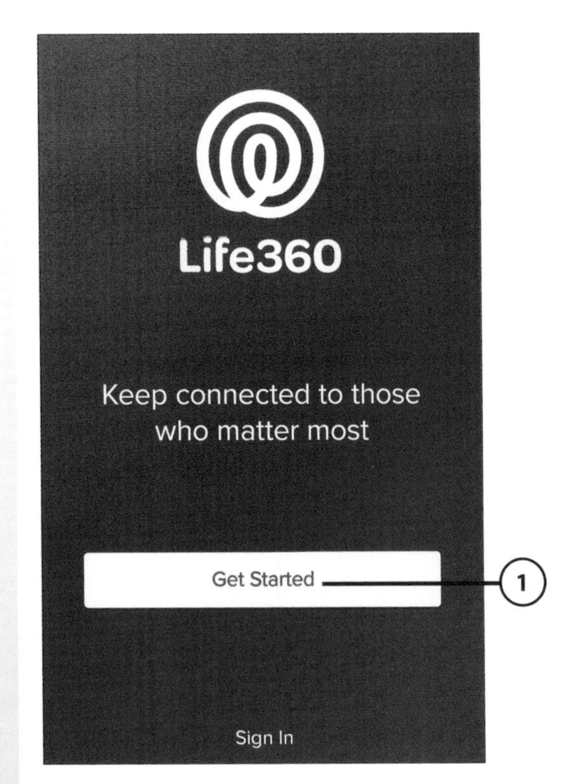
Life360
Keep connected to those who matter most
Get Started
1
Sign In

2. Create an account by entering your information, and then tap the Forward key on the keyboard. A screen opens, prompting you to create your private map.
3. Tap Find Me for the app to use GPS to pinpoint your location on the map. Do this at home to add your home address. The app asks whether you want to see others on the map.

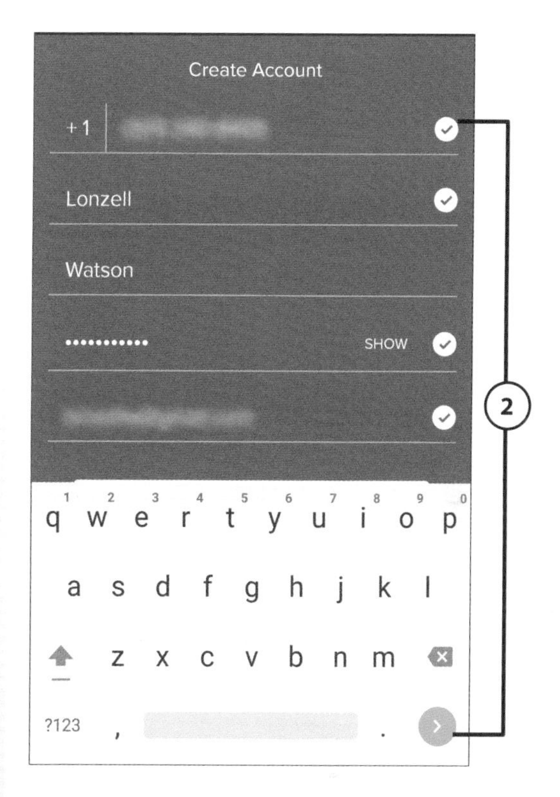

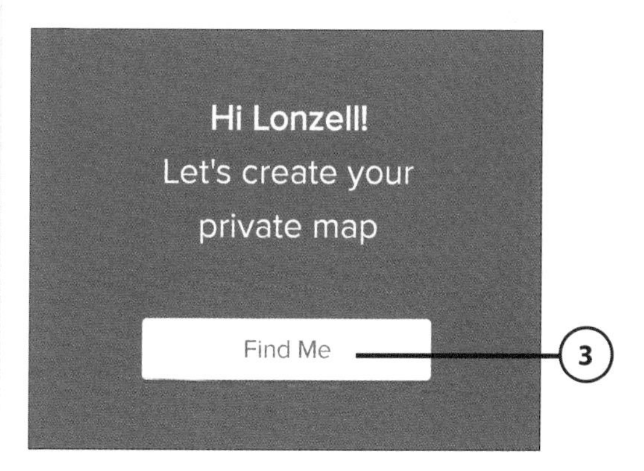

4. Tap Yes. The app compiles a list of suggested people from your address book, and then asks who you want to invite to your Circle.
5. Tap the check box next to the names you want to invite. You can flick the screen from right to left to see your whole address book. You can also tap Skip in the top-right corner to send invites later.
6. Tap Invite (number).

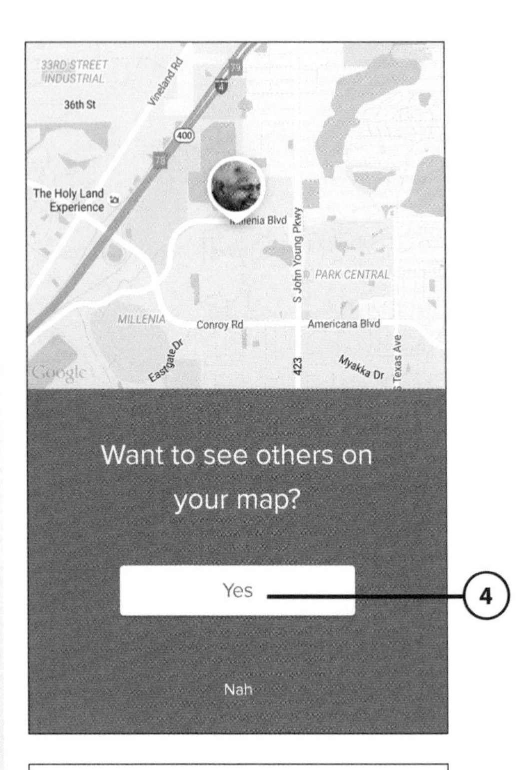

Skip
Add Member
Who do you want to invite to your circle?
RECOMMENDED
ADDRESS BOOK
Connor Watson
Robyn Watson
5
robyn watson
Invite (1)
6

7. Tap Yes to be notified when someone arrives at home.
8. Tap Save to receive a notification when members arrive or leave the address onscreen. Now you have created your first Circle, which by default, is a family Circle. After the invitees respond, you will see their locations on the map.

Add Emergency Contacts and Call a Live Advisor Agent

Tap the icon shaped like an exclamation point to add three emergency contacts. Tap the button shaped like a headset located at the bottom of the screen to learn more about the paid upgrade to the Premium version of Life 360. When you upgrade you get 24/7 help from a live advisor in case of an emergency. You also get instant roadside assistance.

Want to be notified when someone arrives at home?
Yes
7
No

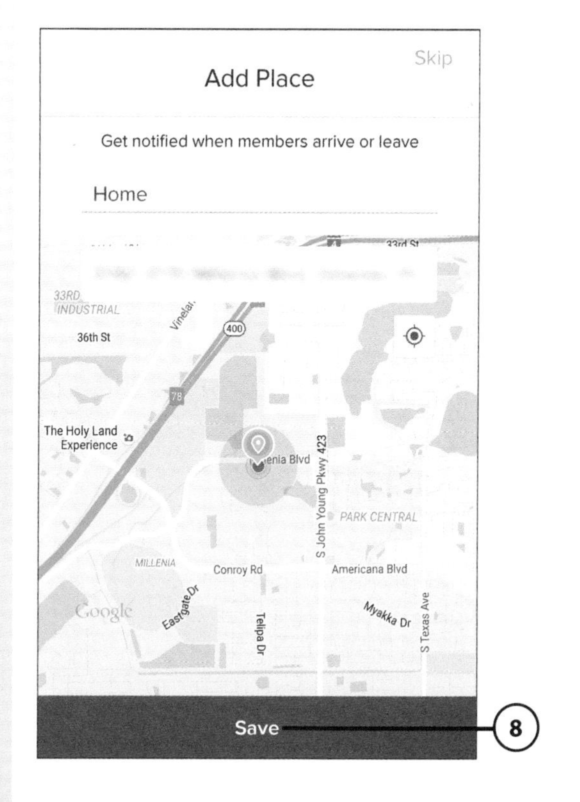

9. Tap the Check In button after you have arrived at a location, so your circle knows you made it safely to your destination.

10. You can tap on the map to receive bits of information about crime in the area, and then tap the X to close the box that pops up.

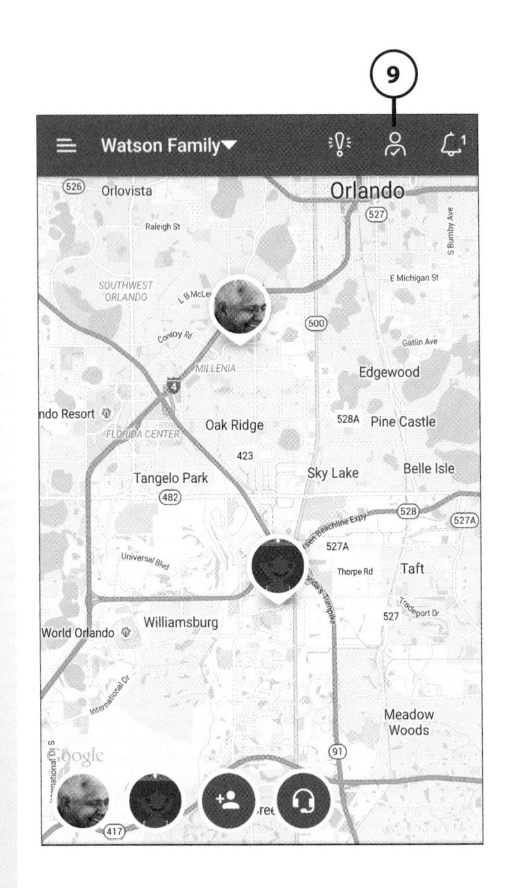

Crime Spot

Theft
October 20, 2015 1:35 AM

Theft By Shoplifting. District:e6

X — 10

(11) To create a new Circle, tap the name of the current Circle—in this case, the Watson Family Circle.

(12) Tap Add Circle.

(13) Tap Add a Circle again.

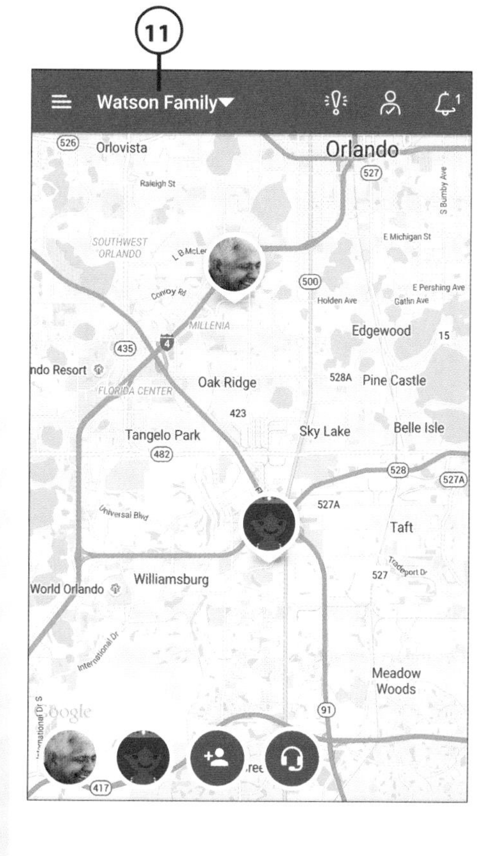

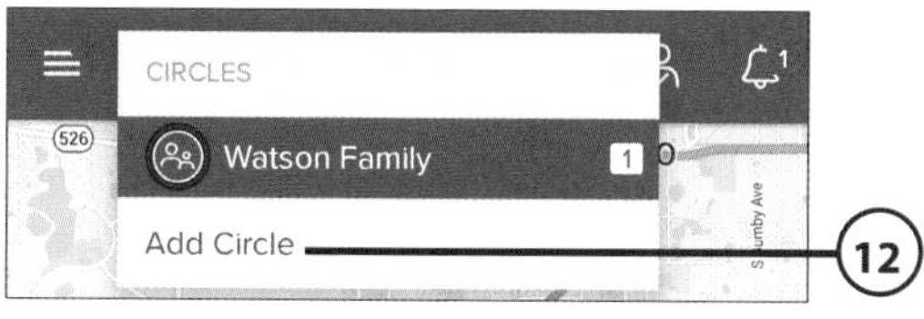

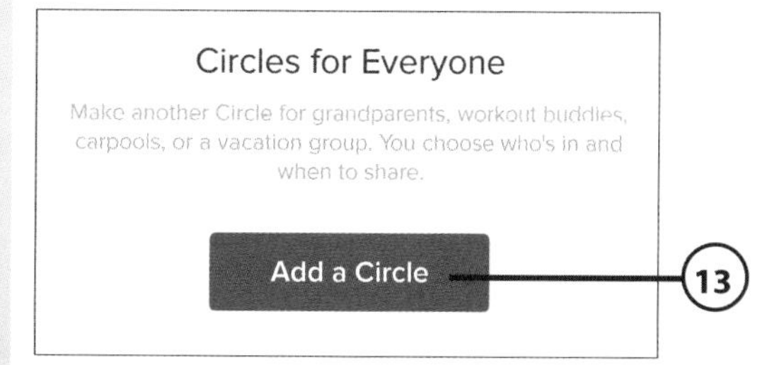

14. Enter the name you want to use for the new Circle. You can tap a suggested Circle name to fill the name field.

15. Tap Done.
16. Tap the names of the individuals you want to add in your Circle, and then tap Invite (number) to send those individuals invites to join your Circle.

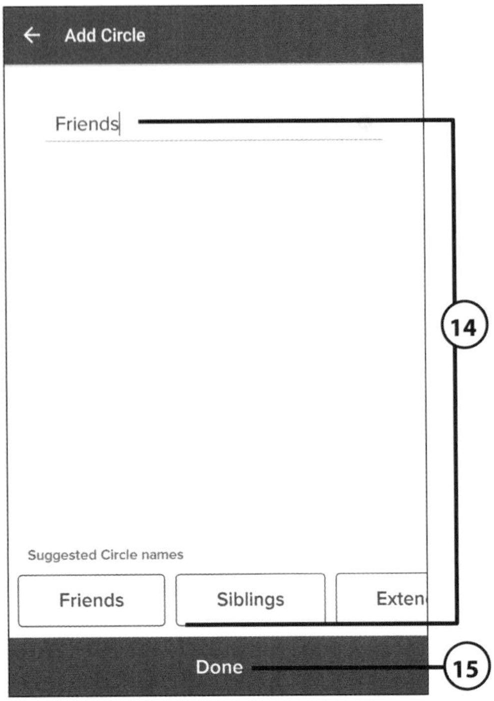

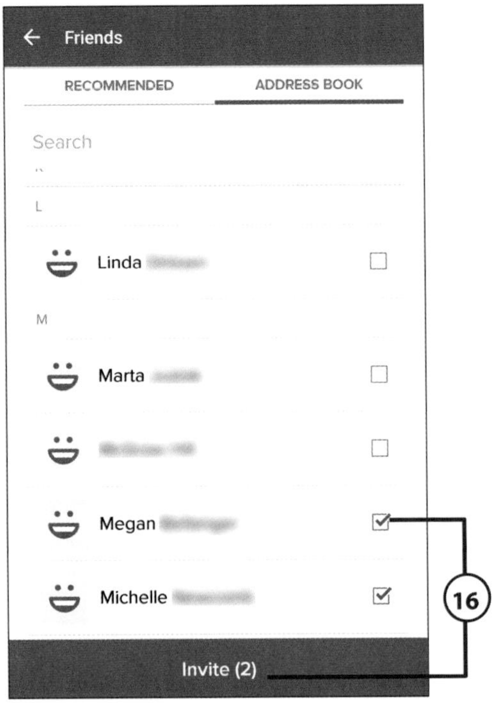

Share Your Location with Those You Choose

You can be selective about with whom you share your location by choosing which Circle(s) can see your location.

1. Navigate to the Circle for which you want to change your location sharing status.
2. Tap the main menu that looks like three horizontal lines in the upper-left corner.
3. Tap Location Sharing in the menu.

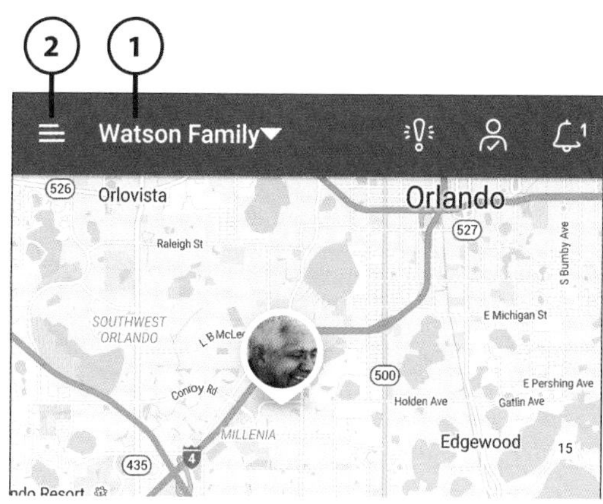

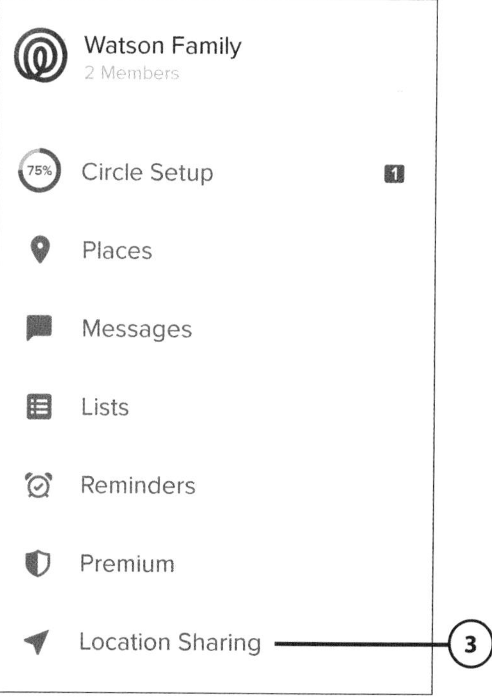

4. Tap My Location Sharing to set the toggle switch to the off position, which turns it gray.

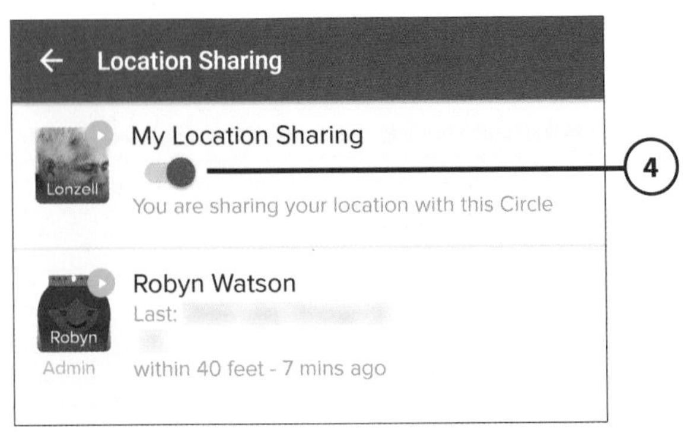

Communicate One on One or with Groups

Life 360 makes it easy for you to send a text message to a single person or share it with a group.

Follow these steps to see how easy it is to communicate with people in your Circles.

1. Navigate to the Circle that includes members to whom you want to send a message.
2. Tap the main menu that looks like three horizontal lines in the upper-left corner.
3. Tap Messages.
4. Tap New Message to send a message to anyone in your circle.

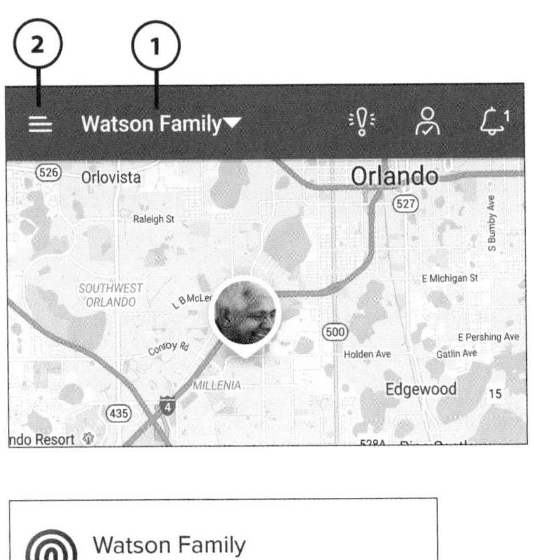

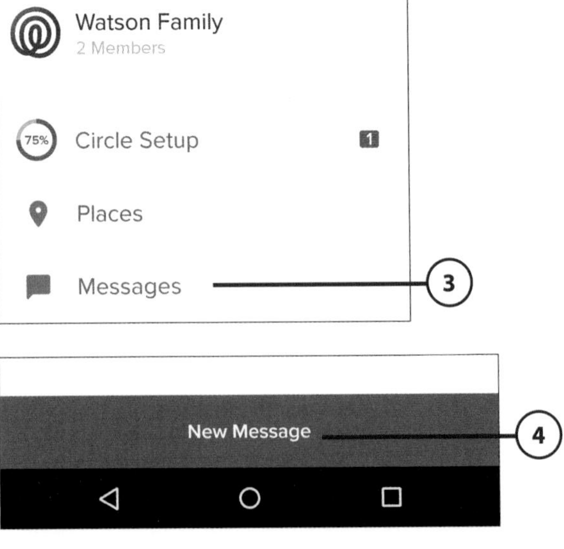

5. Tap the name of an individual to send a message to just that person or tap Everyone to send a message to the entire Circle.
6. Type the message.
7. Tap Send.

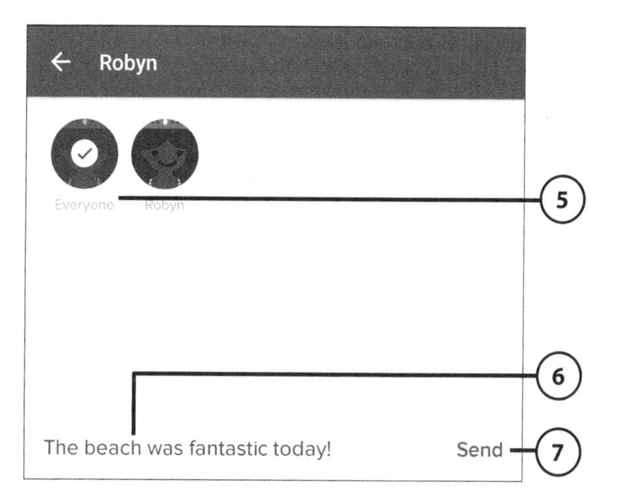

Get Assistance with Alzheimer's with the Comfort Zone Check-In Web Application

Independence can be challenging for those living with Alzheimer's, as family members and caregivers may be concerned for their loved ones' safety. Comfort Zone Check In is an online service that enables families to monitor a person with Alzheimer's using on-demand "Find Me" and "Follow Me" sessions, and scheduled location alerts. Created by the Alzheimer's Association, the service works both outdoors, where GPS can be used, and indoors, where GPS cannot be used.

Here's how it works. Family members and caregivers can track an individual by using one of two devices: any cellphone on the Sprint network, or, for those who either have no cell phone or who use a different cellular carrier, a dedicated tracking device. The dedicated device can be carried in a pocket or purse, or worn on a lanyard.

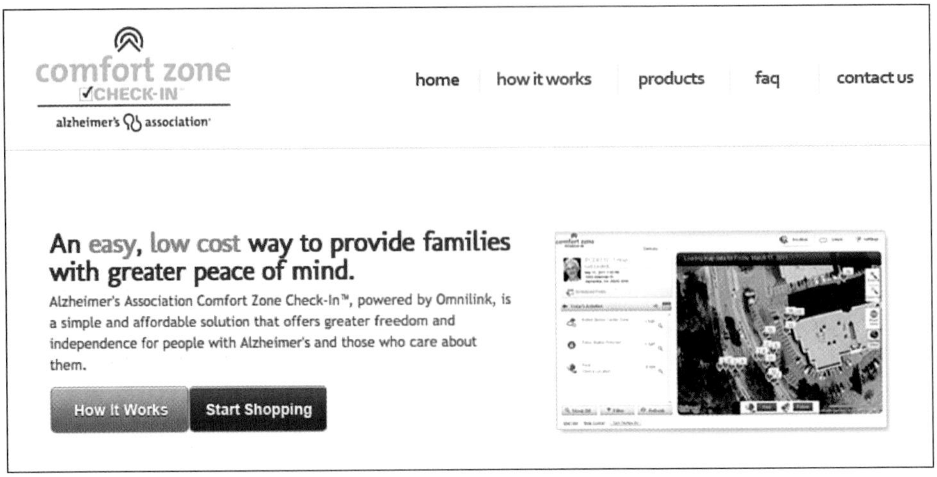

Comfort Zone Check-In allows those who suffer from Alzheimer's to live more freely, while family members and caregivers can have comfort in knowing their whereabouts.

Comfort Zone Check-In's web-based application is a virtual command center. You can manage devices, view location information, set location schedules, request a device's current location, and manage notifications. This service also lets you set up Zones, or pre-determined boundaries, around the home or community in case the individual with Alzheimer's goes beyond an area of safety, at which time the system sends a text or email to alert you. You can also put the device in to a constant tracking state for peace of mind, and access 30 days of location history.

Whether you use a Sprint phone or a dedicated tracking device, you need a Comfort Zone Check-In subscription with cellular coverage. You also need Internet coverage. Before deciding whether this service is right for you, make sure there is coverage in your area by going to comfortzonecheckin.com.

Choosing the Right Medical Alert System

Medical alert systems can make a world of difference in an emergency. A typical medical alert system is comprised of the following components: a base station, medical alert device(s), a call center, and emergency contacts. You or a loved one press a button on a pendant, wristband, or other mobile device, and then the system sends a call to a monitoring service using the base station. You talk with a member of the monitoring center's staff, who assesses the situation and then contacts a neighbor, family member, or appropriate emergency services. These are more robust systems than the apps we discussed earlier, and include multiple hardware devices. Some systems offer comprehensive solutions that combine the aforementioned services, as well as telehealth, health management, activity monitoring, and social engagement features.

Whether you are looking for extra security for a family member living alone or for yourself, read on to see whether a medical alert system is right for you. Some options offer peace of mind not just for in the home, but also while on the go.

This section does not supply a comprehensive look at each system, as a close look at some of these systems would constitute a small book of their own. Prices are not included because they are subject to change. During your consideration of these resources, and if you reach out to these services, here are some questions you should consider asking:

- What are your shipping and activation fees?
- What are the payment plan options? Are they contract-based?
- What is the cancellation policy?
- Does the service accommodate Multi-Person Monitoring without your having to buy a second base station?
- Does the service provide a Check-In Service (a periodic, routine check of the system to make sure it's working)? You don't want the first time you use the device to be during an emergency.

Use the Life Alert Service

Life Alert is an industry leader in 24-hours-a-day, 7-days-a-week service for medical emergencies, including strokes, heart attacks, seizures, and falls that may occur, and even intrusion protection. The system includes a help button in the form of a pendant or a wristband, which are both waterproof and can be worn all the time, including in the shower. The help button is wirelessly connected to a main Unit that acts as a speakerphone, enabling you to speak with an emergency response center dispatcher. The help button range is effective up to 1000 feet from the main Unit. A Life Alert representative stays on the phone with you or your loved one until the emergency has been resolved.

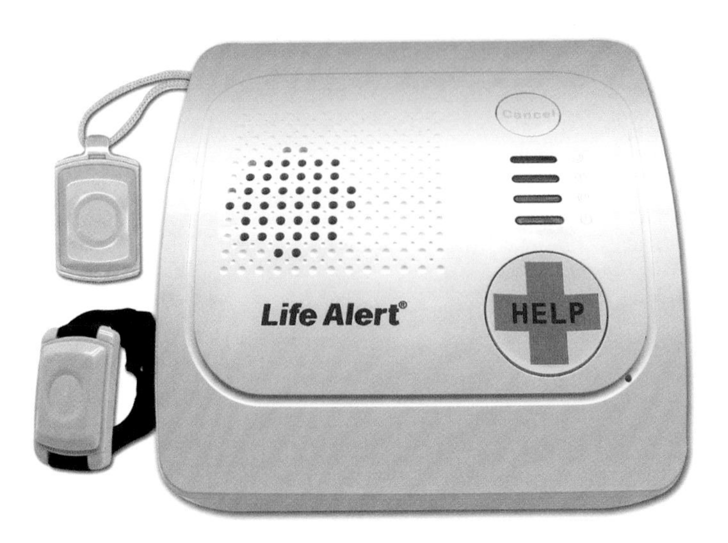

Life Alert's help buttons connect wirelessly to the main unit for 24/7 help in an emergency.

Life Alert offers coverage nationwide, and the service can be provided either over regular analog phone lines (PSTN, Public Switched Telephone Network) or via cellular (3G/WCDMA, Wideband Code Division Multiple Access).

Life Alert also offers optional carbon monoxide and fire detection, which includes the use of more hardware. When carbon monoxide or smoke or fire is detected, an alert sounds to warn you and is also sent to the monitoring center. The dispatcher then communicates with you to assess the situation. If dispatch can't contact you, the dispatcher contacts the proper authorities.

Life Alert is a subscription-based service. Visit lifealert.com to learn all the details and sign up.

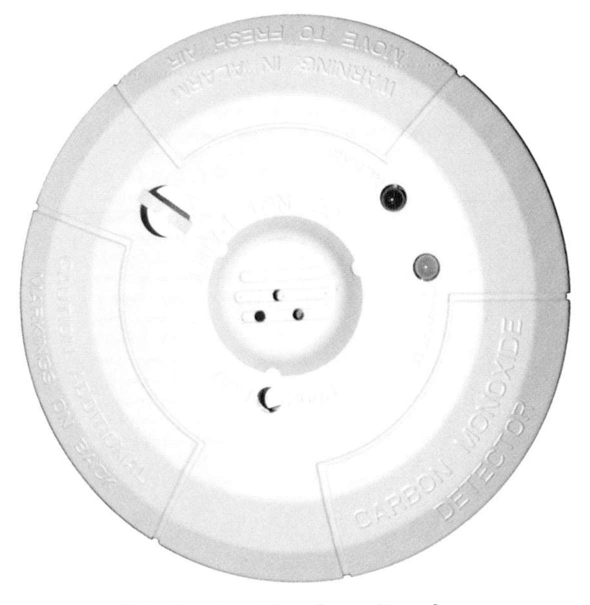

Life Alert's optional monitored carbon monoxide and fire detection

Get the Life Alert Mobile Help Phone and App for Smartphones

Life Alert also offers services that help you remain safe while on the go. The Life Alert Emergency Mobile Help Phone has one large Help button you can press that connects you to Life Alert's Emergency Dispatch Center for immediate help. The Mobile Help Phone has nationwide cellular coverage using AT&Ts 3G network and doesn't require any charging. This service also includes GPS capabilities, so you can be located anywhere in the United States when a GPS signal is available.

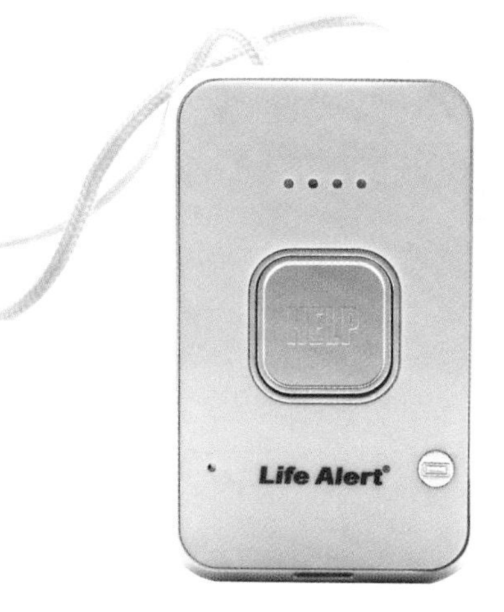

Life Alert's Mobile Help Phone helps you remain safe while on the go.

>>>Go Further

THE LIFE ALERT HELP BUTTON

The Life Alert Help Button is a new edition to the Life Alert cellular connected and two-way voice-enabled devices. This stationary waterproof Help Button is a wall-mounted emergency device for protection, even when in the shower, bathroom, or other enclosed spaces.

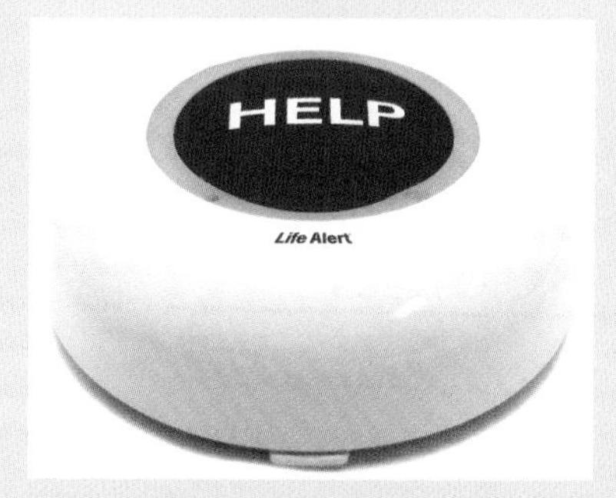

The Life Alert Stationary Help Button

The Life Alert Mobile app also allows you to take the company's services on the go. Just like the Mobile Help Phone, you don't need to wait until an emergency happens to use its services. If you are ever concerned for your safety, for example, walking alone to your car in the dark, press the emergency button on the app to contact Life Alert and speak with a dispatcher. She will stay on the line with you until you feel out of harm's way or send the authorities to your location, if needed. The app also has the ability to use your phone's camera flash as a flashlight and can emit a whistle or yell sound to signal for help. Like with the app's traditional service, you can always use the app for medical emergencies or home intrusion. If you have the carbon monoxide and fire protection service, you can use the app for those services as well. The Life Alert Mobile Help app is available for Android phones and the iPhone. The Life Alert Mobile Help app is available for all cell phone makes and models.

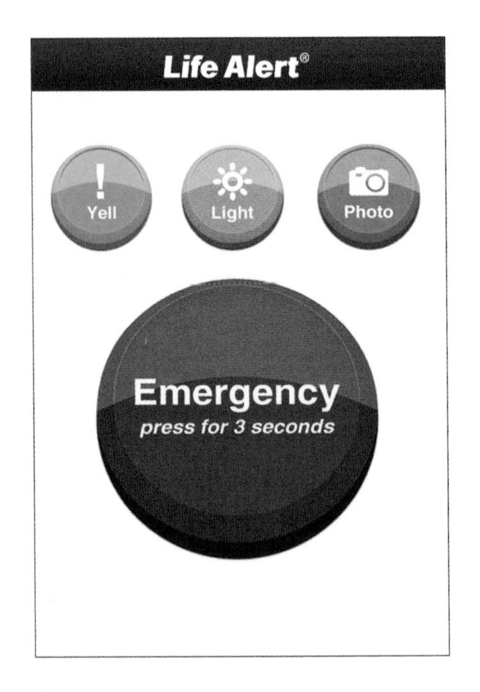

Life Alert's mobile app lets you contact help from home or on the go, even before an emergency may happen.

Use the MobileHelp Medical Alert System

If you are looking for a personal medical alert system that works away from home as well as at home, consider the mobile Medical Alert System. The Cellular Duo system is comprised of a base station, a neck pendant or wrist button, a mobile device, and a pouch to carry it in. When you carry the mobile device, this system uses GPS to enable loved ones and MobileHelp Emergency Operators to see the location of the device on a map.

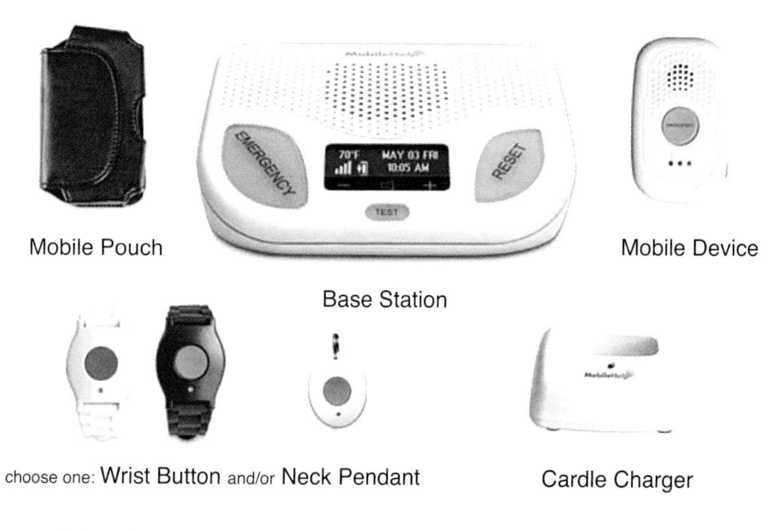

MobileHelp offers emergency response nationwide, indoors and out, without requiring a smartphone.

Here's how it works. When you press the emergency button on your pendant or mobile device, your information and location are sent to the MobileHelp emergency operators. A U.S.-based emergency operator talks to you through the mobile device's speaker to assess the situation. The operator can then contact a neighbor, family member, or emergency service based on your needs. The service can go anywhere you do because it uses cellular technology and offers nationwide coverage, where cellular coverage is available. Satellites constantly transmit the location of the mobile device so operators send the closest paramedics to your location.

There is also a Cellular Classic System that does not include the mobile device, but offers traditional in-home medical alert monitoring. As the name implies, neither the Cellular Duo nor the Cellular Classic System requires a landline. You can also add a Fall Button with Automatic Fall Detect to either system. All are subscription services. Find out more about both of these systems, and decide whether a MobileHelp subscription suits your lifestyle at mobilehelp.com.

Get to Know the Lively 24/7 Emergency Medical Alert System

The Lively system offers a different type of safety net compared to the previous medical alert systems you have explored in this book. The Lively 24/7 Emergency Medical Alert System helps you monitor the healthy living patterns of someone in need of assistance, while respecting her choice for living on her own. The Lively safety watch, in-home hub, and activity sensors can help you monitor whether an individual is taking medication on time, eating regularly, or being active. This system alerts family members quickly by automated notifications, text, and email if your loved one may need help. It also includes 24/7 access to live operators, an online dashboard, and an app so family members can stay informed and connected. As of this writing, a clip for auto fall detection is also being added. Here's how the system works.

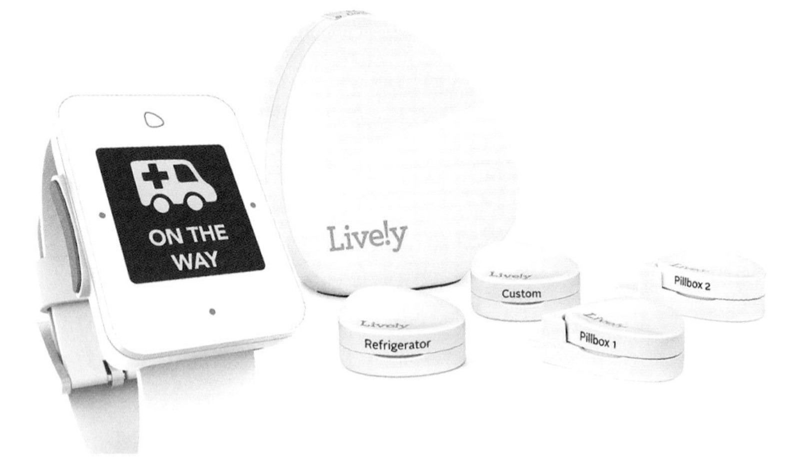

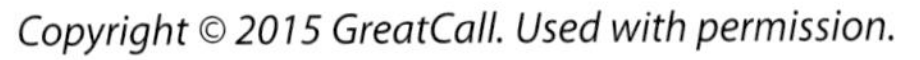

The Lively Emergency Medical Alert System includes a safety watch, in-home hub, and activity sensors.

The hub uses built-in cellular technology; no Internet or extra phone line is needed. It has a range of up to 1,500 feet, so you are covered indoors and outdoors. Pressing the Help button on the waterproof safety watch sends a signal to the in-home hub that initiates a call from the Lively Care Team. It also coordinates all the information gathered from the sensors and the watch, and transmits it to the online dashboard.

The team member then assesses the situation and calls the listed emergency contacts and/or dispatches emergency services, if needed. You can see that help is on the way on the watch face. The safety watch also helps an individual adhere to a medication regimen by providing alerts if a dose is missed. If a medication regimen is not properly adhered to, family members are notified. The watch even acts as a pedometer and tracks numbers of steps taken.

The Lively passive activity sensors can be placed on movable objects or around the home. Attach a sensor on a pillbox to track when a medication is taken. Attach a sensor to the refrigerator to see when an individual may be preparing and consuming food. You can track many other activities, for example, by placing a sensor on the shower door or on their favorite chair.

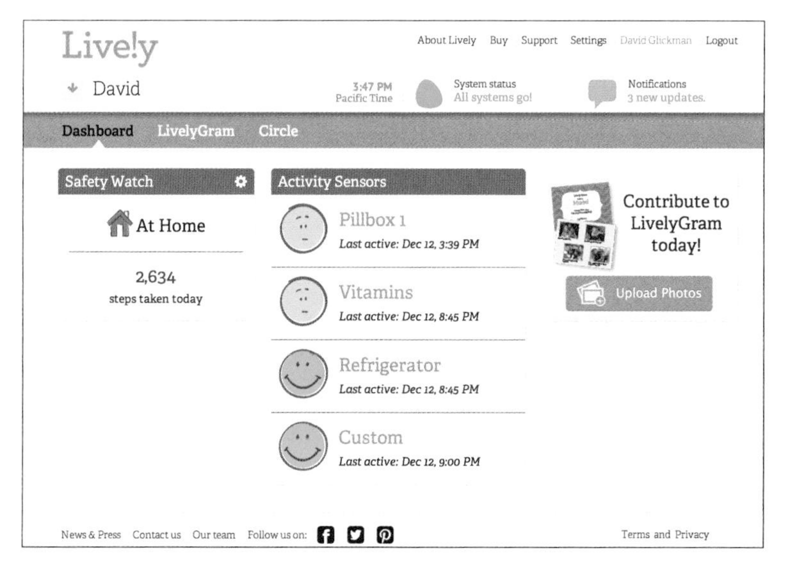

Lively's "At-A-Glance" online dashboard shows notifications, as well as easily accessible information on healthy living patterns.

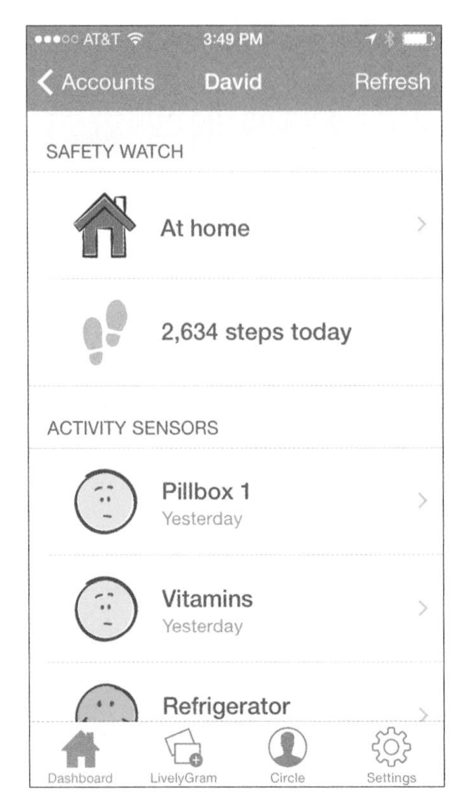

Copyright © 2015 GreatCall. Used with permission.

The Lively app connects to the safety watch so you can see step count, view medication reminders, adjust settings on the watch, and share information with others.

Family members also have online access to monitor their loved one's daily activity pattern data. The online dashboard acts as your virtual command center and lets you give data access to specific family members and caregivers. You can monitor safety watch status, including if it's being worn or not. Set up how notifications are delivered: by email, text, or mobile app, and you can monitor daily activity patterns by viewing details from each activity sensor. The safety watch can also be connected to your Android phone or iPhone so you can stay informed and connected using the Lively app. To learn more about what Lively has to offer and to see how to set up the system, visit mylively.com.

Understand the grandCare Monitoring System

The grandCare Monitoring System is perhaps the most comprehensive system covered in this book. Its features include telehealth, health management, activity monitoring, and social engagement—all conveniently accessible through an easy-to-use touchscreen. The grandCare system is a mix of hardware and software, including sensors for activity tracking. You can't just install the grandCare system onto your own computer. The system can be used with a wired or Wi-Fi Internet connection and can work with telehealth devices.

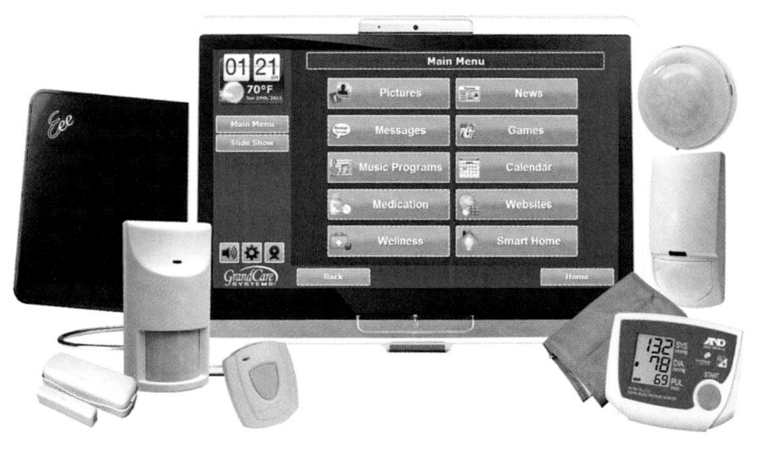

© 2005-2015 GrandCare Systems, LLC

The grandCare Monitoring System includes telehealth, health management, activity monitoring, and social engagement.

It may sound it bit complex, but the grandCare system is designed so the user doesn't have to be technologically savvy to enjoy its benefits. It's very easy for family members and caregivers to stay connected and monitor someone who may require extra help. You should do two things before you purchase the system. Go to us.grandcare.com to schedule a demo to see whether it's right for you. Then, check with your provider to see whether you can get grandCare at a reduced price. The website also helps you pick the best program for you. The system has four basic use purposes: Medical, Non-Medical, Social, or Personal.

If you decide the grandCare system is right for you, installation is easy and was designed so nonprofessional installers can set it up. You are walked through the initial setup step-by-step. Read on and take a look at just some of what grandCare has to offer.

Track Activity Online

The grandCare system is comprised of an activity sensor hub that allows you to set motion, contact, and pressure sensors around the home, and review that information by logging into the Online Care Portal. This discreetly gathered data is good for watching over someone with Alzheimer's. Sensors could be placed on the refrigerator door or kitchen counter to determine whether your loved one is eating meals. Place a sensor in the hallway outside of the bedroom to know what time an individual gets up in the morning. A sensor in the bathroom can determine an increase in bathroom visits. In general, sensors placed in your loved one's kitchen, living room, favorite chair, and usual places provide insight to your loved one's moving around. A substantial decrease in motion or significant change in routine could indicate a problem. Guidelines can be set on the system so that if certain events occur, family members are notified with a phone call, text message, or email.

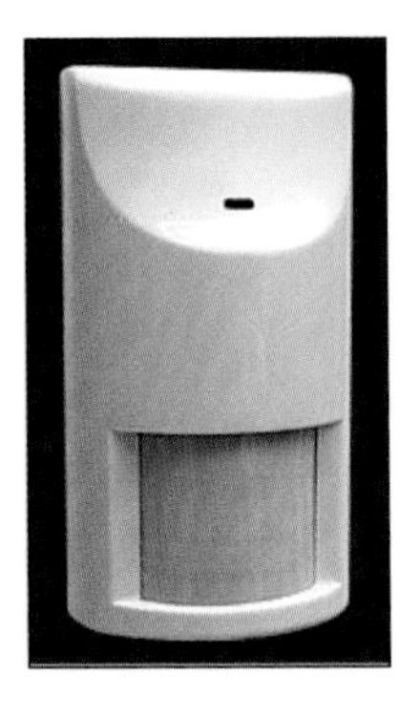

The grandCare motion-activated sensor

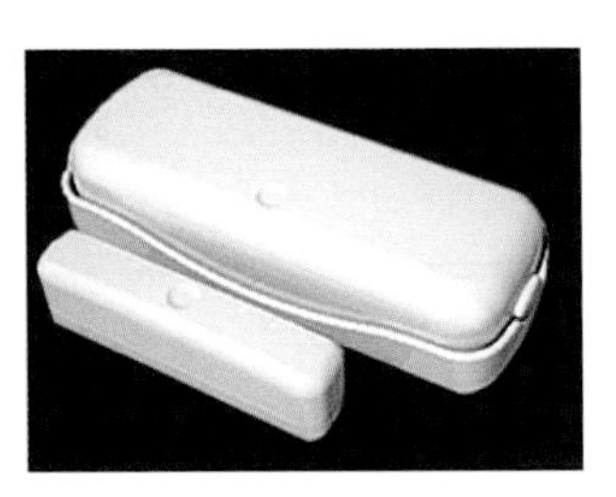

The grandCare contact sensor for doors or windows

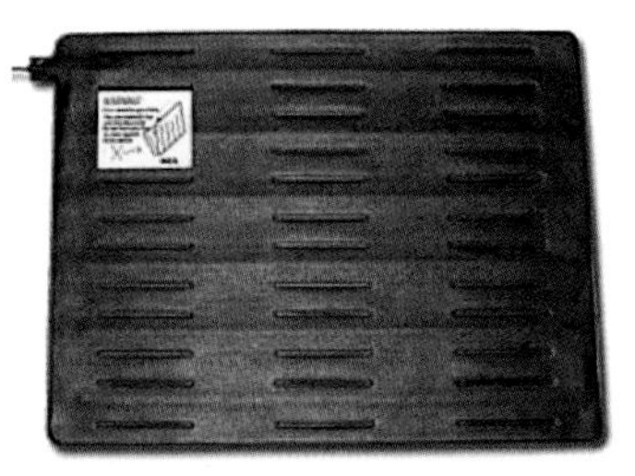

The grandCare pressure sensor for a bed or chair

Monitor Vitals Online

The grandCare system also supports telehealth devices including blood pressure monitors, glucometers, scales, pulse oximeters, and thermometers. Individuals can have discussions about health concerns by video chatting with a health care professional using MediKall, a HIPAA (Health Insurance Portability and Accountability Act) compliant service. HIPAA means your personal data is confidential and secure. grandCare users can place a video call with a simple tap on the touchscreen and contact caregivers who are logged in to the Online Care Portal. Health care providers have remote access to user information and can view health vitals through charts and graphs.

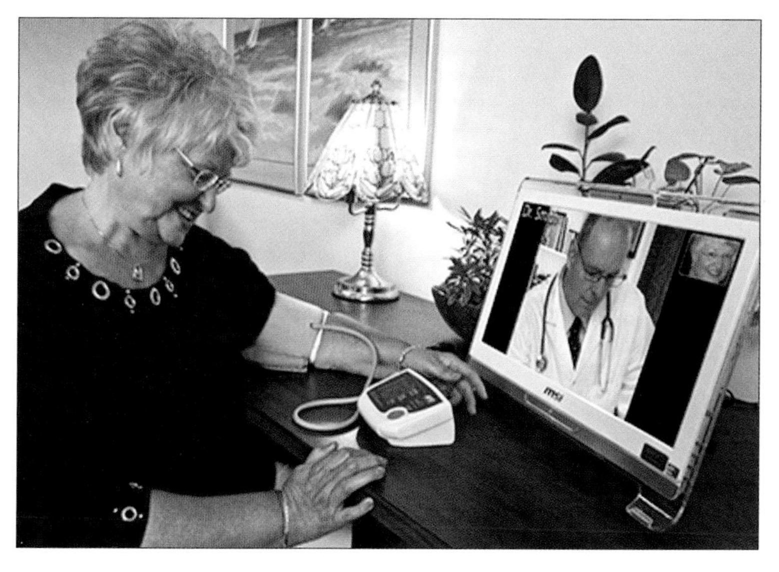

© 2005-2015 GrandCare Systems, LLC

Video chat with doctors and allow them to securely access your health vitals through MediKall, all from within the grandCare online portal.

Turning On Lights in Your Home Remotely

We have spent a lot of time talking about what to do in the event of an emergency. Now it's time to talk about some preventive measures you can take, especially when it comes to falls. The simple precaution of not having to walk in to a dark room and search for a light switch can decrease your chances of tripping. Devices that let you turn on light sources remotely or automatically offer a minor, but added security layer to your home. There are simple solutions, some of which have been around for a long time, that allow you to clap or use voice commands to turn on the lights in the room. Some solutions automatically turn on when it's dark. This section covers some simple and quick solutions that don't require you to use your phone or tablet as a remote to turn on lights.

Control Your Lights with the Clapper

The Clapper is the most well-known remote light activator that we'll cover. It's simple, and it works. Just in case you're not familiar with the commercials, the Clapper is a sound-activated light switch that plugs directly into a power outlet. The switch accommodates up to two devices and features a sound sensitivity dial and clap detection lights. After you plug a light or two into the Clapper, you can turn them on or off depending on the number of times you clap. Clap two times to operate the first light and three times to operate the second. The clapper can also act as a security device when placed in Away mode. In Away mode, the Clapper can turn on the lights at the first sound it picks up to discourage possible intruders.

Visit chia.com/home-goods/the-clapper or search online to purchase the Clapper, or visit your local ACE Hardware, CVS Pharmacy, Rite Aid, True Value, or Walgreens store.

Use the Clapper with Other Appliances

The Clapper can also be used to turn your TV, radio, and many other household appliances on and off.

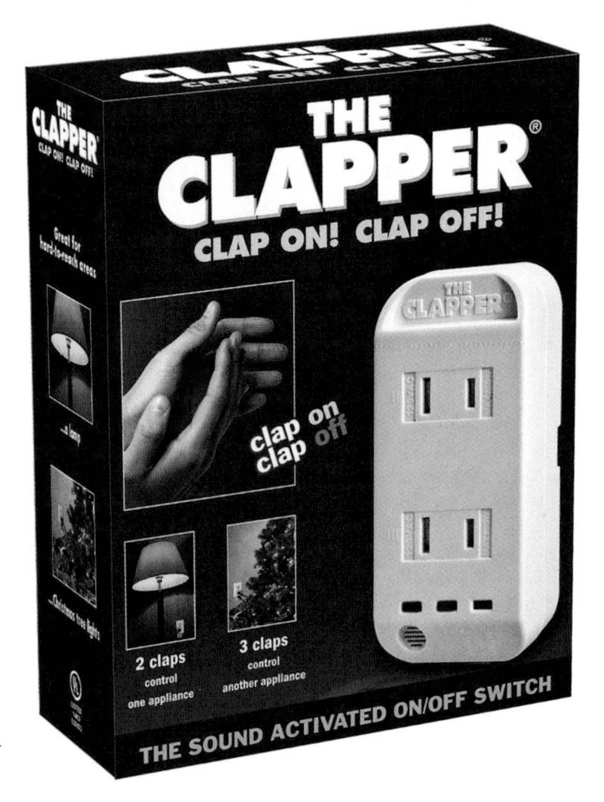

Clapper® is a registered trademark of Joseph Enterprises, Inc. in the United States and other countries. Clapper trademark and image are used with permission.

Known to many, the Clapper's simple solution is still effective.

It's Not All Good

Device Can Be Triggered by Other Sounds

It is possible for the Clapper to be triggered by other sharp sounds when not in Away mode, including closing a door or cabinet, or noises emanating from the television or other speakers.

Light the Way with the Automatic Sensor LED Night Light

The Automatic Sensor LED Night Light from Feit Electric is a little light that you might find useful. This LED light has an automatic sensor that turns on at dusk and turns off at dawn. If you get up in the middle of the night, this little light can light the path to the bathroom without disturbing the whole house. It also serves you well if you like a little light in the bathroom or in the bedroom at night. LED lights like this one use less than 1 watt of energy and have a life of up to 100,000 hours, so you won't have to worry about the light having burnt out in the middle of the night.

Visit feit.com and amazon.com to learn more and to purchase these lights.

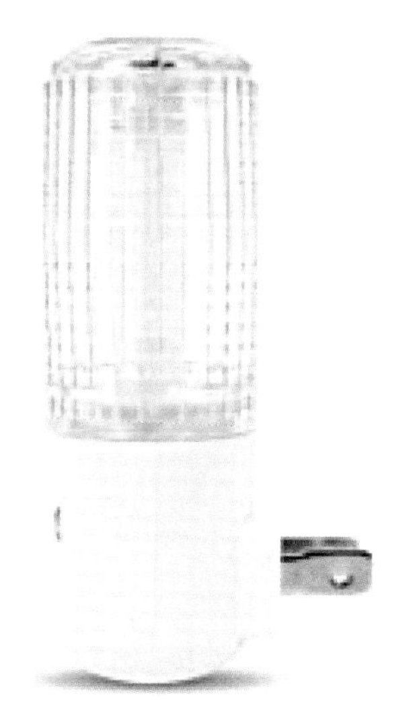

Automatically light your path with a long-lasting LED night light.

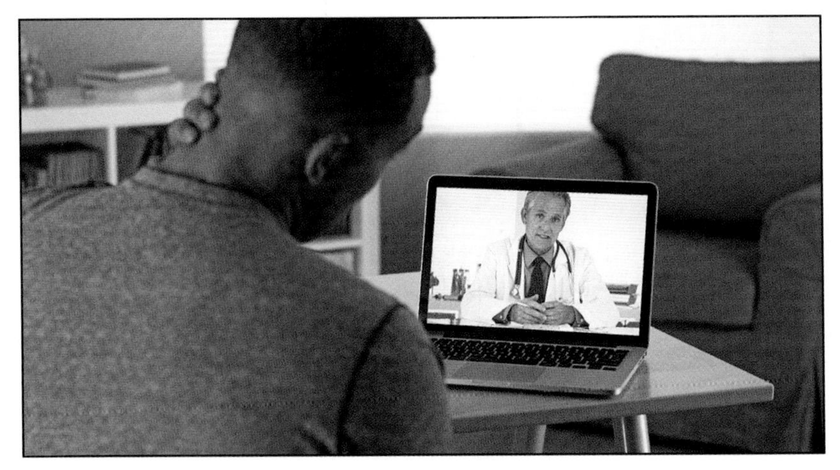

Credit: © rocketclips/fotolia.com

Use convenient online resources to find the health care professionals you need.

In this chapter, you explore online resources that help you find the right caregiver, make appointments, receive treatment online, and save money on medication. You also discover resources that can help your family prepare if something happens to you.

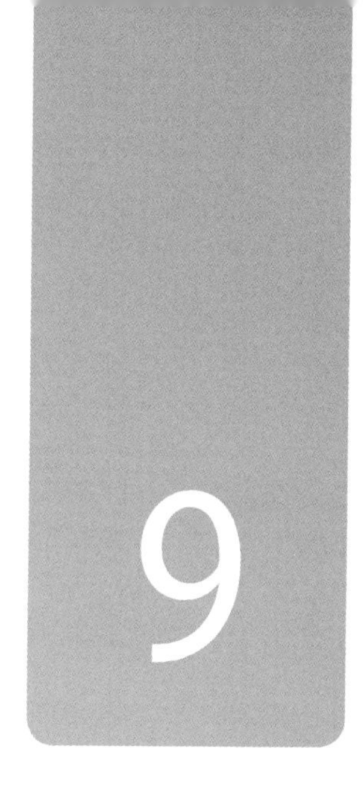

- → Scheduling Doctor Appointments and Finding Doctors
- → Getting Treatment Online
- → Accessing Adult Care Resources
- → Preventing Paying Too Much for Health Procedures and Medication
- → Gathering Your Health Information

Connecting with Your Health Care Professionals and Saving Money on Services

More than ever, web-based services and mobile apps are being used to manage personal health care. The services offered online and through apps varies. It's fine if you don't have a smartphone or tablet; many companies offer the same services on their websites.

Some apps specialize in managing your health care from your home or on the go, including the ZocDoc app. If you are looking for a doctor, Betterdoctor.com provides anonymous reviews so you can find the care provider that best fits your needs.

Getting treatment online has never been easier with services such as Teladoc and Direct Dermatology. These services go beyond being able to make an appointment online and enable you to participate in a doctor's appointment through your computer. Then, resources such as CoPatient and WeRx can help find the best prices for medications.

Checklist for My Family helps you pull together your care providers and medications in one convenient spot and prepare the advance directives you need so your family can know your wishes should something happen to you.

This chapter offers only some of the great resources out there to help you better manage your health care. Hopefully, one of the following options will be a perfect match for you. If not, use the information in this chapter as a starting point for you to find what's best for you and your family.

Scheduling Doctor Appointments and Finding Doctors

If you get tired of waiting on the phone to make a doctor appointment or want to make a more informed decision about choosing a doctor, many websites can help you achieve both of these goals—efficiently. The following services have both mobile (app) and web-based services. The examples show some in-app, and others on their websites. Some services are not available for both the Android and Apple (iOS) platforms, but you are told which platforms are available for each service. Many doctors' offices also have websites where you can find paperwork for new patients and book and cancel appointments.

Find Doctors and Dentists, and Book Appointments with the ZocDoc App

ZocDoc is not a health care provider. ZocDoc is a free app and service you can use to find a neighborhood doctor who accepts your insurance coverage, or lets you pay out of pocket. Doctors pay a fee to be included in ZocDoc, so you may not find your specific doctor. You can read reviews from patients for listed doctors, see open appointment times, and immediately schedule an appointment. After you have scheduled an appointment, the app enables you to check in online and fill out medical forms ahead of time, saving you time in the office. Before you can make an appointment, you must sign in to your existing ZocDoc account or join ZocDoc as a new patient. Visit ZocDoc.com to sign up for a new

ZocDoc account. You can also sign up from your phone, but you might find the web-based option preferable to avoid filling out forms on your phone.

The app is available for Android phones and the iPhone. Download the app and use these instructions to explore the ZocDoc app. The following screenshots are from an iPhone.

Navigate the ZocDoc App

Navigating the ZocDoc app is as simple as tapping the main menu, which shows information including upcoming appointments, notifications, recommended treatments, and the ability to change your profile and insurance information.

1. Tap the ZocDoc app icon on your phone.
2. Tap the main menu that looks like three horizontal lines to navigate the app.

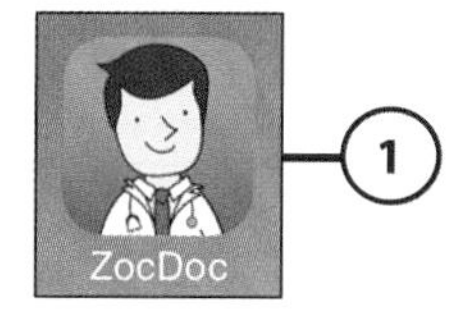

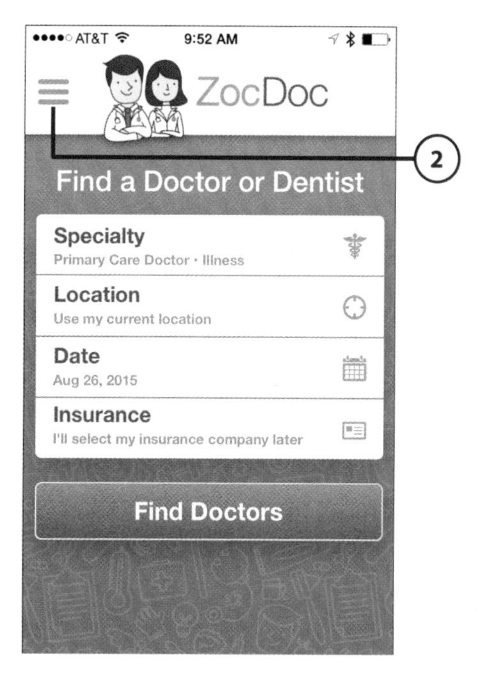

3. Tap Sign In if you already have an existing ZocDoc account.
4. Tap Join Now if you are new to ZocDoc, and create an account. After you sign in or join, the options to Sign In and Join are replaced with Notifications options. The following images display this logged-in view.

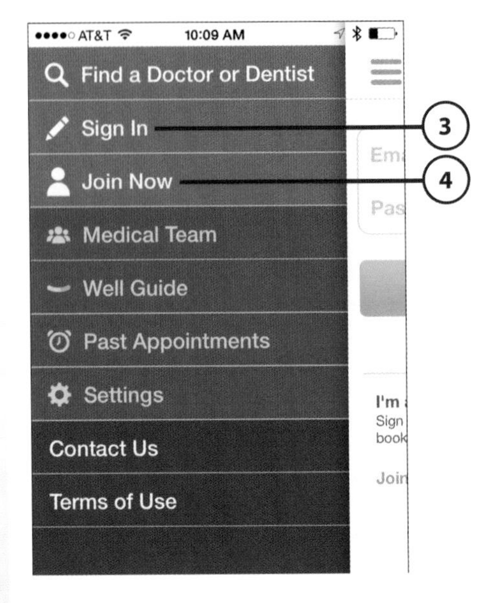

5. Tap in the Notifications area to view scheduled appointments, wellness reminders, and more. Wellness reminders are personalized recommendations based on your gender, age, and medical history to aid you in a healthy lifestyle.
6. Tap Medical Team to view the list of doctors you have scheduled through ZocDoc.
7. Tap Well Guide to book recommended treatments for health maintenance such as vision exams, skin screenings, annual physicals, and dental cleanings.
8. Tap Past Appointments to see a comprehensive list of the appointments you scheduled through ZocDoc.
9. Tap Settings to tweak your profile and password information. You can also change notification settings, insurance information, and demographic information.
10. Tap Sign Out to sign out of your ZocDoc account.

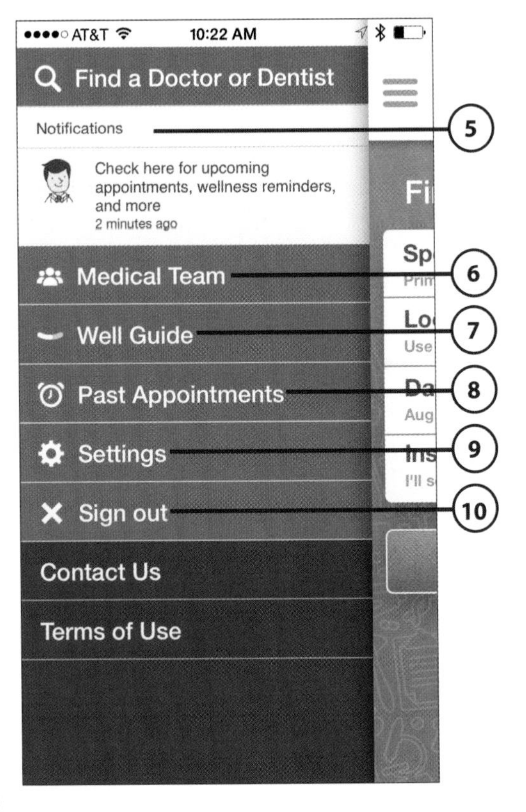

Find a Doctor with ZocDoc

ZocDoc makes it easy for you to find a doctor with the specialty you need. After you find a doctor who is nearby and accepts your insurance plan, you can immediately make an appointment. Doctor reviews are also provided and moderated to offer you information you need to make an informed decision. After you make an appointment, you can check in online, fill out any paperwork a particular doctor might require, and conveniently add the appointment to your calendar.

1. Tap Find a Doctor or Dentist.
2. Tap Specialty.

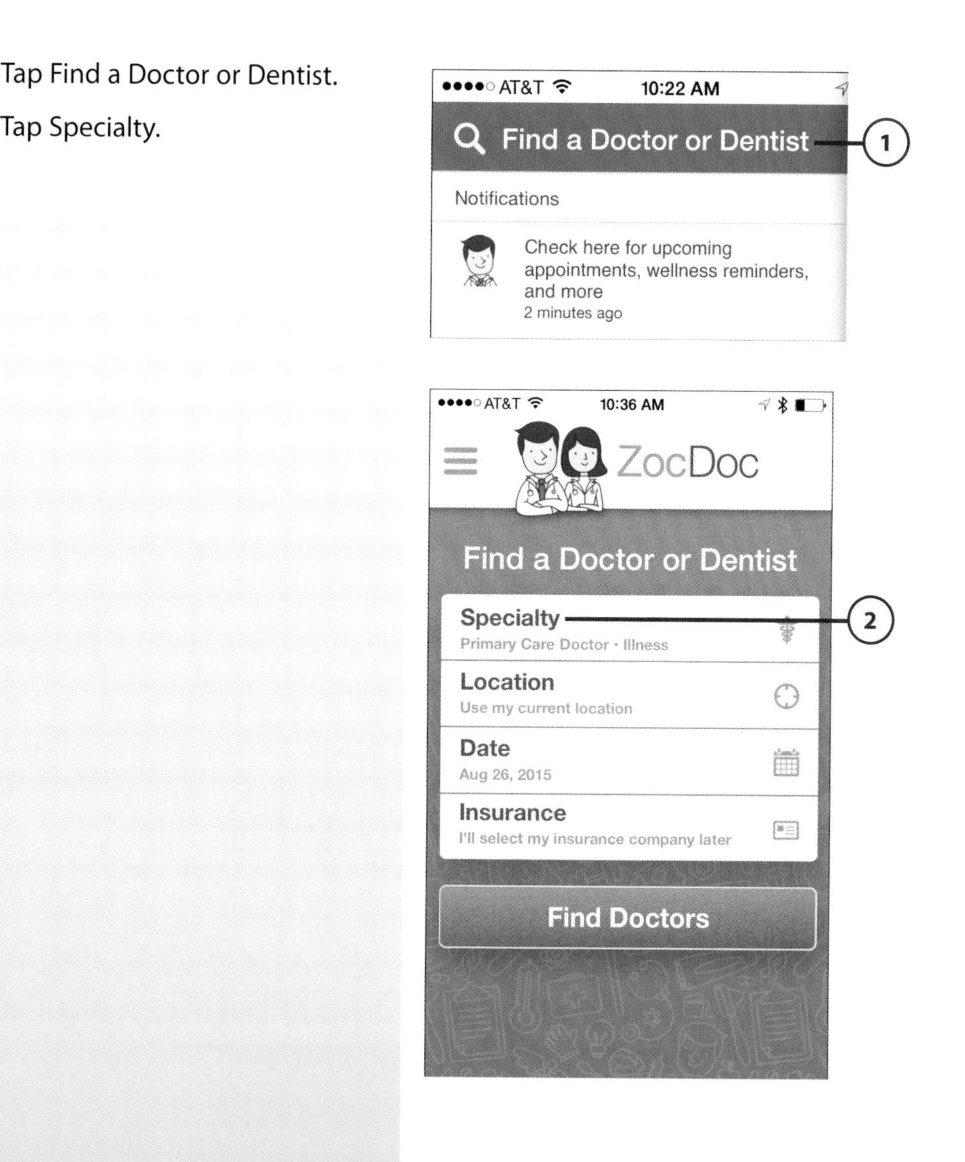

3. Scroll to a desired specialty and tap it to select it.
4. Tap to select a reason for your visit.
5. Tap Location.

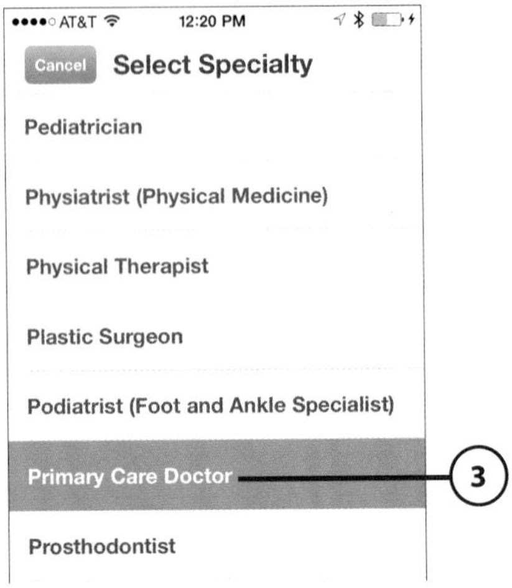

AT&T 12:20 PM
Cancel Select Specialty
Pediatrician
Physiatrist (Physical Medicine)
Physical Therapist
Plastic Surgeon
Podiatrist (Foot and Ankle Specialist)
Primary Care Doctor (3)
Prosthodontist

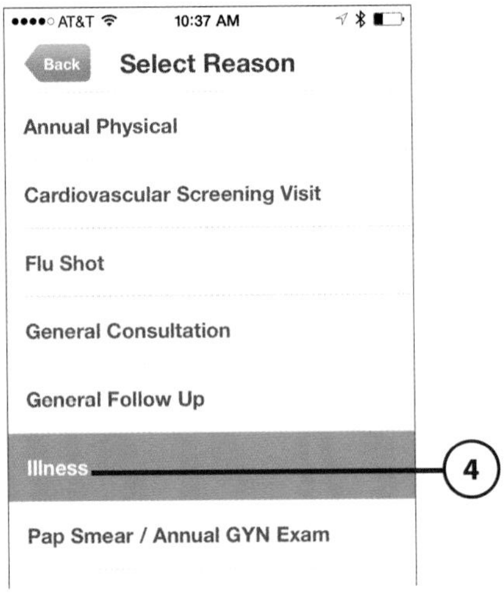

AT&T 10:37 AM
Back Select Reason
Annual Physical
Cardiovascular Screening Visit
Flu Shot
General Consultation
General Follow Up
Illness (4)
Pap Smear / Annual GYN Exam

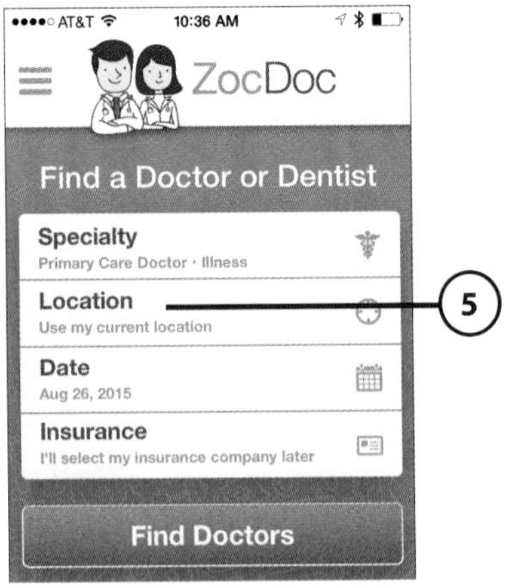

AT&T 10:36 AM
ZocDoc
Find a Doctor or Dentist
Specialty
Primary Care Doctor · Illness
Location (5)
Use my current location
Date
Aug 26, 2015
Insurance
I'll select my insurance company later
Find Doctors

Get to Know Location Settings

Location settings can use a combination of GPS, cellular, and Wi-Fi to pinpoint your location. Apps and websites can then access this information. You access location settings in the Settings menu on your Android phone. On an iPhone, tap Settings, and then choose Privacy to locate the Location Services setting.

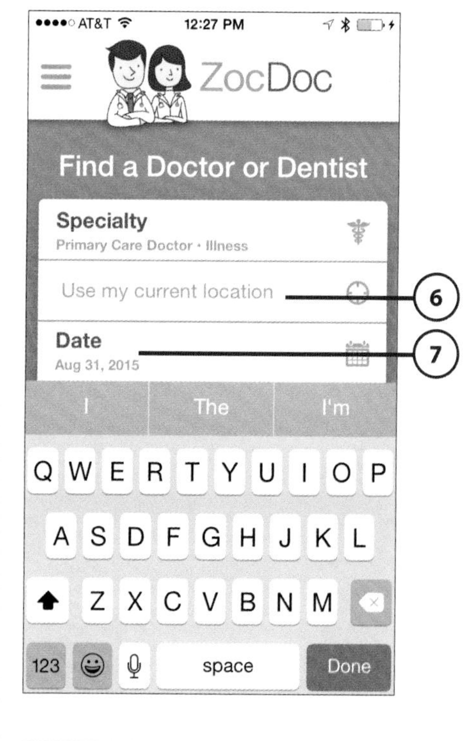

6. Enter a Zip code or city. You can simply move on to the next field (Date) to have ZocDoc automatically pinpoint your current location. This option only works if your location settings are enabled on your smartphone.
7. Tap Date.
8. Select a date for the appointment.
9. Tap Done.

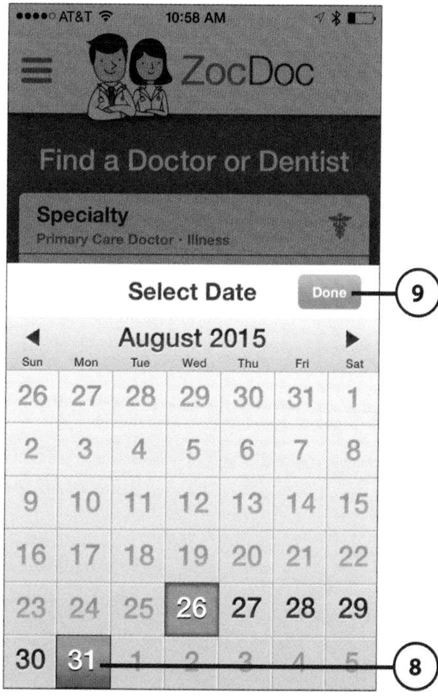

10. Tap Insurance.
11. Scroll through the list using your finger, and then tap to select an insurance carrier.
12. Scroll through the list, and then tap to select an insurance plan.

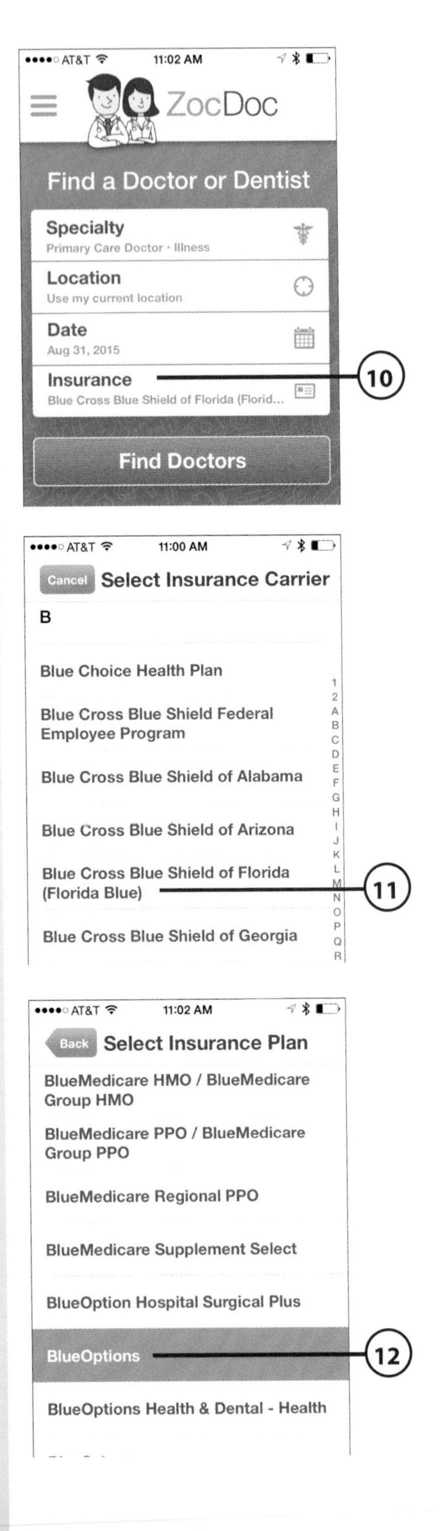

Let ZocDoc Access Your Location

A dialog box might appear asking permission for ZocDoc to access your location while you use the app. Tap Allow to find doctors closest your location.

13. Tap Find Doctors. A list of doctors and appointment times appears.
14. Tap the arrow to learn more about a doctor.
15. Tap to read reviews. You can tap Back in the upper-left corner to go back to the list of doctors.
16. Tap a time that works with your schedule.

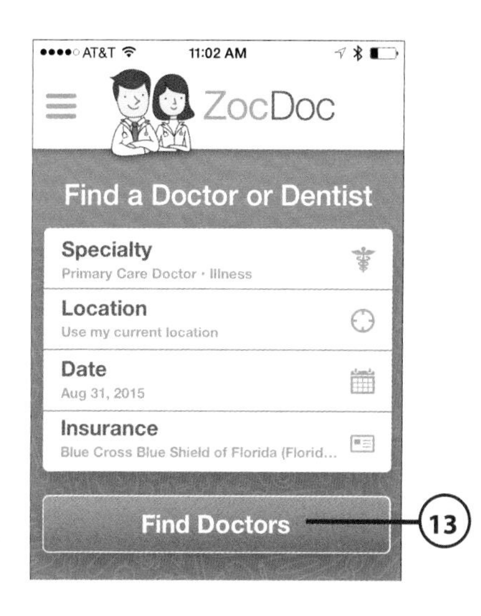

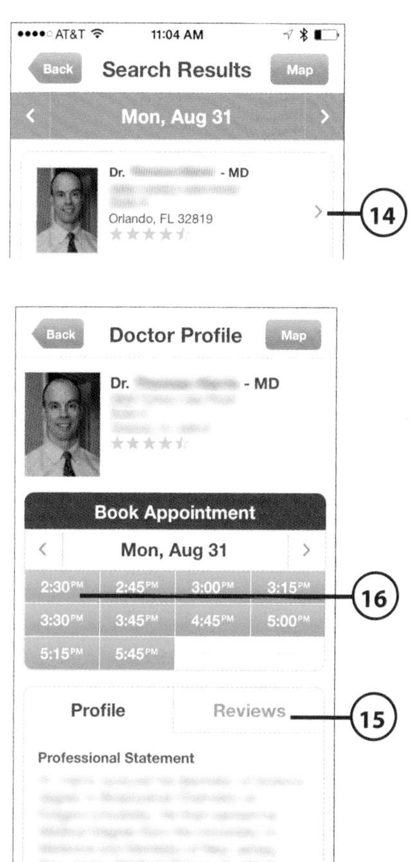

17. Tap Book this Appointment. The Book Appointment screen opens.
18. Scroll down to the bottom of the page, and then tap the appropriate option to designate whether you are a new patient or have seen this doctor before.
19. Tap Continue.
20. Tap to select who will be seeing the doctor. If you are making the appointment for someone else, choose Add a New Patient.
21. Tap Continue.

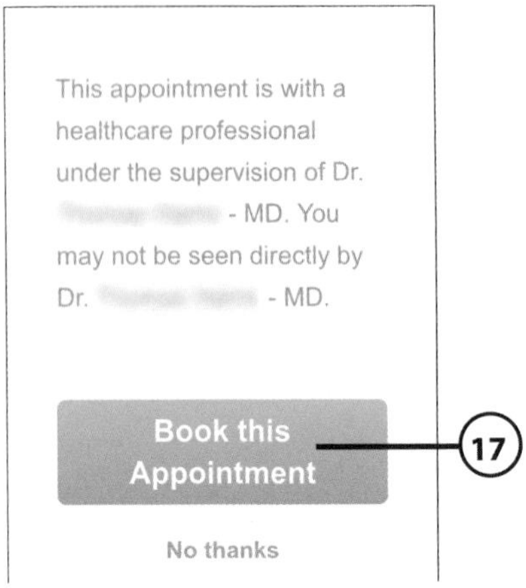

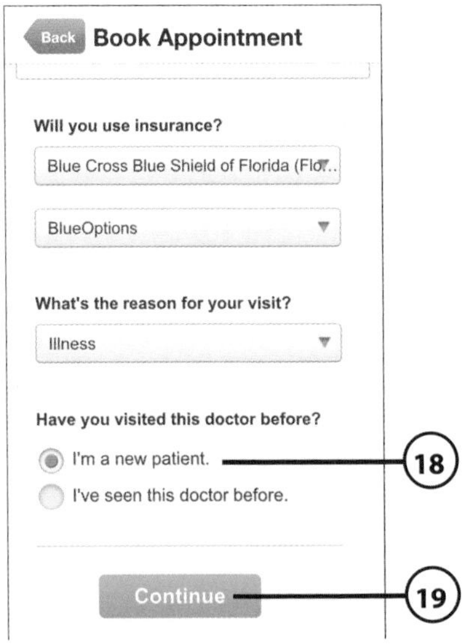

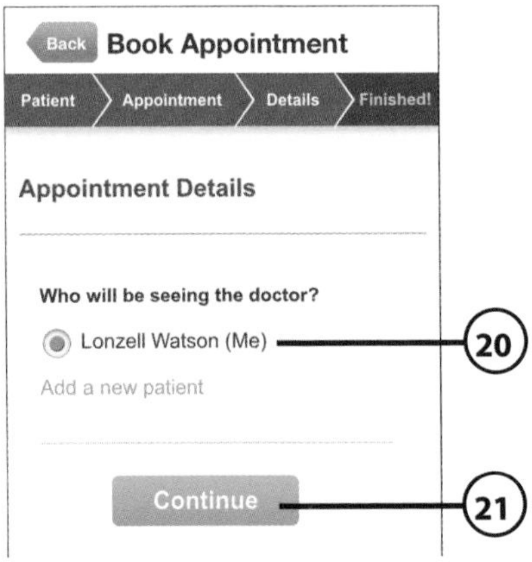

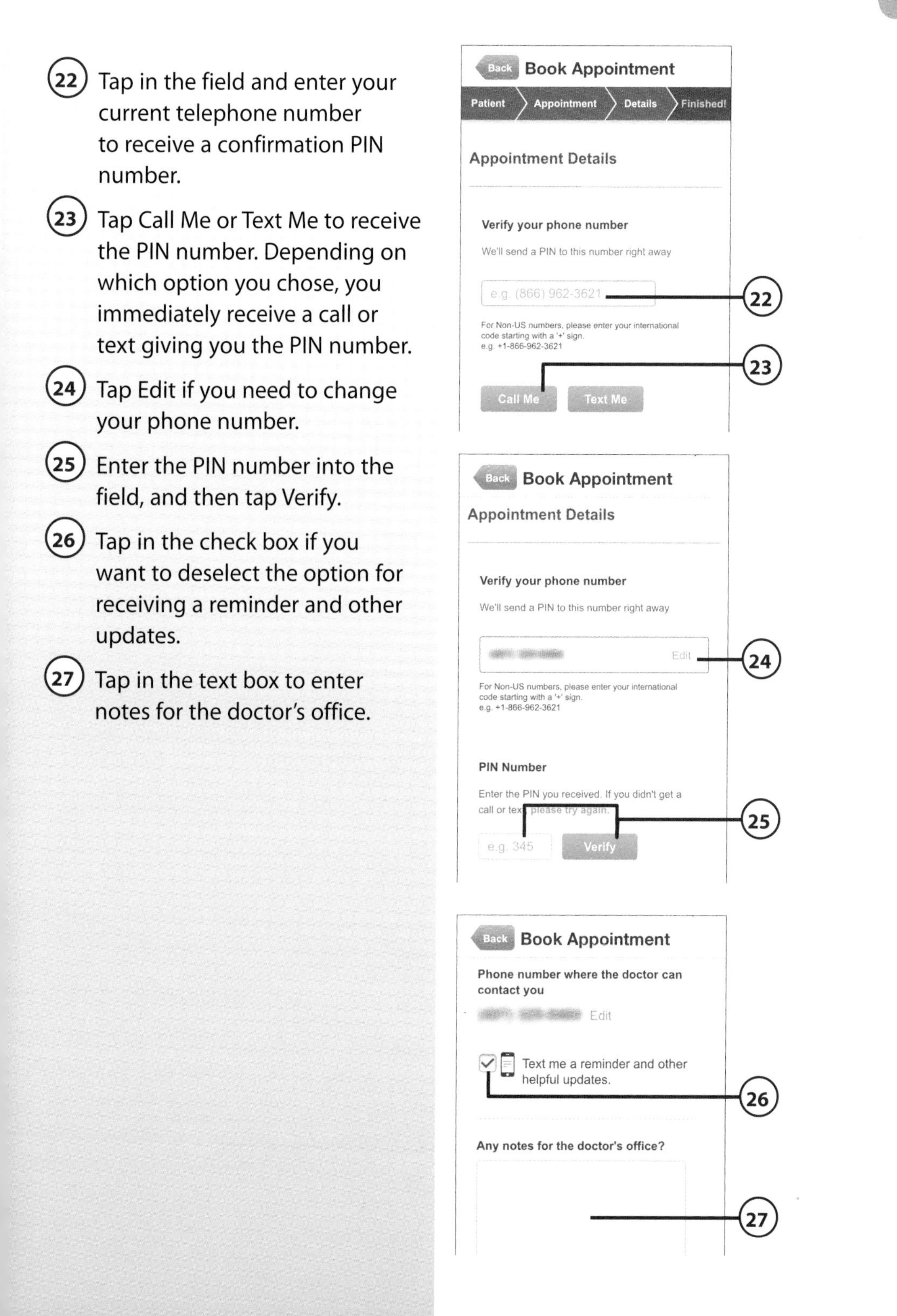

22. Tap in the field and enter your current telephone number to receive a confirmation PIN number.
23. Tap Call Me or Text Me to receive the PIN number. Depending on which option you chose, you immediately receive a call or text giving you the PIN number.
24. Tap Edit if you need to change your phone number.
25. Enter the PIN number into the field, and then tap Verify.
26. Tap in the check box if you want to deselect the option for receiving a reminder and other updates.
27. Tap in the text box to enter notes for the doctor's office.

28. Scroll further down the page and tap Book Appointment.
29. Tap Check-In Online or No thanks.
30. Scroll down the page to see a number for the doctor's office, add the appointment to your calendar, or view your scheduled appointments.

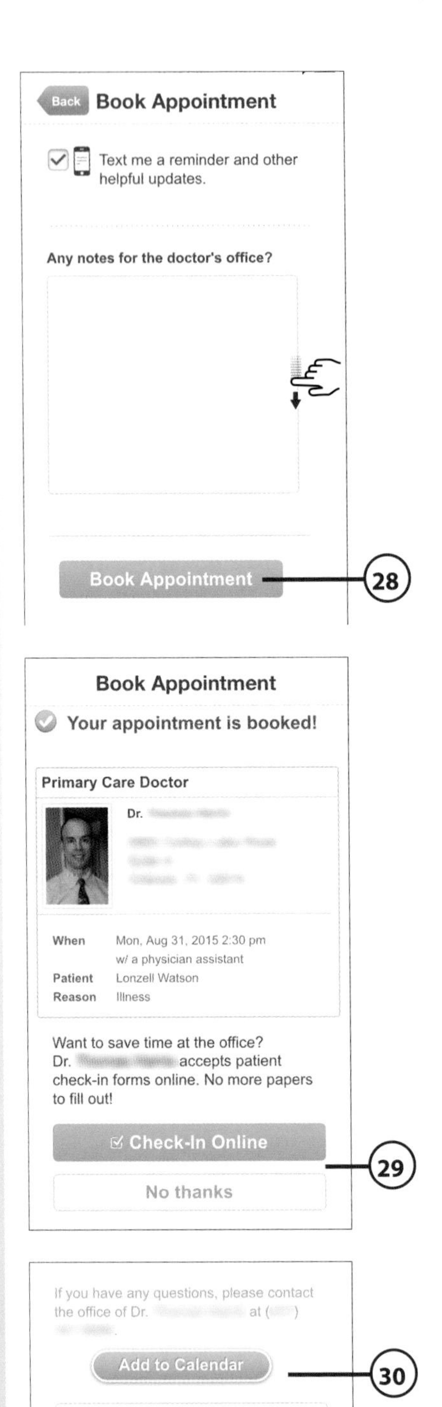

Cancel an Appointment with ZocDoc

If you have a change in schedule, ZocDoc makes it easy for you to cancel your appointment.

1. Tap the main menu button, which looks like three horizontal bars.
2. In the screen that appears, tap the appointment you want to delete under Upcoming Appointments.
3. Tap Cancel. A dialog box appears asking whether you are sure you want to delete the appointment.

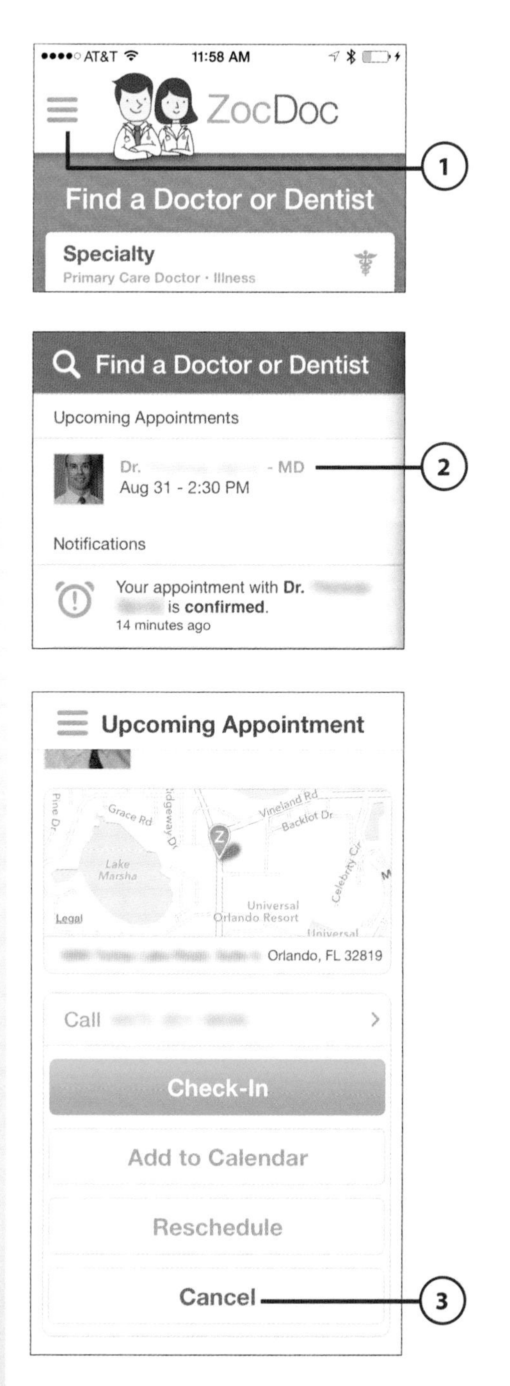

4. Tap Yes. The appointment is cancelled. Your cancelled appointments now appear under the Notifications area under the main menu.

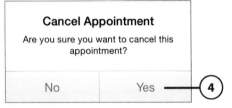

Find a Doctor You'll Love at BetterDoctor

BetterDoctor is a free web-based service that helps to simplify the search for top doctors in your area. This service provides a data-driven approach that includes doctors' education, experience, and referral network. They try to include every doctor in the U.S. There is also a BetterDoctor app. As of this writing, the app is only available for the iPhone through the App Store. With Better Doctor, you can search 1 million doctors—rated by education and experience—by name or by specialty. By setting up an account, you can save doctors to your profile, and save your insurance information while you search doctors. The following steps are performed on the betterdoctor.com website.

1. Go to betterdoctor.com on your desktop's web browser. By default, the website can pinpoint your city.
2. Click Sign Up to create a profile.
3. Click Sign Up with Facebook to create a profile using your existing Facebook account.
4. Click Sign Up with Google to create a profile using your existing Google+ account.
5. Click Sign Up with Email to create a profile using an existing email account. For these instructions, the Sign Up with Email option is selected.

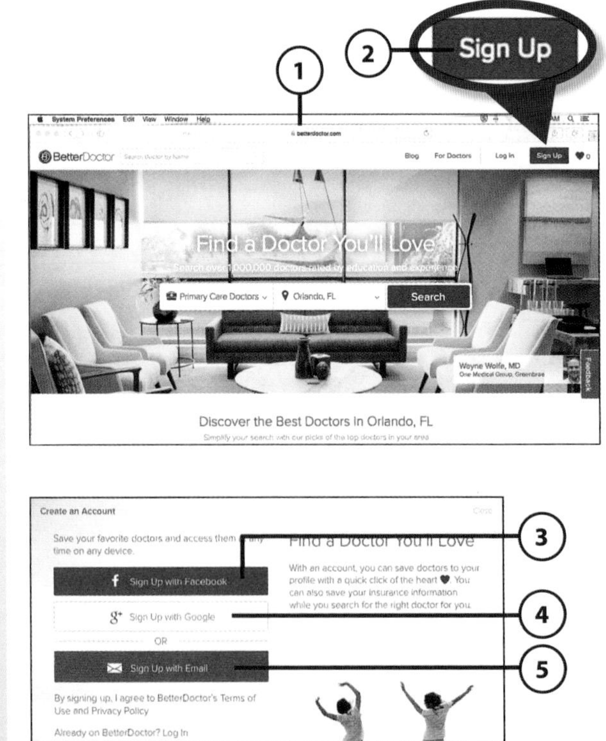

Social Media Privacy Issues

Logging in via Facebook or any website can pose privacy issues by giving the app access to your social media data. Consider signing up using an email account instead.

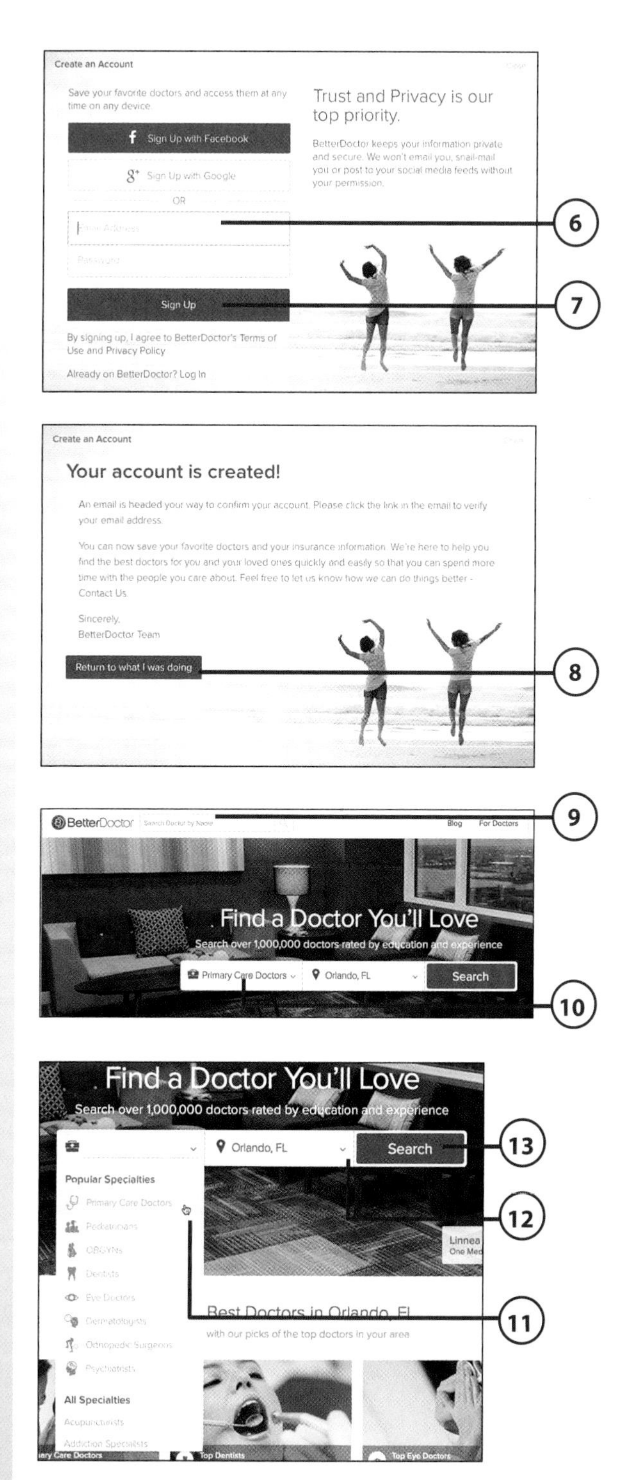

6. Type in your email address and a password.
7. Click Sign Up.
8. Click Return to What I was doing. At the top-right corner of the screen, you can see that you are now logged in.
9. Type if you want to search for a doctor by name.
10. To search by specialty, click the drop-down arrow in the Primary Care Doctors field.
11. Scroll up and down in the menu, and then click on a specialty. You can also type in a specialty in the field above the list.
12. Click in the location field to designate the location. By default, your browser might automatically detect your current location.
13. Click Search. BetterDoctor compiles a list of doctors in your area, complete with excerpts from bios, ratings, and their location on a map.

14. Click Select your Insurance to further filter the list by insurance.
15. Click the heart shape to save a doctor to your profile for later review.
16. Click on a doctor to see more information.
17. Scroll down to view background information. This page also has the contact information and directions to the office.

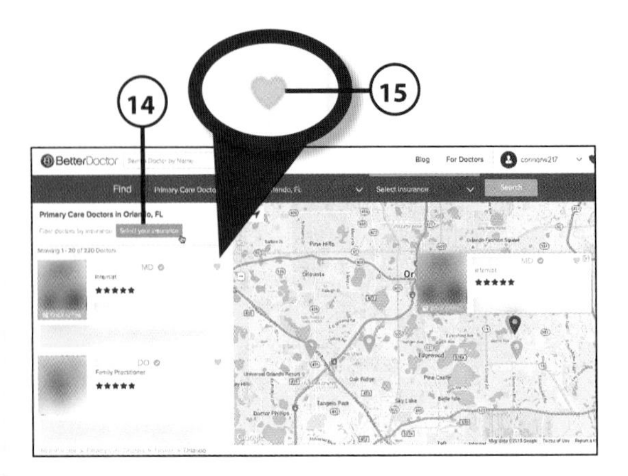

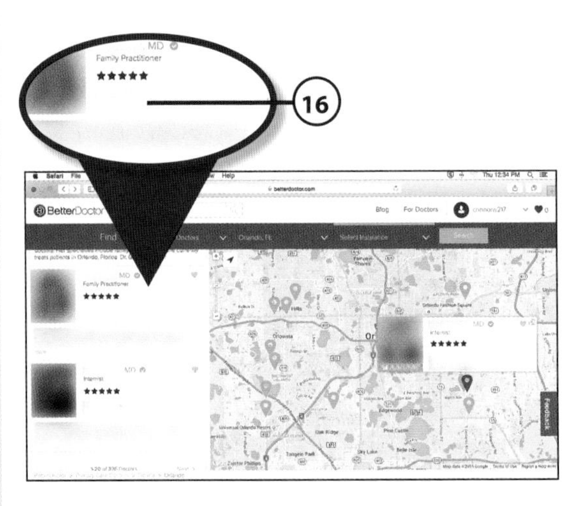

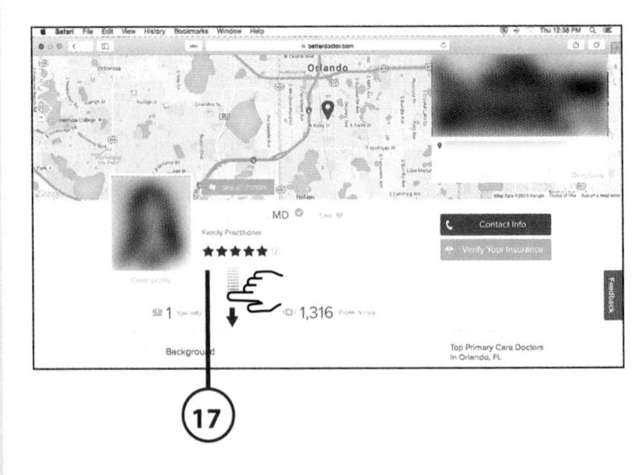

Getting Treatment Online

Services such as Teladoc and Direct Dermatology provide options for you to have video visits with a doctor in the comfort of your own home. You book an appointment online, and then have a two-way video conversation with a specialist on your computer, tablet, or phone. Upload pictures of skin problems for a dermatologist to review. The physicians can diagnose and treat most medical conditions, and can even write prescriptions. There are many online alternatives to the services you learn about here. Take a look at these services and see whether any of them are convenient for you.

Get a Doctor by Phone or Video with Teladoc

Teladoc is an alternative to traditional office visits. You can download the app on the Google Play Store and the App Store. Whether you are traveling, your physician is unavailable, or it's the middle of the night, you can meet with a board-certified doctor who is licensed in your state, twenty-four hours a day, seven days a week. Simply request a consult on the web, phone, or on your Android or Apple (iOS) device, and the doctor will call you back. Teladoc's national network of doctors can make diagnoses, prescribe medications, and send the prescriptions to your local pharmacy. Teladoc is a qualified expense for HSA, FSA, and HRA accounts and can provide you a receipt for deductibles or reimbursement, if needed. Some health plans and employers also cover Teladoc, so check to see whether you might have this type of coverage. To begin, you must first download the app or go online and set up your account with Teladoc. Complete your medical history after the setup process so that the doctors have the information they need. Use the following steps to access a doctor via phone or online video after you have set up your account and filled out your medical history. These steps show the Teladoc app on an iPad.

Common Treatments

Teladoc is NOT equipped to handle medical emergencies. Some of the common conditions patients receive treatment for with Teladoc are cold and flu symptoms, allergies, bronchitis, sinus problems, respiratory infections, pink eye, and ear infections.

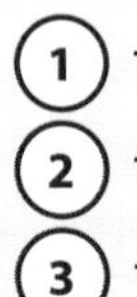

1. Tap the Teladoc app to launch it.
2. Tap Skip to skip the intro.
3. Tap Login on the screen that appears.

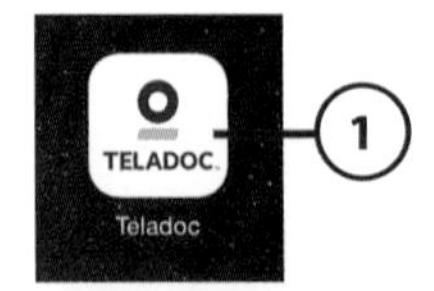

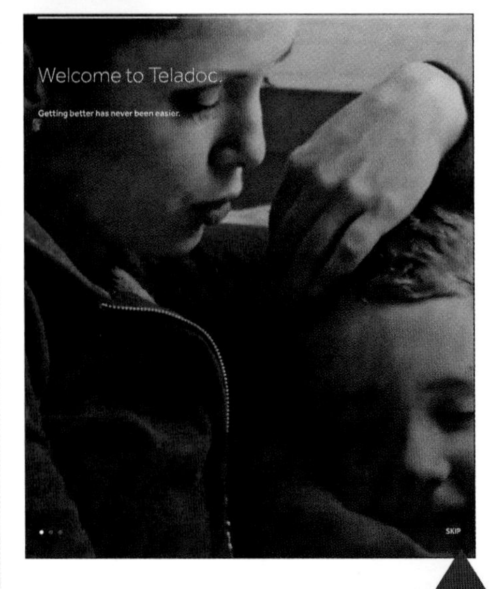

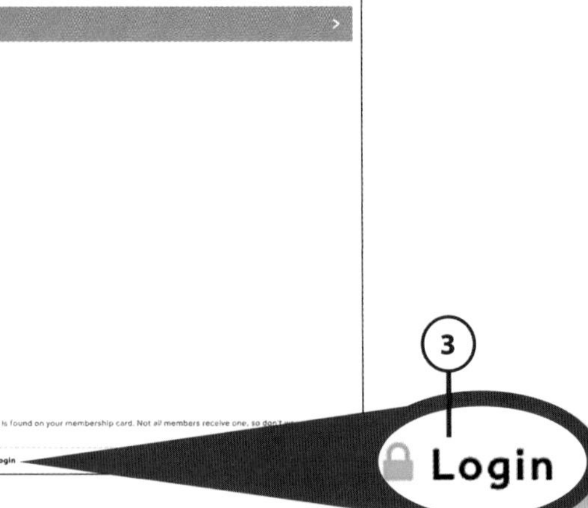

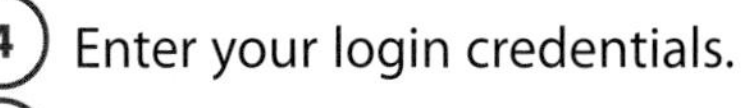

4. Enter your login credentials.
5. Tap Log In.
6. Enter a four-digit code to replace using a password to enter the mobile app, or skip this step. The option to enter a code is skipped in this example.
7. Tap Request a Consult in the screen that appears.
8. Tap I Do in the Who Needs Help Today? screen. You can also tap the dropdown menu to choose a different patient.

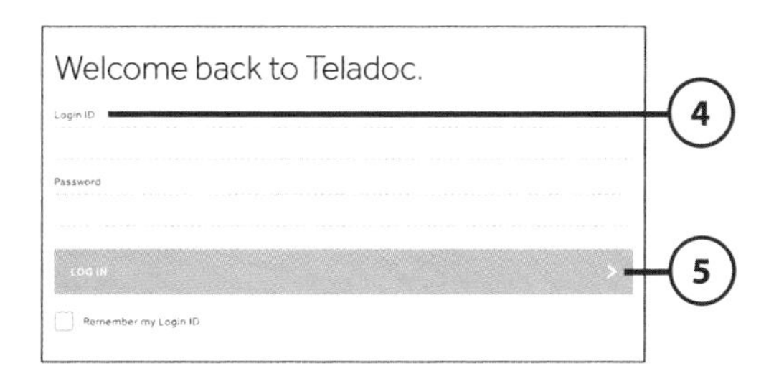

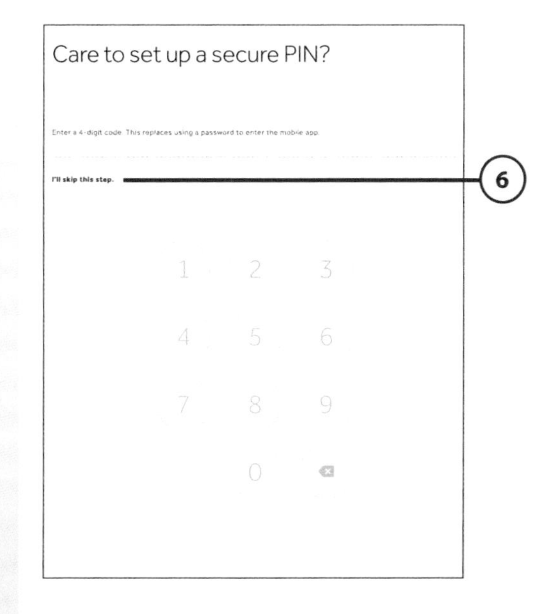
Care to set up a secure PIN?
Enter a 4-digit code. This replaces using a password to enter the mobile app.
I'll skip this step.
1 2 3
4 5 6
7 8 9
0
6

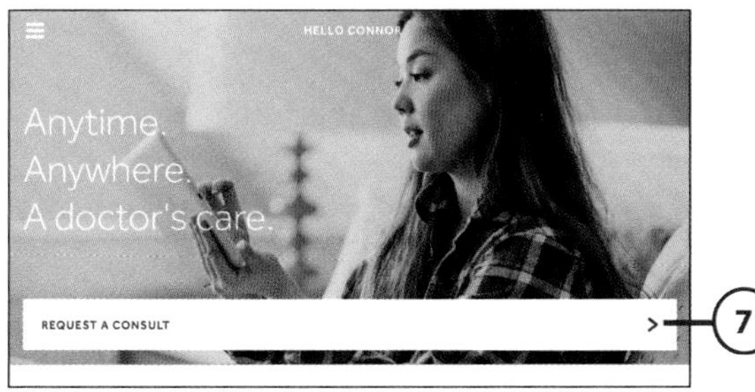
Anytime.
Anywhere.
A doctor's care.
REQUEST A CONSULT
7

Who needs help today?
I DO
8

9. Tap in the Select State field, and then select a state.
10. Tap Next.
11. Tap your preferred way to connect with a doctor. Video Call is chosen in this example.
12. Schedule a time to speak with a doctor by filling out the information on the When Is a Good Time? page.

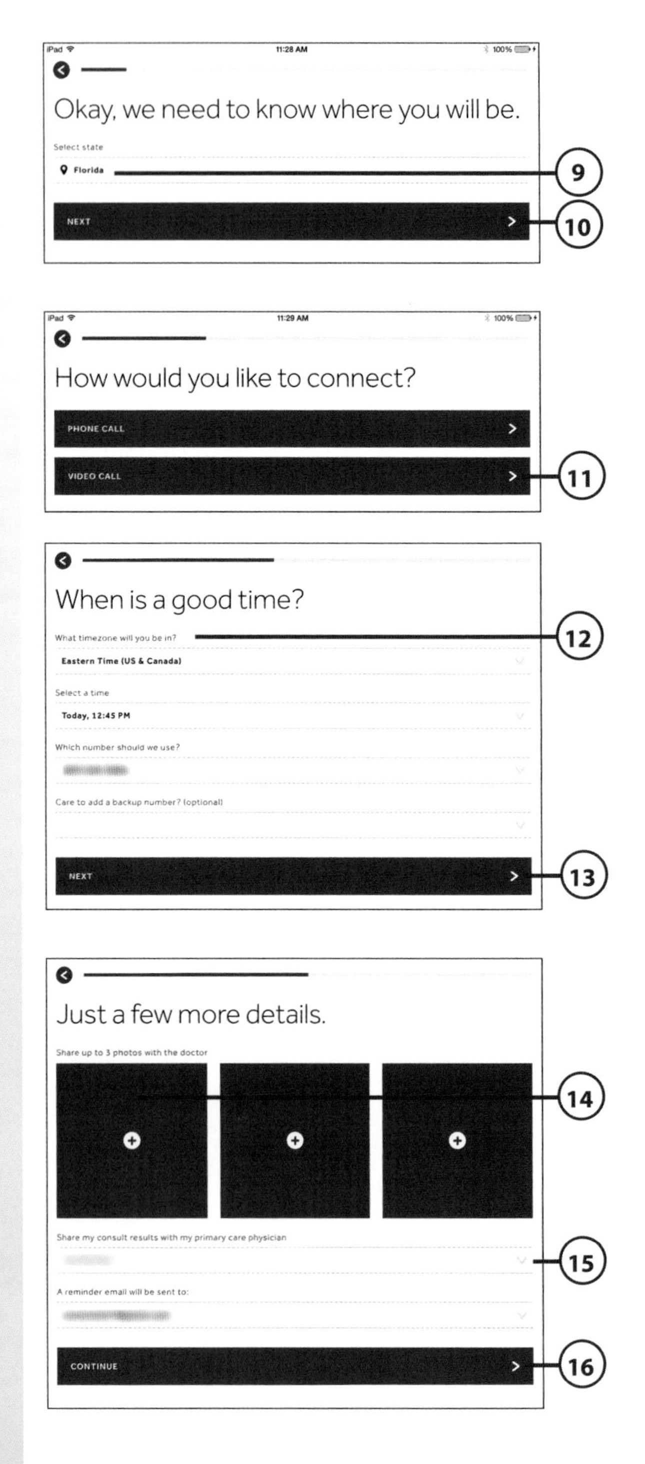

Scheduling Restrictions

You cannot schedule an appointment earlier than an hour before the current time you log in.

13. Tap Next.
14. Tap a square to upload up to three photos from your tablet that may help the doctor to make a diagnosis.
15. Tap the drop-down arrow to share your results with your primary physician.
16. Tap Continue.

17. On the Now, Choose a Pharmacy screen, tap to designate your pharmacy for prescriptions.
18. On the How will you be paying today? screen, tap to choose your method of payment. Credit/Debit Card is used in this example, but you can also pay via PayPal.
19. Enter your payment information.
20. Tap Next.

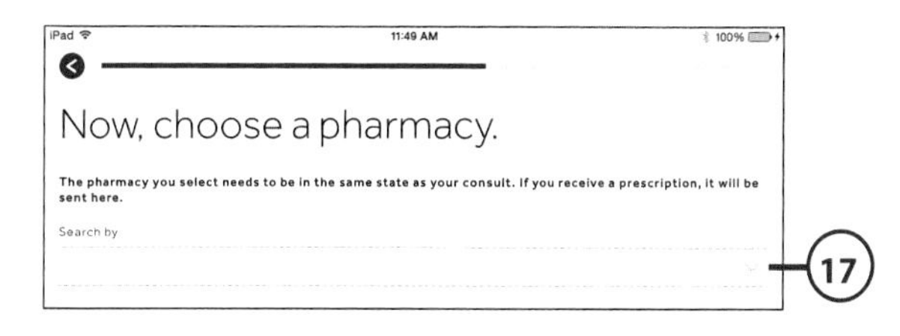

21. At the bottom of the Submit screen, tap the drop-down arrow to let Teladoc know where you would have sought medical help if Teladoc were not an option.
22. Tap Terms and Conditions, and then tap Privacy Policy. Read them both and then tap in the box to certify that you have read each item.
23. Tap Confirm to confirm the appointment. A confirmation code is automatically sent to your email address. A reminder will be sent to you by text message and/or email address 10 minutes before the consult.
24. Tap Continue to return to the main screen.

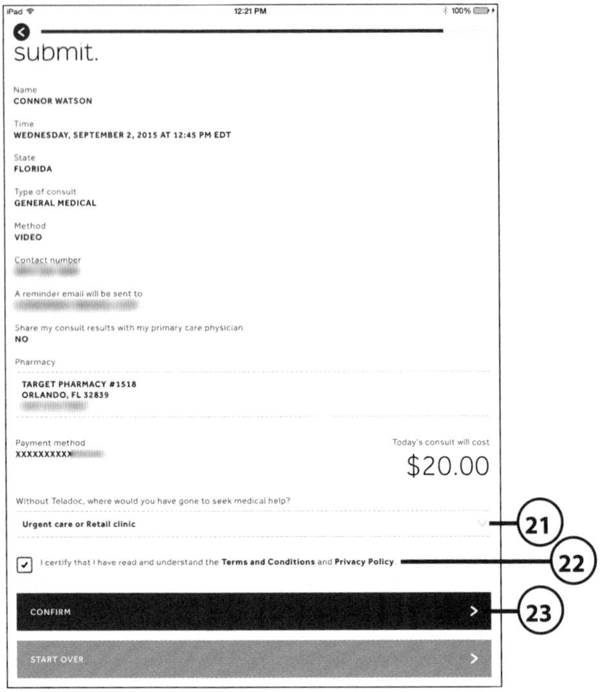

iPad 12:21 PM 100%
submit.
Name
CONNOR WATSON
Time
WEDNESDAY, SEPTEMBER 2, 2015 AT 12:45 PM EDT
State
FLORIDA
Type of consult
GENERAL MEDICAL
Method
VIDEO
Contact number
A reminder email will be sent to
Share my consult results with my primary care physician
NO
Pharmacy
TARGET PHARMACY #1518
ORLANDO, FL 32839
Payment method
XXXXXXXXX
Today's consult will cost
$20.00
Without Teladoc, where would you have gone to seek medical help?
Urgent care or Retail clinic
I certify that I have read and understand the **Terms and Conditions** and **Privacy Policy**
CONFIRM
START OVER
21
22
23

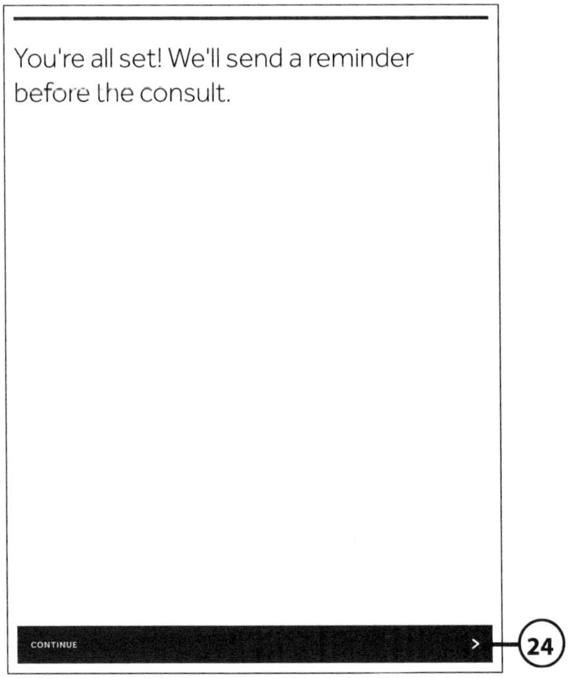

You're all set! We'll send a reminder before the consult.
CONTINUE
24

25. Tap Reschedule to change your current appointment time.
26. Tap the main menu (the three horizontal bars) to access your messages, which can include summaries of your visits, doctor's notes, and your prescriptions. You can also edit your medical history from the main menu.

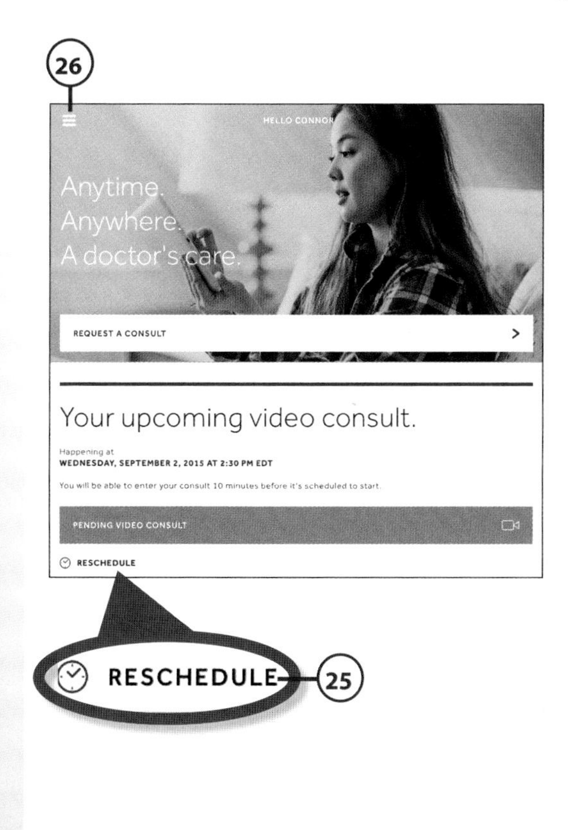

Cancelling a Consultation or Changing a Consultation Type

You can cancel a scheduled consultation or change a consultation type by calling 1-855-835-2362. Check your email and have your confirmation number ready before you call.

Get a Diagnosis and Treatment from Direct Dermatology

Can't get in to see your dermatologist anytime soon? Direct Dermatology is a 24/7, web-based service of online, board-certified dermatologists who can help you with your skin condition. Their dermatologists can also write prescriptions and have them sent to your designated pharmacy. The whole Direct Dermatology process is simple. Sign up for an account, which includes entering your medical history, and then complete a skin evaluation form. Take a photo of your skin problem with a digital camera and upload it to the website. Within two business days, you will receive a notification that your consult report is ready, at which point you can log in to your account to access the report. Direct Dermatology provides services through insurance plans and self-pay. At the time of this writing, Direct Dermatology services are only available to the residents of California and Hawaii. There is currently no app for this service. After you have signed up for an account and filled out the medical history and skin evaluation form, use these steps to receive a consultation.

1. Go to directdermatology.com on your desktop's web browser.
2. Click Patient Login.
3. Enter your login credentials.
4. Click Sign in.
5. Click Start New Case.

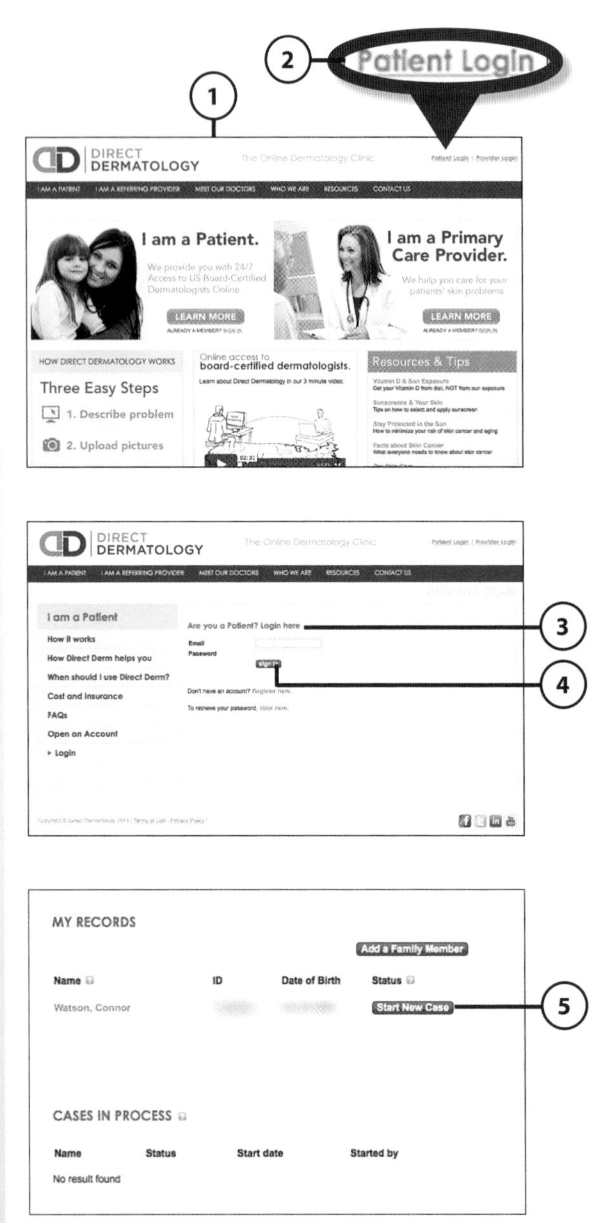

6. Fill out your Demographics info, and then click Save and Continue.
7. Fill out your Insurance info, and then click Save and Continue.
8. Fill out your medical history, and then click Save and Open New Case.

DEMOGRAPHICS

- Please confirm patient's demographics.

* Country of Residence: United States of America
Prefix: ---Select---
* First Name: Connor
Middle Name:
* Last Name: Watson
* Address:
Address 2:
* City:
* State: California
* Zip Code:
Email: com
* Phone:
* Date of Birth:
* Gender: Male Female

* Ethnicity: (Check all that applies)
American Indian Or Alaska Native
Asian
Black Or African American
Hispanic Or Latino
Native Hawaiian Or Pacific Islander
Not Specified
White

Guardian or Emergency contact:
(Required if the patient is a dependent)
Name:
Phone:
Relation to Patient:

Pharmacy: (for prescription pickup)
Pharmacy Search
* Name:
* Address:
* Phone:

<=== Save and Go Back | Save | Save and Continue ===>

1. PATIENT INFO

INSURANCE

Primary Care Physician info (optional)
First Name:
Last Name:
Address:
Address 2:
City:
State: California
Zip Code:
Country: United States of America
Phone:
Fax:

Do we have permission to contact your PCP with your results?
Yes No

* Insurance Plan: ---Select---
Plan name:
Insured ID #:
Prior Auth. #:
Valid Dates:

Secondary Insurances (optional)
Plan name:
Insured ID #:

Insured person is different from patient

<=== Save and Go Back | Save | Save and Continue ===>

Medical Problem List

* Please list your current medical problems (OTHER than for the current skin problem)
(or click 'None' if you have none)
None

Drug Allergies

Are you allergic to the following drugs?
No Allergies

* Penicillin: Yes No
* Cephalosporin: Yes No
* Sulfa: Yes No
* Tetracycline: Yes No
* Aspirin: Yes No
* Other: Yes No

History Of Skin Condition

Do you or your parents or siblings have a history of any of the following skin conditions?

	You	Your Family
Skin Cancer:	Yes No	Yes No
Melanoma:	Yes No	Yes No
Eczema:	Yes No	Yes No
Psoriasis:	Yes No	Yes No

<=== Save and Return to My Account | Save | Save and Open New Case ===>

9. Fill out the information for your current skin complaint, and then click Save and Continue.
10. Read the instructions for uploading pictures, and then take two photos of your skin condition with a digital camera: one close-up and one showing a larger area of your body. You can do this with your phone if it meets the specifications listed on the Direct Dermatology website. Make sure you upload those digital photos to your computer.
11. Click Choose File and upload both photos to the website.
12. Click Upload Pictures. The uploaded pictures appear at the bottom of the screen.

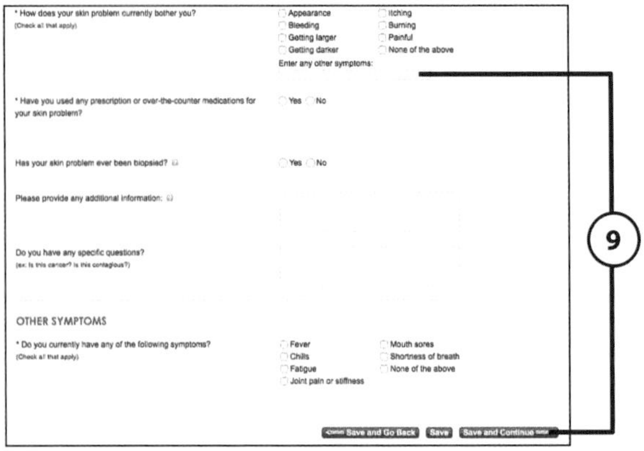

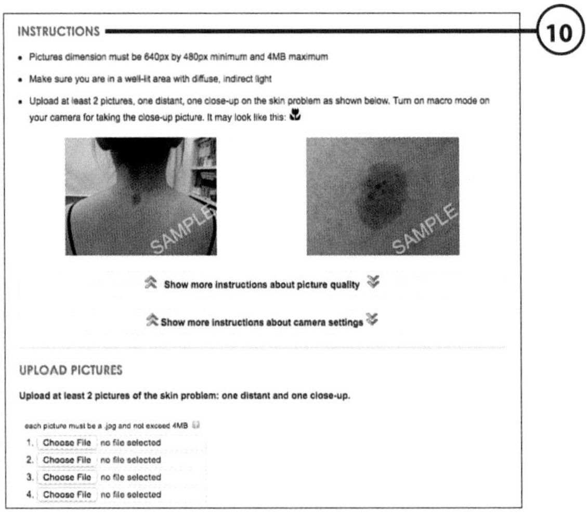

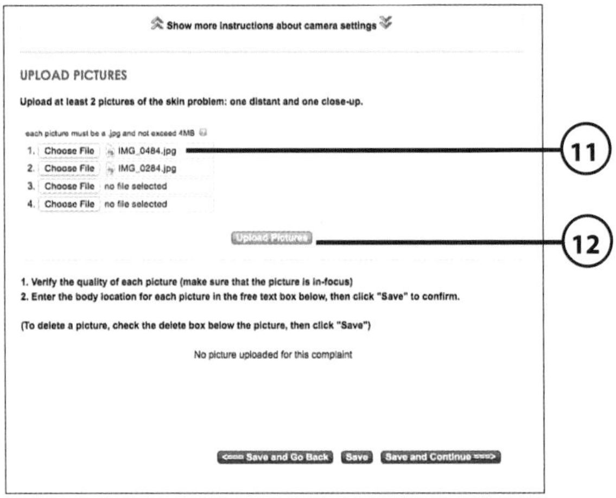

13. Click in the boxes, and then enter the body location for each photo. Make sure you read all the onscreen instructions.
14. Click Save and Continue.
15. Read the Terms of Service, and then click I Accept.
16. Click Submit and Proceed to Payment.
17. Enter your payment information, and then click Continue and follow the prompts to complete your case. You will receive a doctor's report regarding your case within two business days.

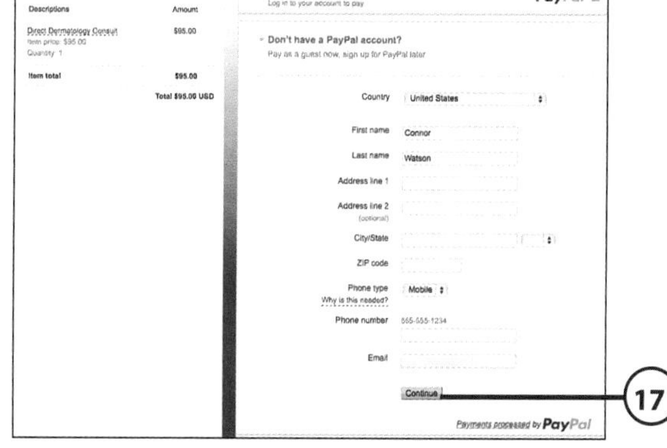

>>>Go Further

ASK A DERMATOLOGIST WITH FIRST DERM

First Derm enables you to receive professional input about a skin condition from a board-certified dermatologist. This paid service is available online and also has a free First Derm app for Android Phones and the iPhone. First Derm is available wherever you are, and your case is answered by a dermatologist in your area. No login information is required. Simply take two pictures of the affected area and upload them on the website (firstderm.com) or by using the app. Describe the affected area and provide some personal details, including city and country. First Derm offers a 24-hour response time. As of this writing, First Derm cannot write prescriptions. Many cases reviewed by First Derm can be treated with over-the-counter drugs. If you need a doctor's visit, the website and app can direct you to the nearest dermatologist and pharmacist. Visit firstderm.com to learn more and download the First Derm app from the Google Play Store and the App Store.

Accessing Adult Care Resources

Many online resources can help you take the guesswork out of finding the right care options. Whether it's finding the right hospital or doctor or finding someone to run errands, do light housekeeping, provide companionship, or provide 24-hour care, sites such as Care.com and CareLinx.com can help you find quality care. Each site offers a unique set of care services. Care.com and CareLinx.com offer in-home and holistic care options including exercise/mobility, mental stimulation, meal preparation, housekeeping, and other personal care needs. These are but a mere fraction of the care resources available to you. All you need to do is perform an Internet search, ask a friend or family member, or discuss adult care resources in online communities to see that there are many. Here are a few very efficient ways to find quality care.

Search for Adult Care, Reviews, and Resources

Do a quick search on the Internet, and you can find many websites that offer adult care, reviews for services and providers, resources, and so-called "diagnoses." But are they credible? How do their services really measure up to others?

Let's first take a look at the Internet search as a means of gathering information about your health.

A common practice for many of us is to start entering symptoms into a search engine in an attempt to learn more about what ails us. What we tend to find on the Internet is that we could be either suffering from the common cold or have some life-threatening illness. My primary care physician has frustratingly referred to this type of self-diagnosing as consulting "Dr. Internet." Although it is empowering and useful to have so much health information at the tip of your fingers, it is no substitute for seeing a real physician. The problem with "Dr. Internet" is that the information you receive can be incomplete and untrustworthy. It can be hard to tell whether real doctors have vetted the information you are receiving. When taken out of context, the information you find can sometimes prove unnecessarily scary. It's okay to share your findings on the Internet with your doctor, but by all means, let a doctor do the diagnosing.

Searches on health-related conditions are among the most popular searches performed on Google. To aid consumers in finding fact-based information on specific conditions, Google has taken big steps toward making sure that doctors have vetted the medical information they return to you. Google is working closely with the Mayo Clinic and its own medical doctors to curate and review the accuracy of the information you receive from Google during a search.

In 2015, Google also more than doubled its ever-expanding health conditions database to around 900 conditions and improved its health information pages so that you can view the information that you need in a quick glance on your desktop or mobile device. Google now uses medical illustrations and offers downloadable PDFs that you can take with you to your doctor's visit. Just know that this information is not exhaustive and should not be used as a substitute for a real doctor examination.

1. Go to Google.com, or open the Google app on your iOS or Android device. These steps are shown on a computer browser.
2. Type in the health-related condition you want to search, and press Enter or click the magnifying glass icon. Google's results are shown as a card directly beneath the first ad on a mobile device or as a panel on the right side of the screen on a computer's browser. Note that Google's results appear differently than the rest of the search results.

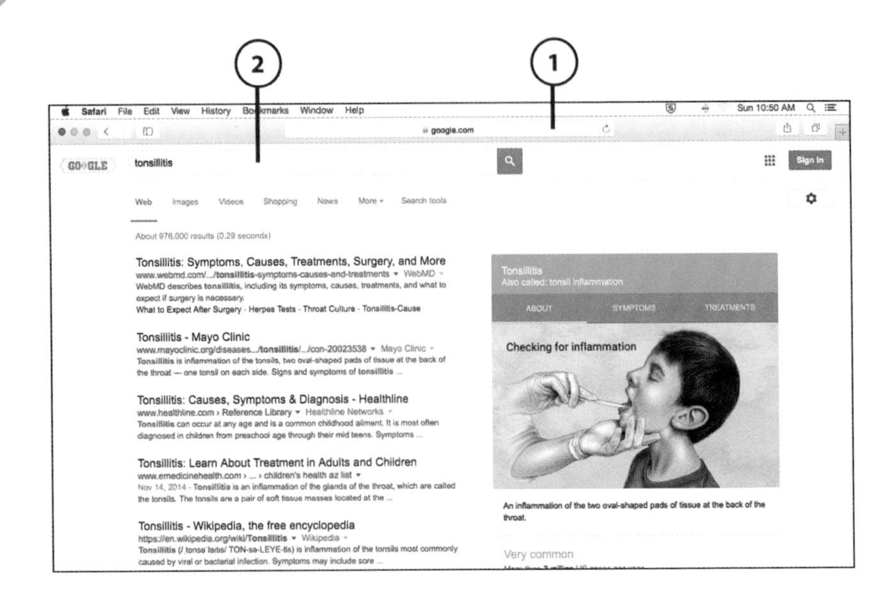

The AARP online community is full of real people with whom you can talk about products and services you might be considering. The AARP website is not only a great place to start your search for health care-related topics, but also might prove to be your home base for any other topics you want to research.

AARP website resources

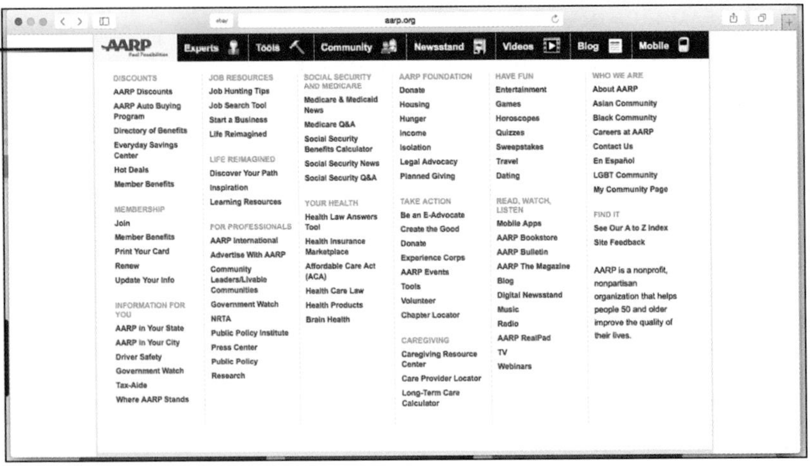

The aarp.org website is filled with many resources of its own, including health tools, money tools, work and retirement resources, home and family resources, and caregiving tools. Get to know some of the latest health products on AARP's

Health Products blog. If you have become a caregiver and need some advice in juggling life, work, and caregiving, AARP's Caregiving Resource Center offers many resources to help you not neglect your own mental and physical health, while caring for those you love. Their Care Provider Locater can help you find the right care for your loved one. The options listed provide ratings and many customer reviews that can help you make an informed decision. This example screen is located at the bottom of the aarp.org main webpage.

AARP Provider Locator

search.seniorliving.aarp.org
Search Results
Caring.com
Find another community
In-Home Care Providers
32839
Search
★★★★★
1 review
Visiting Angels
Orlando, FL 32809
No Photo
0 reviews
Seniors First, Inc.
Orlando, FL 32811
No Photo
Assisted Home Care, Inc
Orlando, FL 32806
No Photo
Learn More
Daytona Beach
New Smyrna Beach
Sanford
Kissimmee
Cape Canaveral
Cocoa Beach
Melbourne
Palm Bay
Sebastian
Map
Satellite
Map data ©2015 Google
Terms of Use

Senior Resource Alliance website

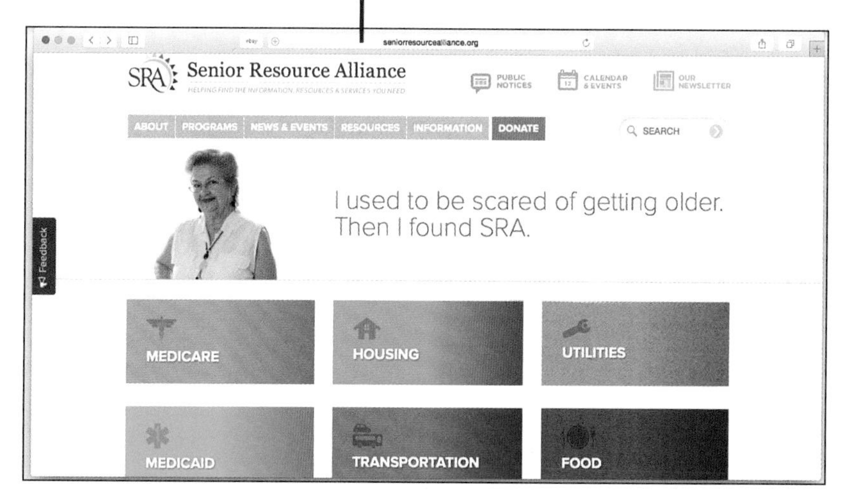

The Senior Resource Alliance is another great resource for aging with vitality. Visit seniorresourcealliance.org to access many solutions for health care, caregiving, nutrition, lifelong learning, transportation, and many other programs.

Discover the Adult Care Options Available at Care.com

Care.com is an online marketplace for finding and managing family care. Among their specialties is adult care. If you are looking for a more holistic approach to care, care.com offers categories such as Companion care and Personal care. These services range from errand help, light housekeeping, and transportation, to bathing and dressing, exercise and mobility needs, and medication reminders. Care.com can also help with dementia and Alzheimer's care, including companionship, mental stimulation, and 24-hour care. To look for a caregiver you must create a job, review the candidates who contact you, hire a caregiver, and then pay for your care.

Care.com is web-based and also has apps available for Android phones, the iPhone, and tablets. The apps are free to download. Regardless of how you access care.com, you first need to create an account. After you have created an account, use the following steps to take advantage of care.com's adult care resources. These steps show the care.com website via computer access.

1. Go to care.com on your desktop's web browser.
2. Click Log In.
3. Enter your login credentials. You can also log in using an existing Facebook account by clicking Sign In with Facebook. Click in the Remember me box to deselect this option if you don't want care.com to remember your password whenever you go to the site.
4. Click Log In.
5. View your current location to see whether it is correct. Care.com should automatically detect your current location. If it does not, click in the field to enter a new Zip code. If you scroll down, this page has many helpful articles that you might find useful concerning adult care. A blog on all things adult care also offers expert advice from a licensed social worker.

6. Click Seniors. Under this tab you find resources for senior housing, home care agencies, home care individuals, special needs caregivers, transportation needs, and more.
7. Click Senior Care Start Here.

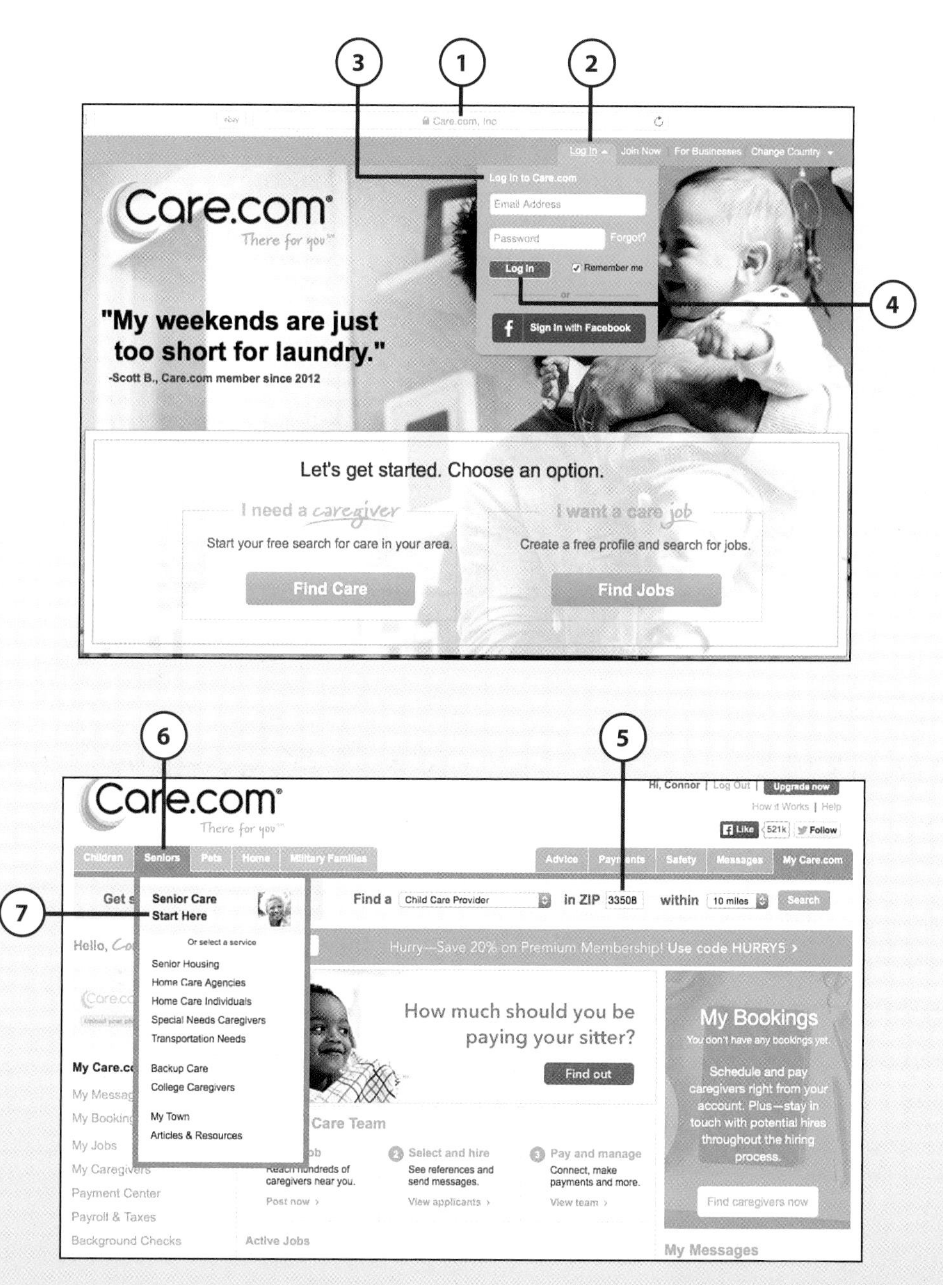

Social Media Privacy Issues

Logging in via Facebook can pose privacy issues by giving the app access to your social media data. Consider creating new login credentials.

Upgrade Your Membership by Subscribing

To take full advantage of care.com, you must pay to upgrade your membership. If you don't have a membership, you cannot message caregivers or post jobs. Tap the orange Upgrade now button in the upper-right corner of the screen to view the Standard, All Access, and Concierge subscription benefits.

8. Click Post a Job in the screen that appears.

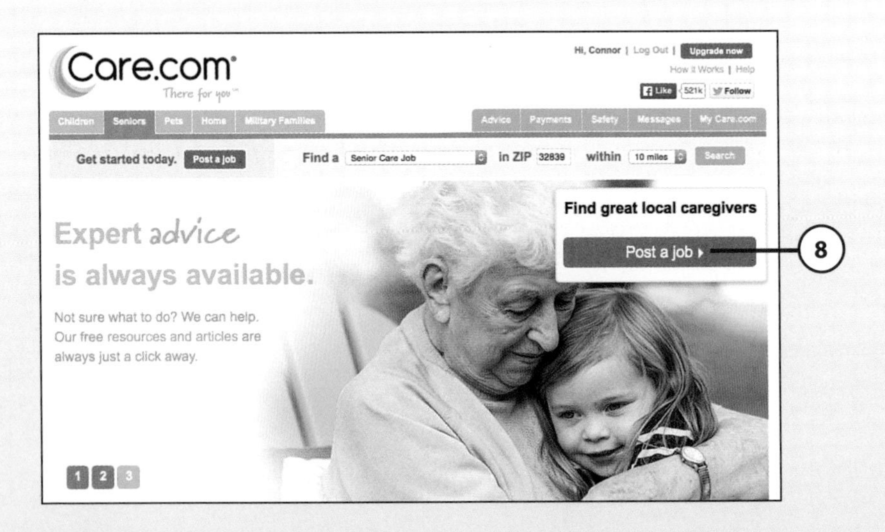

9. Click Senior Care. A screen opens that enables you to create a job.

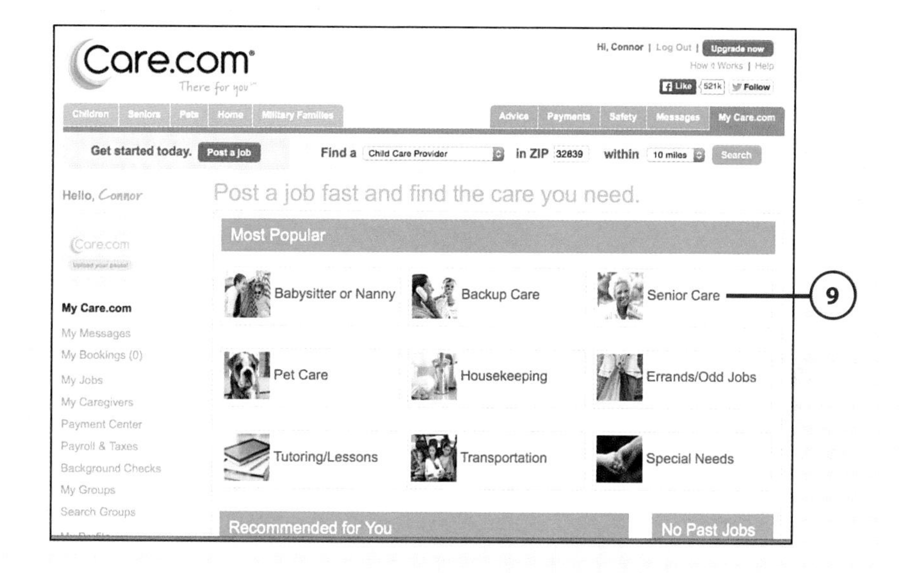

10. Fill out the information to create a job for the care you need. This is where you can choose specific job details including Errands/Shopping, Light Housekeeping, Meal Preparation, and more.

Payment Center
Payroll & Taxes
Background Checks
My Groups
Search Groups
My Profile
Account & Settings
My Stats

My caregivers online
Add caregivers to your list of favorites or maybes. You'll be able to contact them right from here when they're online!

Available Unavailable

	Sun.	Mon.	Tue.	Wed.	Thu.	Fri.	Sat.
Select All	☐	☐	☐	☐	☐	☐	☐
Early Morning (6am-9am)	☐	☐	☐	☐	☐	☐	☐
Late Morning (9am-12pm)	☐	☐	☑	☐	☐	☑	☐
Early Afternoon (12pm -3 pm)	☐	☐	☐	☐	☐	☐	☐
Late Afternoon (3pm-6pm)	☐	☐	☐	☐	☐	☐	☐
Early Evening (6pm-9pm)	☐	☐	☐	☐	☐	☐	☐
Late Evening (9pm-12am)	☐	☐	☐	☐	☐	☐	☐
Overnight (12am-6am)	☐	☐	☐	☐	☐	☐	☐

Where do you need care: 32839

JOB DETAILS *

The person who needs care is in his / her: 70s

The person who needs care is my: Father

My loved one suffers from Alzheimer's / Dementia: ○ Yes ◉ No

Type of Caregiver
◉ Companion Care ○ Hands-on Care
○ Live-in Home Care ○ Respite Care

Services needed:
☐ Feeding ☐ Meal Preparation ☐ Light Housekeeping
☐ Bathing / Dressing ☐ Transportation ☐ Medication Management
☐ Companionship ☑ Errands / Shopping

10

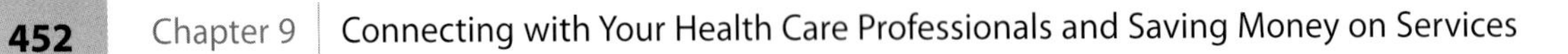

11. Scroll down the page to continue filling out all fields, and then click Save & Continue.

Feeding
Bathing / Dressing
Companionship
Meal Preparation
Transportation
Errands / Shopping
Light Housekeeping
Medication Management

My Ideal Caregiver:
Has Own Transportation
Non-smoker
Comfortable with Pets

High school degree

PAY RATE
$15 - $25 /hr
$10 $15 $20 $25 $30 $35 $40 $45 $50

PAYMENT PREFERENCES
How do you plan to pay your caregiver? (Check any that might apply.)
Credit Card
Cash
Payroll Service
Check

**With limited exceptions (such as casual babysitters) virtually all caregiver jobs are subject to federal, state and local (where applicable) minimum wage laws. Families are responsible as household employers for complying with all applicable minimum wage laws, plus payroll, tax and other labor laws regarding employment of care providers.

Save & Continue ▸ (11)

12. Click in the fields and personalize your job post.

13. Click Submit. Your home page reappears, where you can manage your account and jobs.

Hello, Connor

Post a job and find the care you need, fast

Personalize your job post.
Stand out from other families looking for help! Share additional details about what you're looking for, and you're more likely to attract the perfect caregiver!

My Care.com
My Messages
My Bookings (0)
My Jobs
My Caregivers
Payment Center
Payroll & Taxes
Background Checks
My Groups
Search Groups
My Profile
Account & Settings
My Stats

Job Post Title
Companion Care-Orlando

Description
We need companion care to take care of my father in Orlando. Part of your responsibilities will include running errands.

(12)

120/2,500

My caregivers online
Add caregivers to your list of favorites or maybes. You'll be able to contact them right from here

**With limited exceptions (such as casual babysitters) virtually all caregiver jobs are subject to federal, state and local (where applicable) minimum wage laws. Families are responsible as household employers for complying with all applicable minimum wage laws, plus payroll, tax and other labor laws regarding employment of care providers.

Submit ▸ (13)

14. Look under the Active Jobs section to view the caregivers who apply to the job you posted.

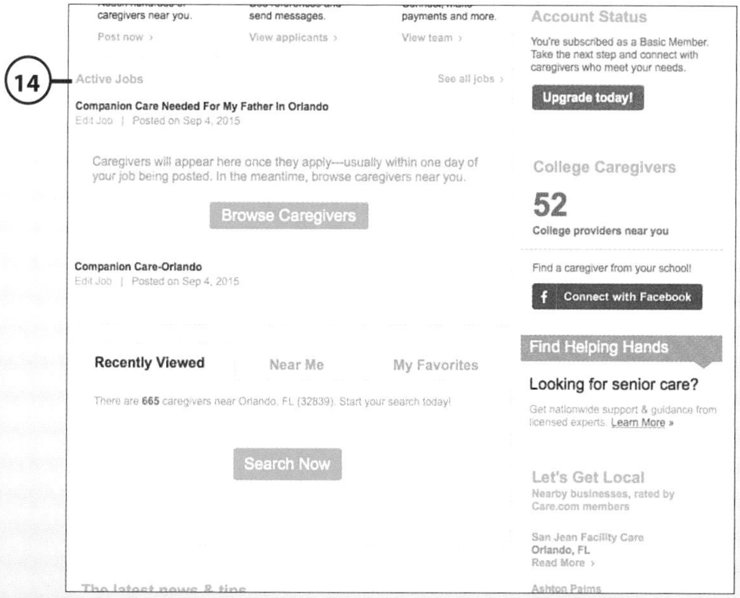

>>>Go Further

VETTING PROSPECTIVE CAREGIVERS

After caregivers apply to the job you posted, handle the process like you would a job interview. You can access caregivers' background checks directly from their profile. Schedule a time to talk with them on the phone and to meet with them in person. Care.com provides a lot of information on what types of questions you can ask during an interview, including posing hypotheticals to see how a caregiver might respond in specific situations. Whenever you hire someone, you can pay through the care.com website or app.

Find Your Caregiver at CareLinx.com

CareLinx is a nationwide network of home care providers that makes it easy and efficient to find as well as manage ongoing employment with the perfect caregiver for less than what it would cost through a traditional agency. You can find professionals at all levels including part-time visiting nurses, live-in caregivers, and companion care. Every caregiver has gone through a screening process and is insured and bonded. You can also choose to use CareLinx Verified Caregivers, who have been interviewed by the CareLinx team, have had references checked, have had complete background checks completed, and have profile pictures included so you have confidence in the person you are hiring. The CareLinx site enables you to filter caregivers by criteria including certifications, experience, and more. The process is simple: Fill out a brief survey to find a caregiver who fits your needs in a given location. Work with a Care Advisor who will walk you through the interview process and handle the paperwork to hire a caregiver. You can then easily manage all your scheduling and payments online.

Carelinx.com is web-based, and as of this writing, does not offer any apps. There is a mobile version of the site, so you can go to carelinx.com on your phone and browse an optimized version of the website. To start using CareLinx, you first need to create an account. To take full advantage of all CareLinx services, you must pay to upgrade your membership. Use the following steps to find the perfect caregiver. These steps are performed on the carelinx.com website.

1. Go to carelinx.com on your desktop's web browser.
2. Click the drop-down menu to specify who needs care.
3. Click the drop-down menu to specify where the person who needs care is located.
4. Click Get Started.

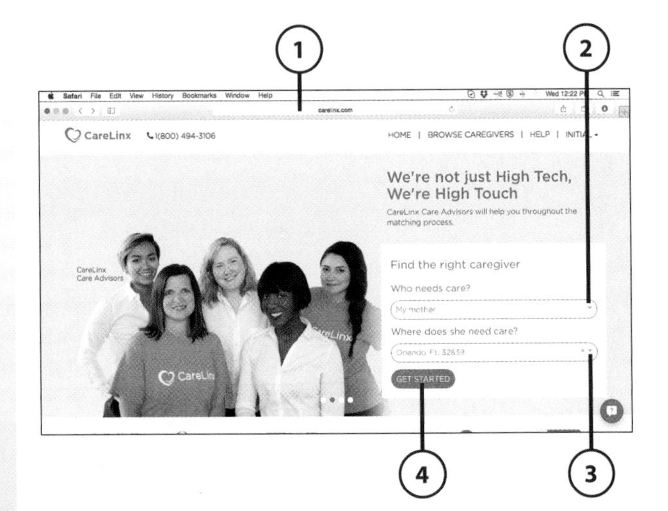

5. Click Start.
6. Click on the icons of the daily activities for which help is needed.
7. Enter any special concerns a caregiver needs to be aware of and describe the person who needs care. These sections are optional, but help to clarify the care needed.
8. Click Next at the bottom of the screen to proceed to the next screen.
9. Tell CareLinx about your care schedule.
10. Click Next at the bottom of the screen.

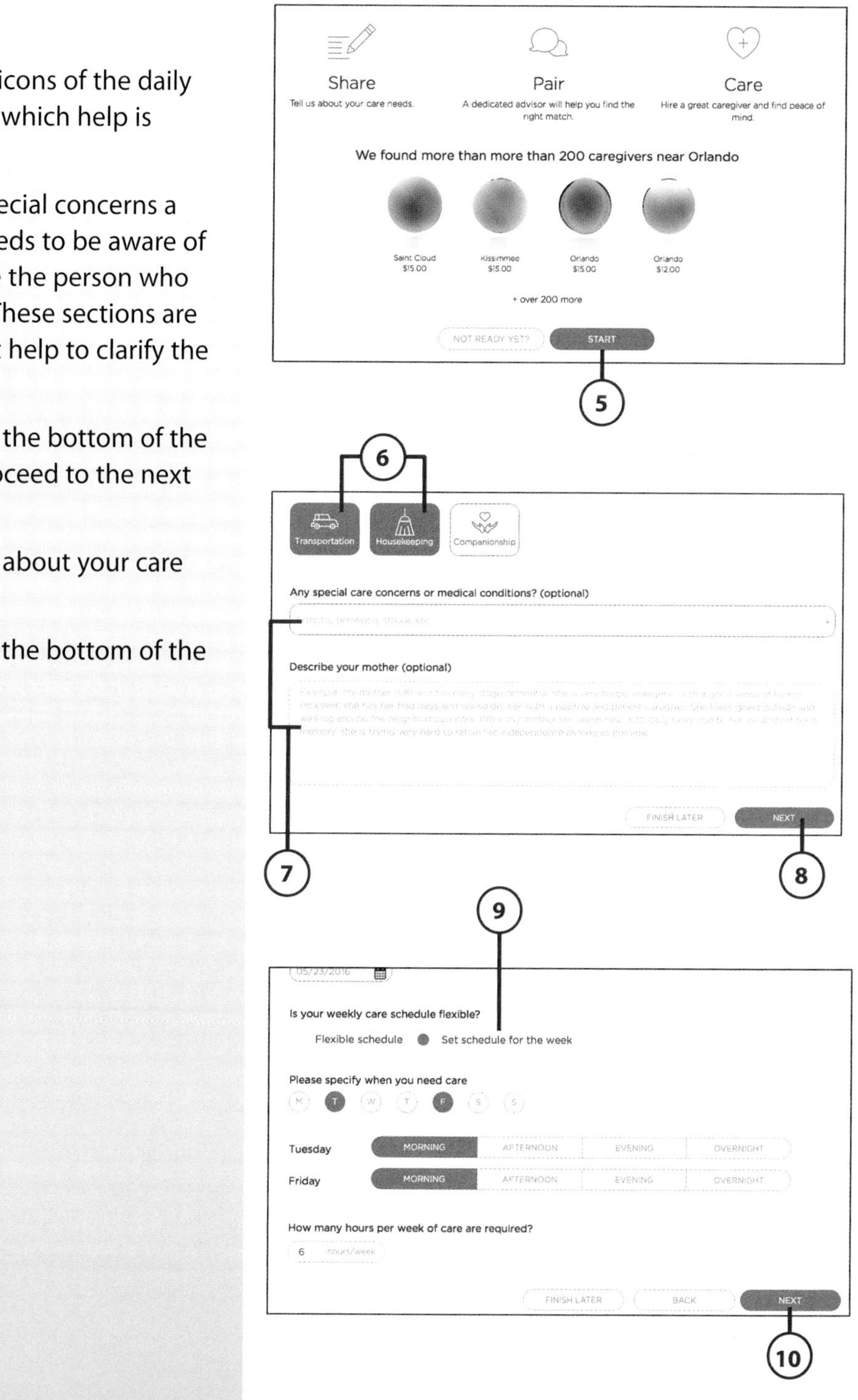

11. Specify what you want in a caregiver by filling out the information.
12. Tap Next.
13. Review your care summary details, and then click Next.

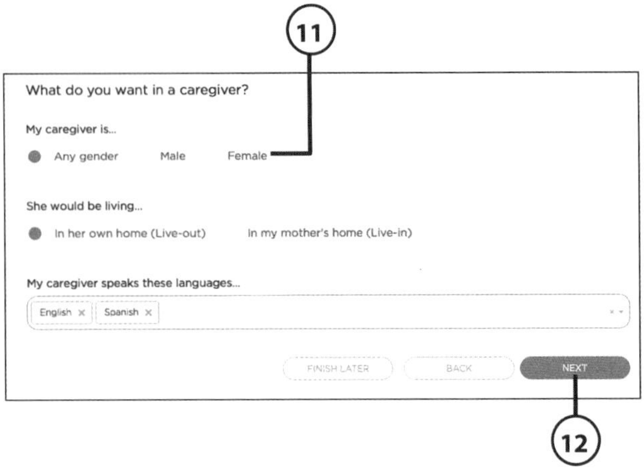

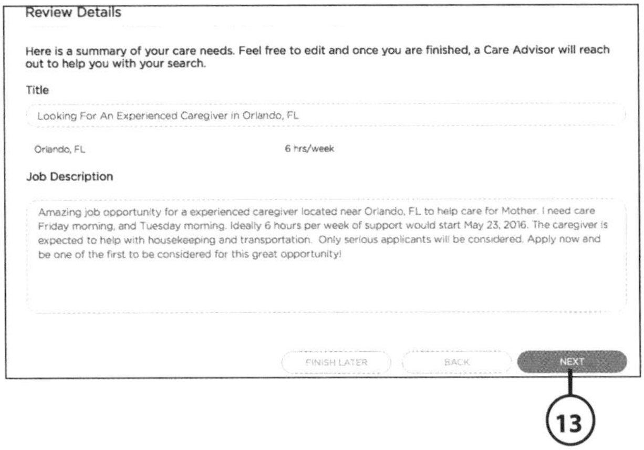

What do you want in a caregiver?

My caregiver is...

Any gender Male Female

She would be living...

In her own home (Live-out) In my mother's home (Live-in)

My caregiver speaks these languages...

English × Spanish ×

FINISH LATER BACK NEXT

Review Details

Here is a summary of your care needs. Feel free to edit and once you are finished, a Care Advisor will reach out to help you with your search.

Title

Looking For An Experienced Caregiver in Orlando, FL

Orlando, FL 6 hrs/week

Job Description

Amazing job opportunity for a experienced caregiver located near Orlando, FL to help care for Mother. I need care Friday morning, and Tuesday morning. Ideally 6 hours per week of support would start May 23, 2016. The caregiver is expected to help with housekeeping and transportation. Only serious applicants will be considered. Apply now and be one of the first to be considered for this great opportunity!

FINISH LATER BACK NEXT

Be Aware of Tax Obligations

Hiring an independent caregiver or senior care provider obligates you to certain payroll taxes in the U.S. If you use an agency to find these services, the agency will take care of these details. If you use a service such as Care.com or CareLinx.com to directly hire in-home care, these services offer a lot of assistance to help you understand the taxes, manage payments, and prepare returns. Check out www.carelinx.com/help/payroll-taxes/ for more information.

---

14. Add your contact information to receive potential caregiver matches.
15. Tap Done to view a list of suggested caregivers with rates and bios that include special skills, languages, services, years of experience, and some personal information. A CareLinx Care advisor will contact you shortly to take you through the process of scheduling interviews with pre-screened caregivers.

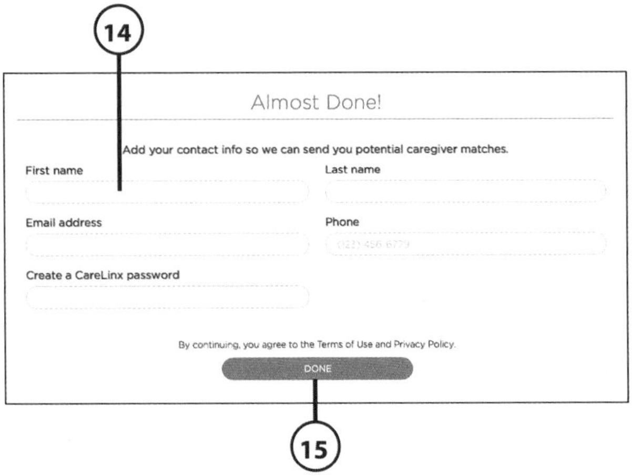

Almost Done!

Add your contact info so we can send you potential caregiver matches.

First name Last name

Email address Phone

Create a CareLinx password

By continuing, you agree to the Terms of Use and Privacy Policy.

DONE

Preventing Paying Too Much for Health Procedures and Medication

Even if you have health insurance or Medicare, hospital stays, required tests, emergency room visits, procedures, and medication regiments can leave you paying exorbitant fees. Resources such as CoPatient and WeRx can help you save money by negotiating unpaid medical bills or by comparing prices for medication, so you can make the most cost-efficient choices. Why pay more than you have to? Take a look at the following services to see whether they can help you save money.

Use Medical Billing Experts at CoPatient to Ensure You're Not Paying Too Much for Unpaid Bills

CoPatient is a medical bill review and negotiation service whose goal is to help you save money. Expert medical bill advocates analyze your bills using software programs to detect billing and coding errors, and then negotiate with hospitals to lower what you pay. To get started, all you need to do is create a CoPatient Account, and then send in your unpaid bills by uploading to the CoPatient website by email, by fax, or by traditional mail. CoPatient analyzes and reviews your bills, and then delivers you a free report. After you receive your free savings report, you can decide whether you want to pay for CoPatient's services to negotiate and secure the savings with your provider(s).

CoPatient.com is a web service and has an app available for the iPhone and iPad. The app is free to download, but the services provided online and in the app have a fee. You must first sign up for a CoPatient account. After you have signed up, use the following steps to have medical billing experts working to save you money. These steps show accessing the copatient.com website via computer.

1. Go to copatient.com on your desktop's web browser.
2. Click Sign In/Up, and then click Sign In.
3. Sign in using your credentials, and then click Sign In. If this is your first time logging in, the Welcome to the CoPatient Dashboard! dialog box appears. If it isn't your first time logging in, go to step 5.

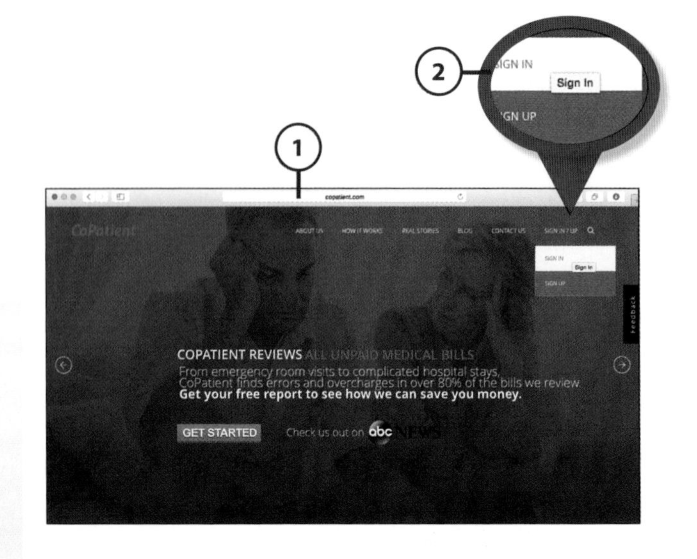

Get to Know the CoPatient Dashboard

The Dashboard contains all the tools you need to manage your health care bills. You can interact with your billing advocate, manage health care expenses, create new cases to be investigated, and allow your Billing Advocate to access to your health information.

Sign In

Username:

Password:

Forgot Password?

Sign In

3

4. Read the Welcome to the CoPatient Dashboard! dialog box to learn more about what you can do in the Dashboard, and then click the X in the upper-right corner to close the box. The CoPatient Dashboard appears.

Welcome to the CoPatient Dashboard! X 4

Everything you need to manage your healthcare bills can be found in one place.

To Do / Notifications
Interact with your Billing Advocate if you have questions about your medical bills or health benefits.

Cases
Don't understand your medical bills? Create a case, then track progress as your Billing Advocate investigates your bills.

Patients
Use one CoPatient Account to manage healthcare expenses for your entire family.

Authorization (!)
Allow your Billing Advocate to access your personal health information by filling out this form

5. Click Add Case to begin the submission process for your unpaid medical bills.
6. Click to choose how you want to submit your documents (upload files, mail documents, fax documents). Upload Files was chosen for this example.

7. Click Upload Files.
8. Browse to the desired file(s), select it, and then click Choose on a Mac or Open on a PC. The file(s) upload.
9. Click Upload More if you have more files to upload, or click Done. Done is chosen in this example.
10. Click Done.

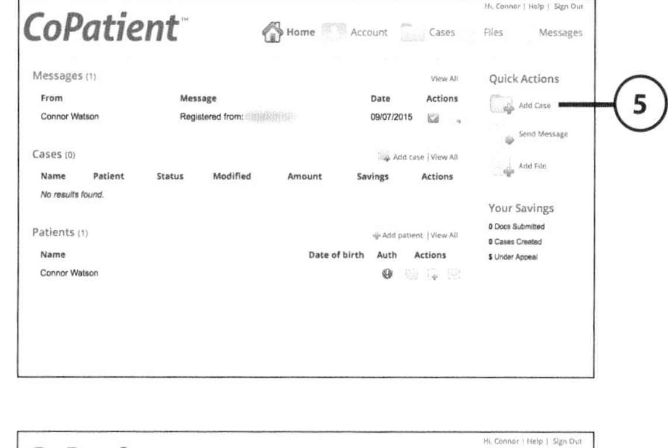

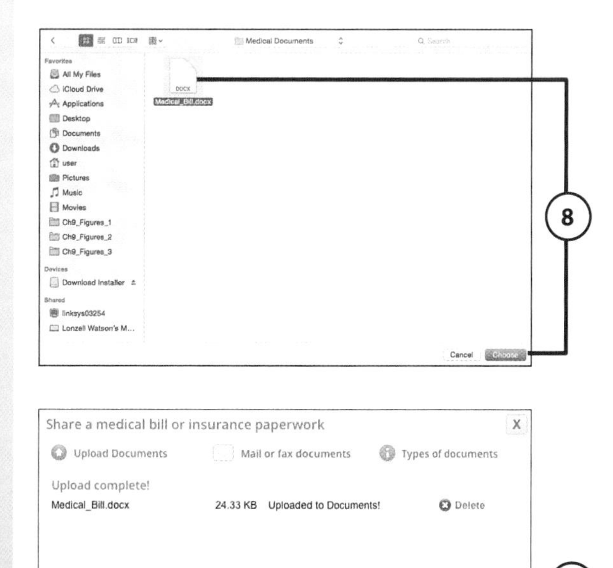

11. Click one of the empty circles to choose whom this bill applies to.
12. Enter the birth date for the individual in the Date of Birth field.
13. Select the Gender.
14. Enter an optional expiration date to limit the time period you authorize CoPatient to access your personal health information.
15. Click Finish Authorization.
16. Fill out the Authorization Form, and then click Sign at the bottom of the page.

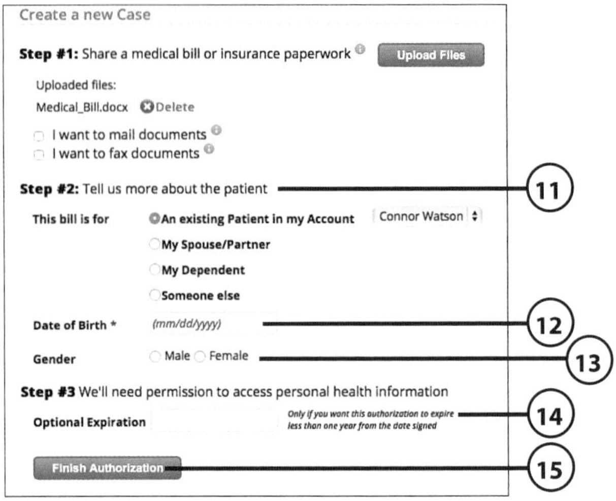

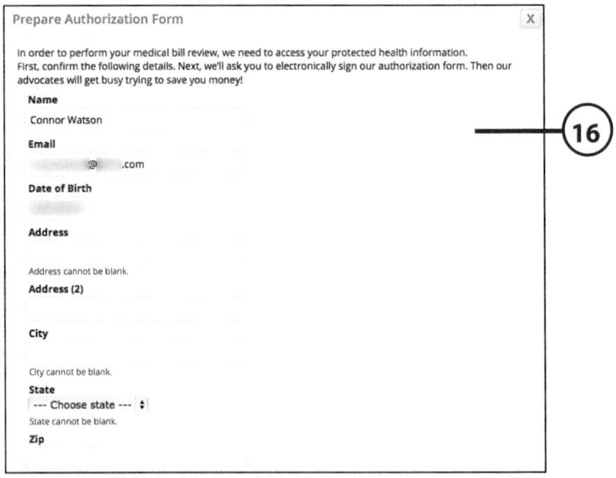

17. Read the Authorization Form, and then sign with your mouse on the signature pad at the bottom.
18. Click Submit Signature to have advocates start the process of trying to save you money.

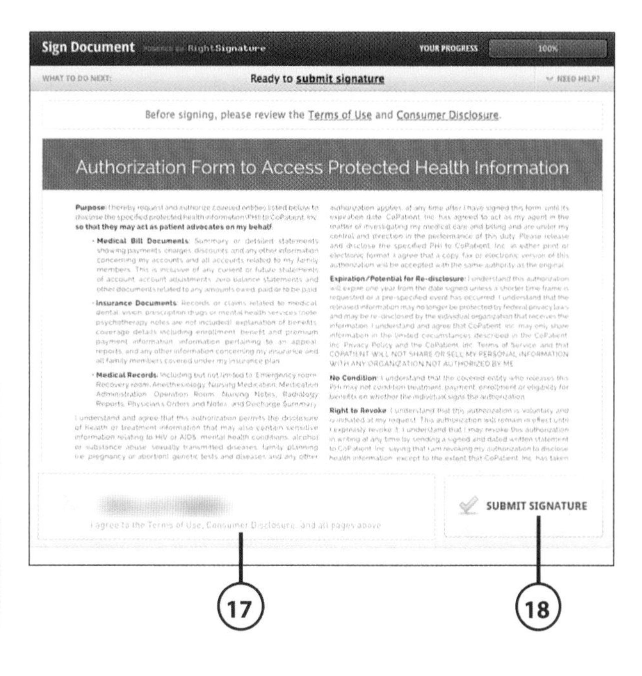

Compare Prescription Prices and Get Prescription Coupons at WeRx

WeRx is a free tool that helps you find a better price for the same prescription medication you take. Users report and compare prices between pharmacies right in your neighborhood so you can find the best price. Simply enter in a medication (brand name or generic), and then enter your location information. WeRx displays the different price points on a map of your vicinity so you can compare local and online prices and share prices with others. You also have access to cost-saving coupons that you can redeem.

WeRx.com is web-based and also has a mobile app available for Android devices and the iPhone and iPad. The app is free to download. You must sign up to join the WeRx community and to start spreading the word about more affordable medication. After you have joined the community and created your profile, use these steps to compare prices, get prescription coupons, and start saving money on your medications. These steps show the WeRx.org website accessed on a computer.

1. Go to werx.org on your desktop's web browser.
2. Click Login.
3. Enter your login credentials, and then click Login.

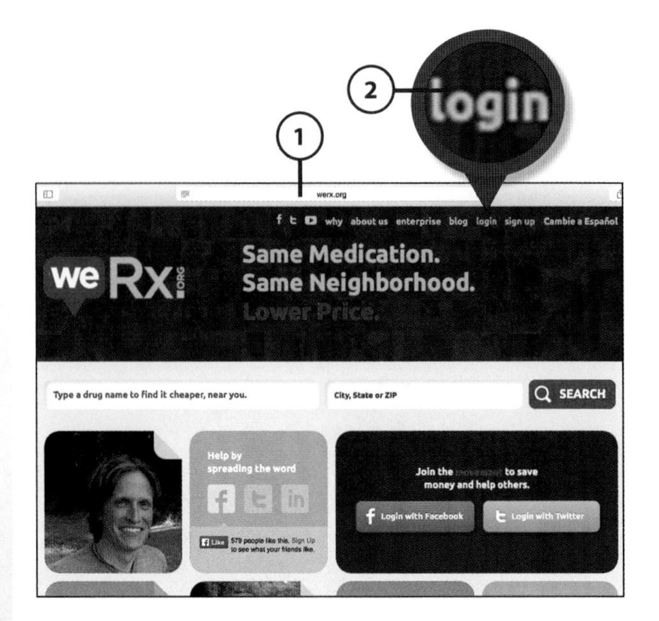

Community Participation Is Key

Reporting what you have paid for medications at your local pharmacy is very important to the WeRx community. The more you contribute, the more helpful the website.

---

4. In the first text box, type in the name of the drug you want to find cheaper, near you.
5. In the second text box, type in your current location using the City, State, or Zip.
6. Click Search. A list of prices for the drug you searched appear along with pharmacy information and a map indicating the location of the pharmacy.

7. Adjust the Strength and Quantity of your medication at the top of the page.
8. Scroll down to view the prices found for the drug.
9. Click the printer icon to take advantage of the WeRx Instant Savings Program and print out an Instant Savings Card for this drug. Present the card to the pharmacist to redeem your savings.
10. Click the envelope icon to have your Instant Savings Card sent to you by email.
11. Click the Report a Cash/Retail Price button to report the amount you paid for this drug at your pharmacy.

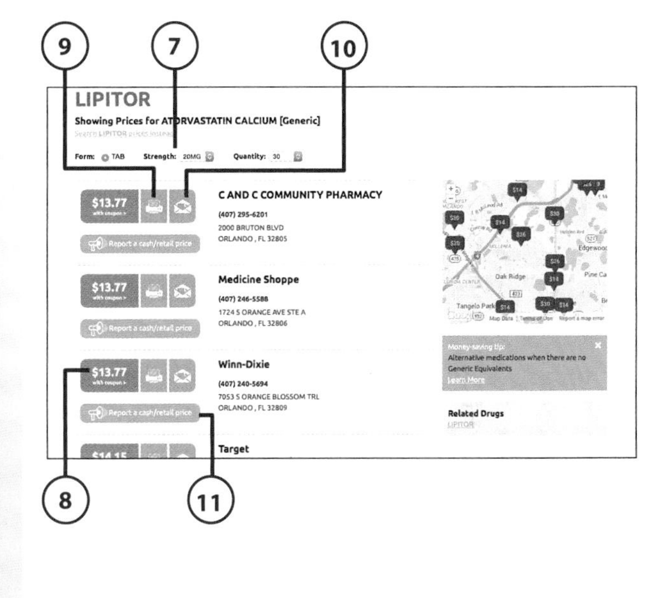

Gathering Your Health Information

Gathering your medical information and your instructions for what to do should something happen to you provides you and your family peace of mind, while also ensuring that your wishes are carried out. Resources provided by the ABA/AARP's *Checklist for My Family*—a book with a digital component—can guide you through the creation and collection of medical care information, wishes, and legal documents you need to plan your estate. Let's take a closer look.

Organize Your Life with the Digital Component of AARP/ABA *Checklist for My Family*

AARP and the American Bar Association have put together a resource to help you collect, organize, and communicate the important information in your life. *Checklist for My Family: A Guide to My History, Financial Plans and Final Wishes* is a bestselling book that has an accompanying set of downloadable PDFs (digital documents) that walk you through the process of gathering your legal documents, finances, online accounts, wishes, medical care, and more into one place. Although gathering the details can be time-consuming and considering end-of-life matters can be difficult, checklists such as these can simplify and organize your life now while sparing your loved ones significant frustration and stress in a difficult time. After you purchase the book, you'll get instructions for downloading the PDFs.

Index

Symbols

A

B

E

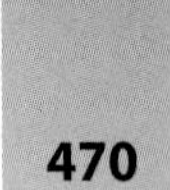

I

J–K–L

N

O

P

Q–R

S

T

X–Y–Z